OBESITY EPIDEMIOLOGY, PATHOGENESIS, AND TREATMENT

A Multidisciplinary Approach

OBESITY EPIDEMIOLOGY, PATHOGENESIS, AND TREATMENT

A Multidisciplinary Approach

Edited by

Rexford S. Ahima, MD, PhD

Apple Academic Press

TORONTO NEW JERSEY

Apple Academic Press Inc.
3333 Mistwell Crescent
Oakville, ON L6L 0A2
Canada

Apple Academic Press Inc.
9 Spinnaker Way
Waretown, NJ 08758
USA

Printed in the United States of America on acid-free paper

International Standard Book Number-13: 978-1-77188-008-4 (Hardcover)

Library of Congress Control Number: 2013954652

Library and Archives Canada Cataloguing in Publication

Obesity epidemiology, pathogenesis, and treatment: a multidisciplinary approach/edited by Rexford S. Ahima, MD, PhD.

Includes bibliographical references and index.
ISBN 978-1-77188-008-4
1. Obesity--Epidemiology. 2. Obesity--Pathogenesis. 3. Obesity--Treatment. I. Ahima, Rexford S., editor of compilation

RC628.O245 2014   616.3'98   C2013-907694-8

Apple Academic Press also publishes its books in a variety of electronic formats. Some content that appears in print may not be available in electronic format. For information about Apple Academic Press products, visit our website at **www.appleacademicpress.com** and the CRC Press website at **www.crcpress.com**

ABOUT THE EDITOR

REXFORD S. AHIMA, MD, PhD

Dr. Rexford S. Ahima is a Professor of Medicine at the University of Pennsylvania. He received his BSc training at the University of London, MD at the University of Ghana, and PhD in neuroscience at Tulane University in New Orleans, Louisiana, internship and residency training in internal medicine at the Albert Einstein College of Medicine, New York, and clinical and research fellowships in Endocrinology, Diabetes and Metabolism at the Beth Israel Deaconess Medical Center, and Harvard Medical School, Boston. Dr. Ahima's research is focused on the actions of adipose hormones on energy homeostasis, and glucose and lipid metabolism. He is an elected member of the American Society for Clinical Investigation (ASCI), and the Association of American Physicians (AAP), and a fellow of the American College of Physicians (ACP), and The Obesity Society (TOS).

CONTENTS

Acknowledgment and How to Cite .... *xi*

List of Contributors .... *xiii*

Introduction .... *xxiii*

1. **Population Trends and Variation in Body Mass Index from 1971 to 2008 in the Framingham Heart Study Offspring Cohort** **1**

   Jason P. Block, S.V. Subramanian, Nicholas A. Christakis, and A. James O'Malley

2. **Community Energy Balance: A Framework for Contextualizing Cultural Influences on High Risk of Obesity in Ethnic Minority Populations** **19**

   Shiriki Kumanyika, Wendell C. Taylor, Sonya A. Grier, Vikki Lassiter, Kristie J. Lancaster, Christiaan B. Morssink, and André M.N. Renzaho

3. **A Genome-Wide Association Study on Obesity and Obesity-Related Traits** **57**

   Kai Wang, Wei-Dong Li, Clarence K. Zhang, Zuoheng Wang, Joseph T. Glessner, Struan F. A. Grant, Hongyu Zhao, Hakon Hakonarson, and R. Arlen Price

4. **Differences between Adiposity Indicators for Predicting All-Cause Mortality in a Representative Sample of United States Non-Elderly Adults** **71**

   Henry S. Kahn, Kai McKeever Bullard, Lawrence E. Barker, and Giuseppina Imperatore

5. **A New Body Shape Index Predicts Mortality Hazard Independently of Body Mass Index** **101**

   Nir Y. Krakauer and Jesse C. Krakauer

6. **Metabolically Healthy and Unhealthy Obesity Phenotypes in the General Population: The FIN-D2D Survey** **127**

   Pia Pajunen, Anna Kotronen, Eeva Korpi-Hyövälti, Sirkka Keinänen-Kiukaanniemi, Heikki Oksa, Leo Niskanen, Timo Saaristo, Juha T. Saltevo, Jouko Sundvall, Mauno Vanhala, Matti Uusitupa, and Markku Peltonen

7. Liver and Muscle in Morbid Obesity: The Interplay of Fatty Liver and Insulin Resistance 145

Mariana Verdelho Machado, Duarte M. S. Ferreira, Rui E. Castro, Ana Rita Silvestre, Teresinha Evangelista, João Coutinho, Fátima Carepa, Adília Costa, Cecília M. P. Rodrigues, and Helena Cortez-Pinto

8. Sarcopenia Exacerbates Obesity-Associated Insulin Resistance and Dysglycemia: Findings from the National Health and Nutrition Examination Survey III 175

Preethi Srikanthan, Andrea L. Hevener, and Arun S. Karlamangla

9. Prevalence of Obesity and Associated Cardiovascular Risk: The DARIOS Study 191

Francisco Javier Félix-Redondo, María Grau, José Miguel Baena-Díez, Irene R. Dégano, Antonio Cabrera de León, Maria Jesús Guembe, María Teresa Alzamora,Tomás Vega-Alonso, Nicolás R. Robles, Honorato Ortiz, Fernando Rigo, Eduardo Mayoral-Sanchez, Maria José Tormo, Antonio Segura-Fragoso, and Daniel Fernández-Bergés

10. Obstructive Sleep Apnea Is a Predictor of Abnormal Glucose Metabolism in Chronically Sleep Deprived Obese Adults 213

Giovanni Cizza, Paolo Piaggi, Eliane A. Lucassen, Lilian de Jonge, Mary Walter, Megan S. Mattingly, Heather Kalish, Gyorgy Csako, and Kristina I. Rother, for the Sleep Extension Study Group

11. Cluster Analysis of Obesity and Asthma Phenotypes 233

E. Rand Sutherland, Elena Goleva, Tonya S. King, Erik Lehman, Allen D. Stevens, Leisa P. Jackson, Amanda R. Stream, John V. Fahy, and Donald Y. M. Leung

12. Diet, Physical Exercise and Cognitive Behavioral Training as a Combined Workplace Based Intervention to Reduce Body Weight and Increase Physical Capacity in Health Care Workers: A Randomized Controlled Trial 251

Jeanette R. Christensen, Anne Faber, Dorte Ekner, Kristian Overgaard, Andreas Holtermann, and Karen Søgaard

13. Reduction in Adiposity, β-Cell Function, Insulin Sensitivity, and Cardiovascular Risk Factors: A Prospective Study among Japanese with Obesity 275

Maki Goto, Akemi Morita, Atsushi Goto, Kijo Deura, Satoshi Sasaki, Naomi Aiba, Takuro Shimbo, Yasuo Terauchi, Motohiko Miyachi, Mitsuhiko Noda, and Shaw Watanabe, for the SCOP Study Group

14. Bariatric Surgery: The Challenges with Candidate Selection, Individualizing Treatment and Clinical Outcomes 291
K. J. Neff, T. Olbers, and C. W. le Roux

Author Notes 327

Index 337

ACKNOWLEDGMENT AND HOW TO CITE

The editor and publisher thank each of the authors who contributed to this book, whether by granting their permission individually or by releasing their research as open source articles. To cite the work contained in this book and to view the individual permissions, please refer to the "How to Cite" box at the beginning of each chapter. The chapters in this book were previously published in various places in various formats. Each chapter was read individually and carefully selected by the editor in order to give the reader a comprehensive perspective on the subject of obesity epidemiology. The book presents a series of insightful articles on the epidemiology, pathophysiology, and management of obesity. Together these articles provide a better understanding of obesity and related diseases and offer an integrative framework for individualized dietary and exercise programs, behavior modification, pharmacological approaches, surgery, and population interventions to reduce the burden of obesity.

- Chapter 1 examines BMI trajectories and finds that individual BMI levels, especially at baseline, are the main determinants of rising BMI levels.
- Chapter 2 determines that research and intervention programs targeting ethnic minorities should consider the context of food and physical activity relevant to the sociocultural perspectives and the circumstances of social disadvantage and rapid cultural changes influencing these communities.
- Chapter 3 reports the results of a GWAS and candidate SNP genotyping study of obesity. The authors found significant signals between BMI and FTO (strongest signal at rs17817449), and genome-wide significant signals between waist-to-hip ratio and NRXN3 (rs11624704).
- Chapter 4 examines adiposity as measured by BMI and abdominal adiposity indicators in adults, as well as how predictions of mortality associated with adiposity varied with adiposity indicators, sex, ethnicity, and other population characteristics.
- Chapter 5 studies the relationship of body shape and mortality in adults from the National Health and Nutrition Examination Survey (NHANES) 1999-2004. A Body Shape Index (ABSI) based on waist circumference (WC) adjusted for height and weight: $ABSI \equiv WC/(BMI^{2/3})(height^{1/2})$ was

significantly associated with excess mortality even after adjusting for smoking, diabetes, blood pressure, and cholesterol.

- Chapter 6 showed that while obesity is often associated with abnormal lipid and glucose metabolism, inflammation and cardiovascular morbidity, studies have suggested that some obese people are protected from cardiometabolic complications.
- Chapter 7 examines the relationship of liver and muscle lipid metabolism in obese patients with non-alcoholic fatty liver disease (NAFLD) undergoing bariatric surgery. In this cohort, the presence of intra-myocellular lipids was associated with non-alcoholic steatohepatitis (NASH) and liver fibrosis. However, muscle mitochondrial dysfunction did not appear to be a major contributor to intramyocellular lipid accumulation, liver disease or insulin resistance.
- Chapter 8 illustrates that muscle loss (sarcopenia) often co-exists with obesity and increases the risk for type 2 diabetes.
- Chapter 9 determines the relationship of obesity and cardiovascular risk in Spain. Overweight, large waist circumference and waist-to-hip ratio, and abdominal obesity were significantly associated with diabetes, hypertension, hypercholesterolemia and coronary risk.
- Chapter 10 describes a study that connects sleep abnormalities, including obstructive sleep apnea (OSA), with obesity and insulin resistance. The severity of OSA was significantly associated with higher fasting glucose, insulin, ACTH, proinflammatory cytokines, and C-reactive protein, indicating increased inflammation, insulin resistance and cardiovascular risk.
- Chapter 11 examines asthma characteristics and identifies significant associations with obesity, inflammatory biomarkers, and response to glucocorticoids.
- Chapter 12 describes a randomized controlled lifestyle intervention among female obese health care workers. They show that diet, exercise, and behavior modification are essential for successful weight loss and maintenance
- Chapter 13 studies obese Japanese subjects for one year. Body fat is positively associated with HbA1c and fasting plasma glucose, and reductions in BMI and visceral fat are associated with reduced insulin resistance, increased insulin secretion, and reduced CVD risk factors.
- Chapter 14 discusses the types of bariatric surgery, criteria for selecting patients, post-surgical care, complications and outcomes, and the psychosocial and economic effects of bariatric surgery.

LIST OF CONTRIBUTORS

Naomi Aiba
Department of Nutrition and Life Science, Kanagawa Institute of Technology, Kanagawa, Japan

María Teresa Alzamora
Centro de Salud Riu Nord- Riu Sud, Santa Coloma de Gramenet, Barcelona and USR Metropolitana Nord, IDIAP Jordi Gol, Mataró, Spain

José Miguel Baena-Díez
Grupo de Epidemiología y Genética Cardiovascular, Programa de Investigación en Procesos Inflamatorios y Cardiovasculares, IMIM (Institut Hospital del Mar d'Investigacions Mèdiques), Barcelona, Spain and Centre d'Atenció Primària La Marina. Unitat de Recerca Barcelona Ciutat, Institut de Recerca en Atenció Primària Jordi Gol, Institut Català de la Salut, Barcelona, Spain

Lawrence E. Barker
Division of Diabetes Translation, U. S. Centers for Disease Control and Prevention, Atlanta, Georgia, United States of America

Jason P. Block
Obesity Prevention Program, Department of Population Medicine, Harvard Medical School/Harvard Pilgrim Health Care Institute, Boston, Massachusetts, United States of America

Kai McKeever Bullard
Division of Diabetes Translation, U. S. Centers for Disease Control and Prevention, Atlanta, Georgia, United States of America

Fátima Carepa
Departamento de Cirurgia, Hospital Santa Maria, Lisbon, Portugal

Rui E. Castro
Research Institute for Medicines and Pharmaceutical Sciences (iMed.UL), Faculty of Pharmacy, University of Lisbon, Lisbon, Portugal

Nicholas A. Christakis
Department of Health Care Policy, Harvard Medical School, Boston, Massachusetts, United States of America

Jeanette R Christensen
Department of Sport Science, Aarhus University, Aarhus, Denmark

Giovanni Cizza
Section on Neuroendocrinology of Obesity, National Institute of Diabetes, Digestive, and Kidney Disease, Bethesda, Maryland, United States of America

Helena Cortez-Pinto
Departamento de Gastrenterologia, Unidade de Nutrição e Metabolismo, Hospital Santa Maria, Faculdade de Medicina de Lisboa, IMM, Lisbon, Portugal

Adília Costa
Departamento de Anatomia Patológica, Hospital Santa Maria, Lisbon, Portugal

João Coutinho
Departamento de Cirurgia, Hospital Santa Maria, Lisbon, Portugal

Gyorgy Csako
Department of Laboratory Medicine, Clinical Center, National Institutes of Health, Bethesda, Maryland, United States of America

Irene R Dégano
Grupo de Epidemiología y Genética Cardiovascular, Programa de Investigación en Procesos Inflamatorios y Cardiovasculares, IMIM (Institut Hospital del Mar d'Investigacions Mèdiques), Barcelona, Spain

Lilian de Jonge
Section on Neuroendocrinology of Obesity, National Institute of Diabetes, Digestive, and Kidney Disease, Bethesda, Maryland, United States of America

Antonio Cabrera de León
Unidad de Investigación de Atención Primaria y del Hospital Universitario Señora de Candelaria. Medicina Preventiva y Salud Pública, Universidad de La Laguna, Santa Cruz de Tenerife, Spain

Kijo Deura
Saku Central Hospital, Nagano, Japan

Dorte Ekner
National Research Centre for the Working Environment, Copenhagen, Denmark

Teresinha Evangelista
Departamento de Neuropatologia, Hospital Santa Maria, Lisbon, Portugal

Anne Faber
National Research Centre for the Working Environment, Copenhagen, Denmark

John V. Fahy
Department of Medicine, University of California San Francisco, San Francisco, California, United States of America

Francisco Javier Félix-Redondo
Centro de Salud Villanueva Norte, Servicio Extremeño de Salud, Villanueva de la Serena, Badajoz, Spain and Unidad de Investigación Grimex. Programa de Investigación en Enfermedades Cardiovasculares PERICLES, Villanueva de la Serena, Badajoz, Spain

Daniel Fernández-Bergés
Hospital Don Benito-Villanueva, Don Benito, Badajoz, Spain and Unidad de Investigación Grimex. Programa de Investigación en Enfermedades Cardiovasculares PERICLES, Villanueva de la Serena, Badajoz, Spain

Duarte M. S. Ferreira
Research Institute for Medicines and Pharmaceutical Sciences (iMed.UL), Faculty of Pharmacy, University of Lisbon, Lisbon, Portugal

Joseph T. Glessner
Center for Applied Genomics, Children's Hospital of Philadelphia, Philadelphia, Pennsylvania, United States of America

Elena Goleva
Department of Pediatrics, National Jewish Health, Denver, Colorado, United States of America

Atsushi Goto
Department of Diabetes Research, Diabetes Research Center, National Center for Global Health and Medicine, Tokyo, Japan, Department of Endocrinology and Metabolism, Yokohama City University Graduate School of Medicine, Yokohama, Japan, and National Institute of Health and Nutrition, Tokyo, Japan

Maki Goto
Department of Diabetes Research, Diabetes Research Center, National Center for Global Health and Medicine, Tokyo, Japan, Department of Endocrinology and Metabolism, Yokohama City University Graduate School of Medicine, Yokohama, Japan, and National Institute of Health and Nutrition, Tokyo, Japan

Struan F. A. Grant
Center for Applied Genomics, Children's Hospital of Philadelphia, Philadelphia, Pennsylvania, United States of America and Department of Pediatrics, University of Pennsylvania, Philadelphia, Pennsylvania, United States of America

María Grau
Grupo de Epidemiología y Genética Cardiovascular, Programa de Investigación en Procesos Inflamatorios y Cardiovasculares, IMIM (Institut Hospital del Mar d'Investigacions Mèdiques), Barcelona, Spain

Sonya A. Grier
American University, Kogod School of Business, 4400 Massachusetts Avenue, NW, Washington, D.C. 20016, USA

Maria Jesús Guembe
Grupo de Investigación Riesgo Vascular en Navarra (RIVANA), Servicio de Investigación, Innovación y Formación Sanitaria, Departamento de Salud, Gobierno de Navarra, Pamplona, Spain

Hakon Hakonarson
Center for Applied Genomics, Children's Hospital of Philadelphia, Philadelphia, Pennsylvania, United States of America and Department of Pediatrics, University of Pennsylvania, Philadelphia, Pennsylvania, United States of America

Andrea L. Hevener
Division of Endocrinology, Diabetes, and Hypertension, Department of Medicine, David Geffen School of Medicine, University of California Los Angeles, Los Angeles, California, United States of America

Andreas Holtermann
National Research Centre for the Working Environment, Copenhagen, Denmark

Giuseppina Imperatore
Division of Diabetes Translation, U. S. Centers for Disease Control and Prevention, Atlanta, Georgia, United States of America

Leisa P. Jackson
Department of Pediatrics, National Jewish Health, Denver, Colorado, United States of America

Henry S. Kahn
Division of Diabetes Translation, U. S. Centers for Disease Control and Prevention, Atlanta, Georgia, United States of America

Heather Kalish
Biomedical Engineering and Physical Science Shared Resource, National Institute of Biomedical and Bioengineering, Bethesda, Maryland, United States of America

Arun S. Karlamangla
Division of Gerontology, Department of Medicine, David Geffen School of Medicine, University of California Los Angeles, Los Angeles, California, United States of America

Sirkka Keinänen-Kiukaanniemi
Institute of Health Sciences (General Practice), University of Oulu, Finland and Unit of General Practice, Oulu University Hospital and Health Centre of Oulu, Oulu, Finland

Tonya S. King
Department of Public Health Sciences, Pennsylvania State University College of Medicine, Hershey, Pennsylvania, United States of America

Eeva Korpi-Hyövälti
Department of Internal Medicine, South Ostrobothnia Central Hospital, Seinäjoki, Finland

Anna Kotronen
Diabetes Prevention Unit, Division of Welfare and Health Promotion, National Institute for Health and Welfare, Helsinki, Finland, Department of Medicine, Division of Diabetes, University of Helsinki, Helsinki, Finland, and Minerva Medical Research Institute, Helsinki, Finland

Jesse C. Krakauer
Middletown Medical, Middletown, New York, United States of America

Nir Y. Krakauer
Department of Civil Engineering, The City College of New York, New York, New York, United States of America

Shiriki Kumanyika
Center for Clinical Epidemiology and Biostatistics (CCEB), University of Pennsylvania Perelman School of Medicine, 8 Blockley Hall, 423 Guardian Drive, Philadelphia, PA 19104□6021, Philadelphia, PA 19104, USA

Kristie J. Lancaster
Dept. of Nutrition, Food Studies and Public Health, New York University, 411 Lafayette St., 5th floor New York City, NY 10003, USA

Vikki Lassiter
Center for Clinical Epidemiology and Biostatistics (CCEB), University of Pennsylvania Perelman School of Medicine, 8 Blockley Hall, 423 Guardian Drive, Philadelphia, PA 19104□6021, Philadelphia, PA 19104, USA

Erik Lehman
Department of Public Health Sciences, Pennsylvania State University College of Medicine, Hershey, Pennsylvania, United States of America

C.W. le Roux
Experimental Pathology, UCD Conway Institute, School of Medicine and Medical Sciences, University College Dublin, Belfield, Dublin 4, Dublin, Ireland and Department of Gastrosurgical Research and Education, University of Gothenburg, 5-413 45 Gothenburg, Sweden

Wei-Dong Li
Center for Neurobiology and Behavior, Department of Psychiatry, University of Pennsylvania, Philadelphia, Pennsylvania, United States of America

Eliane A. Lucassen
Section on Neuroendocrinology of Obesity, National Institute of Diabetes, Digestive, and Kidney Disease, Bethesda, Maryland, United States of America and Department of Molecular Cell Biology, Lab for Neurophysiology, Leiden University Medical Center, Leiden, The Netherlands

Mariana Verdelho Machado
Departamento de Gastrenterologia, Unidade de Nutrição e Metabolismo, Hospital Santa Maria, Faculdade de Medicina de Lisboa, IMM, Lisbon, Portugal

Megan S. Mattingly
Section on Neuroendocrinology of Obesity, National Institute of Diabetes, Digestive, and Kidney Disease, Bethesda, Maryland, United States of America

Eduardo Mayoral-Sanchez
Plan Integral de Diabetes de Andalucía, Servicio Andaluz de Salud. CIBER de Fisiopatología de la Obesidad y Nutrición (CIBERobn), Instituto de Salud Carlos III, Madrid, Spain

Motohiko Miyachi
National Institute of Health and Nutrition, Tokyo, Japan

Akemi Morita
National Institute of Health and Nutrition, Tokyo, Japan and Department of Nutrition, College of Nutrition, Koshien University, Hyogo, Japan

Christiaan B. Morssink
Section on Public Health, Department of Family Medicine and Community Health, University of Pennsylvania Perelman School of Medicine, Philadelphia, PA 19104, USA

K.J. Neff
Experimental Pathology, UCD Conway Institute, School of Medicine and Medical Sciences, University College Dublin, Belfield, Dublin 4, Dublin, Ireland

Leo Niskanen
Department of Medicine/Diabetology and Endocrinology, Kuopio University Hospital, Kuopio, Finland

Mitsuhiko Noda
Department of Diabetes Research, Diabetes Research Center, National Center for Global Health and Medicine, Tokyo, Japan and Department of Diabetes and Metabolic Medicine, Center Hospital, National Center for Global Health and Medicine, Tokyo, Japan

Heikki Oksa
Tampere University Hospital, Tampere, Finland

T. Olbers
Department of Bariatric Surgery, Carlanderska Hospital, Gothenburg, Sweden and Department of Gastrosurgical Research and Education, University of Gothenburg, 5-413 45 Gothenburg, Sweden

A. James O'Malley
Department of Health Care Policy, Harvard Medical School, Boston, Massachusetts, United States of America

Honorato Ortiz
Servicio de Epidemiologia, Dirección General de Atención Primaria, Consejería de Sanidad Comunidad de Madrid, Madrid, Spain

Kristian Overgaard
Department of Sport Science, Aarhus University, Aarhus, Denmark

Pia Pajunen
Diabetes Prevention Unit, Division of Welfare and Health Promotion, National Institute for Health and Welfare, Helsinki, Finland

Markku Peltonen
Diabetes Prevention Unit, Division of Welfare and Health Promotion, National Institute for Health and Welfare, Helsinki, Finland

Paolo Piaggi
Obesity Research Center, Endocrinology Unit, University Hospital of Pisa, Pisa, Italy

R. Arlen Price
Center for Neurobiology and Behavior, Department of Psychiatry, University of Pennsylvania, Philadelphia, Pennsylvania, United States of America

André M.N. Renzaho
Migration, Social Disadvantage, and Health Programs, International Public Health Unit, Monash University and Centre for International Health, Burnet Institute, Level 3, Burnet Building, 89 Commercial Road, Melbourne Vic 3004, Australia

Fernando Rigo
Grupo Cardiovascular de Baleares redIAPP, UB Génova. C. S. Sana Agustín, Palma de Mallorca, Baleares, Spain

Nicolás R. Robles
Hospital Universitario Infanta Cristina, Badajoz, Spain and Unidad de Investigación Grimex. Programa de Investigación en Enfermedades Cardiovasculares PERICLES, Villanueva de la Serena, Badajoz, Spain

Cecília M. P. Rodrigues
Research Institute for Medicines and Pharmaceutical Sciences (iMed.UL), Faculty of Pharmacy, University of Lisbon, Lisbon, Portugal

Kristina I. Rother
Section on Pediatric Diabetes and Metabolism, National Institute of Diabetes, Digestive, and Kidney Disease, Bethesda, Maryland, United States of America

Timo Saaristo
Tampere University Hospital, Tampere, Finland and Finnish Diabetes Association, Tampere, Finland

Juha T Saltevo
Department of Medicine, Central Finland Central Hospital, Jyväskylä, Finland

Satoshi Sasaki
Department of Social and Preventive Epidemiology, School of Public Health, University of Tokyo, Tokyo, Japan

Antonio Segura-Fragoso
Instituto de Ciencias de la Salud, Talavera de la Reina, Toledo, Spain

Takuro Shimbo
Department of Clinical Research and Informatics, National Center for Global Health and Medicine, Tokyo, Japan

Ana Rita Silvestre
Departamento de Neuropatologia, Hospital Santa Maria, Lisbon, Portugal

Karen Søgaard
Institute of Sports Science and Clinical Biomechanics, University of Southern Denmark, Odense, Denmark

Preethi Srikanthan
Division of Gerontology, Department of Medicine, David Geffen School of Medicine, University of California Los Angeles, Los Angeles, California, United States of America

Allen D. Stevens
Department of Medicine, National Jewish Health, Denver, Colorado, United States of America

Amanda R. Stream
Department of Medicine, University of Colorado, Denver, Colorado, United States of America

S. V. Subramanian
Department of Social and Behavioral Sciences, Harvard School of Public Health, Boston, Massachusetts, United States of America

Jouko Sundvall
Disease Risk Unit, Department of Chronic Disease Prevention, National Institute for Health and Welfare, Helsinki, Finland

E. Rand Sutherland
Department of Medicine, National Jewish Health, Denver, Colorado, United States of America and Department of Medicine, University of Colorado, Denver, Colorado, United States of America

Wendell C. Taylor
School of Public Health, University of Texas Health Science Center at Houston, 7000 Fannin Street, Suite 2670, Houston, TX 77030, USA

Yasuo Terauchi
Department of Endocrinology and Metabolism, Yokohama City University Graduate School of Medicine, Yokohama, Japan

Maria José Tormo
Servicio de Epidemiología, Consejería de Sanidad y Política Social de Murcia, Departamento de Ciencias Sociosanitarias, Universidad de Murcia.CIBER de Epidemiologia y Salud Pública (CIBERESP), Murcia, Spain

Matti Uusitupa
Institute of Public Health and Clinical Nutrition, Clinical Nutrition, University of Eastern Finland, and Research Unit, Kuopio University Hospital, Kuopio, Finland

Mauno Vanhala
School of Medicine, Unit of Primary Health Care, University of Eastern Finland, Kuopio, Finland and Unit of Family Practice, Central Hospital of Central Finland, Jyväskylä, Finland

Tomás Vega-Alonso
Dirección General de Salud Pública e Investigación, Desarrollo e Innovación, Consejería de Sanidad de la Junta de Castilla y León, Valladolid, Spain

Mary Walter
Section on Neuroendocrinology of Obesity, National Institute of Diabetes, Digestive, and Kidney Disease, Bethesda, Maryland, United States of America

Kai Wang
Center for Applied Genomics, Children's Hospital of Philadelphia, Philadelphia, Pennsylvania, United States of America and Zilkha Neurogenetic Institute, Department of Psychiatry and Department of Preventive Medicine, University of Southern California, Los Angeles, California, United States of America

Zuoheng Wang
Department of Biostatistics, Yale University, New Haven, Connecticut, United States of America

Shaw Watanabe
National Institute of Health and Nutrition, Tokyo, Japan

Clarence K. Zhang
WM Keck Laboratory, Biostatistics Division, Yale University School of Medicine, New Haven, Connecticut, United States of America

Hongyu Zhao
Department of Biostatistics, Yale University, New Haven, Connecticut, United States of America

INTRODUCTION

MUCH ADO ABOUT OBESITY

Overweight and obesity are characterized by excessive fat accumulation in adipose tissue and other organs. The body mass index (BMI), calculated as a person's weight in kilograms divided by the square of the height in meters (kg/m^2), is used for classifying overweight and obesity [1-7]. Based on BMI categories established by the World Health Organization (WHO), a BMI greater than or equal to 25 is considered "overweight," and a BMI greater than or equal to 30 is considered "obese" [1]. The WHO estimated that in 2008, 35% of adults, 34% men and 35% of women, were overweight. The global prevalence of obesity doubled between 1980 and 2008. In 2008, 10% of men and 14% of women were obese, compared with 5% for men and 8% for women in 1980 [1]. Overweight and obesity are the result of an imbalance of ingested and expended calories [8]. Although there are genetic factors underlying obesity [9], the current global trends are mainly due to excessive caloric intake, particularly energy-dense foods rich in fat and sugar, and poor in fiber and micronutrients [10-15]. The global obesity problem is further compounded by low physical activity due to urbanization, changes in transportation, increased leisure, and other environmental structures that promote sedentary lifestyle [16-19].

Higher BMI levels are associated with greater risks of developing type 2 diabetes, dyslipidemia, coronary artery disease, stroke, sleep apnea, osteoarthritis, infertility, cancer and other diseases [1-7; 20, 21]. Obesity is also associated with disability and premature death [22-24]. Obesity and its comorbidities have enormous health care and economic costs, which have spurred local, national and international efforts to limit the burden through prevention. Comprehensive strategies include personal lifestyle changes aimed at reducing total caloric intake, dietary fat, sugar and red meat, increasing intake of fish and white meat, fiber-rich vegetables, legumes, fresh fruit, whole grains and nuts, and increasing physical activity.

The food industry could play a positive role by reducing the contents of fat, sugar and salt in processed foods, promoting healthy foods at affordable prices, and avoiding the marketing of "junk foods" especially aimed at children. Governments and health care providers should offer treatment for obese people affected by various diseases in order to prevent secondary complications. Furthermore, there is a crucial need for agricultural and economic policies that support the production of vegetables and fruits, reduce subsidies of processed foods, and modify transportation and infrastructure to promote physical activity.

The following articles have been chosen to provide an in-depth and insightful look into obesity, providing a better understanding of it, as well as its related diseases.

Chapter 1, by Block and colleagues, examines body mass index (BMI) across place and time to determine the pattern of BMI mean and standard deviation trajectories. The authors included participants in the Framingham Heart Study (FHS) Offspring Cohort over eight waves of follow-up, from 1971 to 2008. After exclusions, the final sample size was 4569 subjects with 28,625 observations. The study used multi-level models to examine population means and variation at the individual and neighborhood (census tracts) levels across time with measured BMI as the outcome, controlling for individual demographics and behaviors and neighborhood poverty. Because neighborhoods accounted for limited BMI variance, they removed this level as a source of variation in final models. The authors examined sex-stratified models with all subjects and models stratified by sex and baseline weight classification. Mean BMI increased from 24.0 kg/m^2 at Wave 1 to 27.7 at Wave 8 for women and from 26.6 kg/m^2 to 29.0 for men. In final models, BMI variation also increased from Waves 1 to 8, with the standard deviation increasing from 4.18 kg/m^2 to 6.15 for women and 3.31 kg/m^2 to 4.73 for men. BMI means increased in parallel across most baseline BMI weight classifications, except for more rapid increases through middle-age for obese women followed by declines in the last wave. BMI standard deviations also increased in parallel across baseline BMI classifications for women, with greater divergence of BMI variance for obese men compared to other weight classifications. Over nearly 40 years, BMI mean and variation increased in parallel across most baseline weight classifications in the sample. Individual-level characteristics, especially baseline BMI, were the primary factors in rising BMI. These findings have important implications not only for understanding the sources of the obesity epidemic in the United States but also for the targeting of interventions to address the epidemic.

Increases in the availability, affordability, and promotion of high-calorie foods and beverages and decreased obligations for routine physical activity have fostered trends of increased obesity worldwide. In high-income, plural societies, above average obesity prevalence is often observed in ethnic minority communities, suggesting that obesity-promoting influences are more prevalent or potent in these communities. In chapter 2, by Kumanyika and colleagues, an interdisciplinary group of scholars engaged in multiple rounds of focused discussion and literature review to develop a Community Energy Balance Framework (CEB). The objective was to explore the nature of the excess obesity risk in African descent and other ethnic minority populations and identify related implications for planning and evaluating interventions to prevent obesity. A key principle that emerged is that researchers and programmers working with ethnic minority communities should contextualize the food and physical activity-related sociocultural perspectives of these communities, taking into account relevant historical, political, and structural contexts. This perspective underscores the fallacy of approaches that place the entire burden of change on the individual, particularly in circumstances of social disadvantage and rapid cultural shifts. The CEB framework is proposed for use and further development to aid in understanding potential health-adverse effects of cultural-contextual stresses and accommodations to these stresses.

Large-scale genome-wide association studies (GWAS) have identified many loci associated with body mass index (BMI), but few studies focused on obesity as a binary trait. In chapter 3, Wang and colleague report the results of a GWAS and candidate SNP genotyping study of obesity, including extremely obese cases and never overweight controls as well as families segregating extreme obesity and thinness. The authors first performed a GWAS on 520 cases (BMI>35 kg/m^2) and 540 control subjects (BMI<25 kg/m^2), on measures of obesity and obesity-related traits. They subsequently followed up obesity-associated signals by genotyping the top ~500 SNPs from GWAS in the combined sample of cases, controls and family members totaling 2,256 individuals. For the binary trait of obesity, they found 16 genome-wide significant signals within the FTO gene (strongest signal at rs17817449, $P = 2.5\times10^{-12}$). The authors next examined obesity-related quantitative traits (such as total body weight, waist circumference and waist to hip ratio), and detected genome-wide significant signals between waist to hip ratio and NRXN3(rs11624704, $P = 2.67\times10^{-9}$), previously associated with body weight and fat distribution. The study demonstrated how a relatively small sample ascertained through extreme phenotypes can detect genuine associations in a GWAS.

Adiposity predicts health outcomes, but this relationship could depend on population characteristics and adiposity indicator employed. In a representative sample of 11,437 US adults (National Health and Nutrition Examination Survey, 1988–1994, ages 18–64) chapter 4, by Kahn and colleagues, estimated associations with all-cause mortality for body mass index (BMI) and four abdominal adiposity indicators (waist circumference [WC], waist-to-height ratio [WHtR], waist-to-hip ratio [WHR], and waist-to-thigh ratio [WTR]). In a fasting subsample the authors considered the lipid accumulation product (LAP; [WC enlargement*triglycerides]). For each adiposity indicator the study estimated linear and categorical mortality risks using sex-specific, proportional-hazards models adjusted for age, black ancestry, tobacco exposure, and socioeconomic position. There were 1,081 deaths through 2006. Using linear models they found little difference among indicators (adjusted hazard ratios [aHRs] per SD increase 1.2–1.4 for men, 1.3–1.5 for women). Using categorical models, men in adiposity midrange (quartiles 2+3; compared to quartile 1) were not at significantly increased risk (aHRs<1.1) unless assessed by WTR (aHR 1.4 [95%CI 1.0–1.9]). Women in adiposity midrange, however, tended toward elevated risk (aHRs 1.2–1.5), except for black women assessed by BMI, WC or WHtR (aHRs 0.7–0.8). Men or women in adiposity quartile 4 (compared to midrange) were generally at risk (aHRs>1.1), especially black men assessed by WTR (aHR 1.9 [1.4–2.6]) and black women by LAP (aHR 2.2 [1.4–3.5]). Quartile 4 of WC or WHtR carried no significant risk for diabetic persons (aHRs 0.7–1.1), but elevated risks for those without diabetes (aHRs>1.5). For both sexes, quartile 4 of LAP carried increased risks for tobacco-exposed persons (aHRs>1.6) but not for non-exposed (aHRs<1.0). Predictions of mortality risk associated with top-quartile adiposity vary with the indicator used, sex, ancestry, and other characteristics. Interpretations of adiposity should consider how variation in the physiology and expandability of regional adipose-tissue depots impacts health.

Obesity, typically quantified in terms of Body Mass Index (BMI) exceeding threshold values, is considered a leading cause of premature death worldwide. For given body size (BMI), it is recognized that risk is also affected by body shape, particularly as a marker of abdominal fat deposits. Waist circumference (WC) is used as a risk indicator supplementary to BMI, but the high correlation of WC with BMI makes it hard to isolate the added value of WC. In chapter 5, Krakauer and Krakauer considered a USA population sample of 14,105 non-pregnant adults from the National Health and Nutrition Examination Survey (NHANES) 1999–2004 with follow-up for mortality averaging 5 year (828 deaths). They developed A Body Shape Index (ABSI) based on WC adjusted for height and weight. ABSI had little correlation with height, weight, or BMI. Death rates increased approximately exponentially with above average baseline ABSI (overall regression coefficient of +33% per standard deviation of ABSI [95% confidence interval: +20% – +48%]), whereas elevated death rates were found for both high and low values of BMI and WC. Twenty-two percent (8% – 41%) of the population mortality hazard was attributable to high ABSI, compared to 15% (3% – 30%) for BMI and 15% (4% – 29%) for WC. The association of death rate with ABSI held even when adjusted for other known risk factors including smoking, diabetes, blood pressure, and serum cholesterol. ABSI correlation with mortality hazard held across the range of age, sex, and BMI, and for both white and black ethnicities (but not for Mexican ethnicity), and was not weakened by excluding deaths from the first 3 years of follow-up. Body shape, as measured by ABSI, appears to be a substantial risk factor for premature mortality in the general population derivable from basic clinical measurements. ABSI expresses the excess risk from high WC in a convenient form that is complementary to BMI and to other known risk factors.

The aim of chapter 6, by Pajunen and colleagues, was to examine the prevalence of different metabolical phenotypes of obesity, and to analyze, by using different risk scores, how the metabolic syndrome (MetS) definition discriminates between unhealthy and healthy metabolic phenotypes in different obesity classes. The Finnish type 2 diabetes (FIN-D2D) survey, a part of the larger implementation study, was carried out in 2007. The present cross-sectional analysis comprises 2,849 individuals aged 45-74 years. The MetS was defined with the new Harmonization definition. Cardiovascular risk was estimated with the Framingham and SCORE risk scores. Diabetes risk was assessed with the FINDRISK score. Non-alcoholic fatty liver disease (NAFLD) was estimated with the NAFLD score. Participants with and without MetS were classified in different weight categories and analysis of regression models were used to test the linear trend between body mass index (BMI) and various characteristics in individuals with and without MetS; and interaction between BMI and MetS. A metabolically healthy but obese phenotype was observed in 9.2% of obese men and in 16.4% of obese women. The MetS-BMI interaction was significant for fasting glucose, 2-hour plasma glucose, fasting plasma insulin and insulin resistance (HOMA-IR)($p < 0.001$ for all). The prevalence of total diabetes (detected prior to or during survey) was 37.0% in obese individuals with MetS and 4.3% in obese individuals without MetS ($p < 0.001$). MetS-BMI interaction was significant ($p < 0.001$) also for the Framingham 10 year CVD risk score, NAFLD score and estimated liver fat %, indicating greater effect of increasing BMI in participants with MetS compared to participants without MetS. The metabolically healthy but obese individuals had lower 2-hour postload glucose levels ($p = 0.0030$), lower NAFLD scores ($p < 0.001$) and lower CVD risk scores (Framingham, $p < 0.001$; SCORE, $p = 0.002$) than normal weight individuals with MetS. Undetected Type 2 diabetes was more prevalent among those with MetS irrespective of the BMI class and increasing BMI had a significantly greater effect on estimates of liver fat and future CVD risk among those with MetS compared with participants without MetS. A healthy obese phenotype was associated with a better metabolic profile than observed in normal weight individuals with MetS.

Nonalcoholic fatty liver disease (NAFLD) can be seen as a manifestation of overnutrition. The muscle is a central player in the adaptation to energy overload, and there is an association between fatty-muscle and -liver. In chapter 7, Machado and colleagues aimed to correlate muscle morphology, mitochondrial function and insulin signaling with NAFLD severity in morbid obese patients. Liver and deltoid muscle biopsies were collected during bariatric surgery in NAFLD patients. NAFLD Activity Score and

Younossi's classification for nonalcoholic steatohepatitis (NASH) were applied to liver histology. Muscle evaluation included morphology studies, respiratory chain complex I to IV enzyme assays, and analysis of the insulin signaling cascade. A healthy lean control group was included for muscle morphology and mitochondrial function analyses. Fifty one NAFLD patients were included of whom 43% had NASH. Intramyocellular lipids (IMCL) were associated with the presence of NASH (OR 12.5, $p<0.001$), progressive hepatic inflammation ($p = 0.029$) and fibrosis severity ($p = 0.010$). There was a trend to an association between IMCL and decreased Akt phosphorylation ($p = 0.059$), despite no association with insulin resistance. In turn, hepatic steatosis ($p = 0.015$) and inflammation ($p = 0.013$) were associated with decreased Akt phosphoryation. Citrate synthase activity was lower in obese patients ($p = 0.047$) whereas complex I ($p = 0.040$) and III ($p = 0.036$) activities were higher, compared with controls. Finally, in obese patients, complex I activity increased with progressive steatosis ($p = 0.049$) and with a trend with fibrosis severity ($p = 0.056$). In morbid obese patients, presence of IMCL associates with NASH and advanced fibrosis. Muscle mitochondrial dysfunction does not appear to be a major driving force contributing to muscle fat accumulation, insulin resistance or liver disease. Importantly, insulin resistance in muscle might occur at a late point in the insulin signaling cascade and be associated with IMCL and NAFLD severity.

Sarcopenia often co-exists with obesity, and may have additive effects on insulin resistance. Sarcopenic obese individuals could be at increased risk for type 2 diabetes. Srikanthan and colleagues performed a study in chapter 8 to determine whether sarcopenia is associated with impairment in insulin sensitivity and glucose homeostasis in obese and non-obese individuals. The authors performed a cross-sectional analysis of National Health and Nutrition Examination Survey III data utilizing subjects of 20 years or older, non-pregnant ($N = 14{,}528$). Sarcopenia was identified from bioelectrical impedance measurement of muscle mass. Obesity was identified from body mass index. Outcomes were homeostasis model assessment of insulin resistance (HOMA IR), glycosylated hemoglobin level (HbA1C), and prevalence of pre-diabetes ($6.0 \leq$ HbA1C<6.5 and not on medication) and type 2 diabetes. Covariates in multiple regression were age, educational level, ethnicity and sex. Sarcopenia was associated with insulin resistance in non-obese (HOMA IR ratio 1.39, 95% confidence interval (CI) 1.26 to 1.52) and obese individuals (HOMA-IR ratio 1.16, 95% CI 1.12 to 1.18). Sarcopenia was associated with dysglycemia in obese individuals (HbA1C ratio 1.021, 95% CI 1.011 to 1.043) but not in non-obese individuals. Associations were stronger in those under 60 years of age. The authors acknowledge that the cross-sectional study design limits our ability to draw causal inferences. Sarcopenia, independent of obesity, is associated with adverse glucose metabolism, and the association is strongest in individuals under 60 years of age, which suggests that low muscle mass may be an early predictor of diabetes susceptibility. Given the increasing prevalence of obesity, further research is urgently needed to develop interventions to prevent sarcopenic obesity and its metabolic consequences.

Chapter 9, by Félix-Redondo and colleagues, aims to estimate the prevalence of overweight and obesity in the Spanish population as measured with body mass index (BMI), waist circumference (WC) and waist to height ratio (WHtR) and to determine the associated cardiovascular risk factors. Pooled analysis with individual data from 11 studies conducted in the first decade of the 21st century. Participants aged 35–74 years were asked about the history of cardiovascular diseases, hypertension, diabetes and hypercholesterolemia. Height, weight, WC, blood pressure, glycaemia, total cholesterol, low-density and high-density lipoprotein cholesterol and coronary risk were measured. The prevalence of overweight (BMI 25–29.9 kg/m^2), general obesity (BMI $\geq$30 kg/m^2), suboptimal WC ($\geq$ 80 cm and < 88 in women, $\geq$ 94 and < 102 in men), abdominal obesity (WC $\geq$88 cm $\geq$102 cm in women and men, respectively) and WHtR $\geq$0.5 was estimated, standardized for the European population. The study included 28,743 individuals. The prevalence of overweight and suboptimal WC was 51% and 30% in men and 36% and 22% in women, respectively; general obesity was 28% in both sexes and abdominal obesity 36% in men and 55% in women. The prevalence of WHtR $\geq$0.5 was 89% and 77% in men and women, respectively. All cardiovascular risk factors were significantly associated with abnormal increased values of BMI, WC and WHtR. Hypertension showed the strongest association with overweight [OR = 1.99 (95% confidence interval 1.81-2.21) and OR = 2.10 (1.91-2.31)]; suboptimal WC [OR = 1.78 (1.60-1.97) and OR = 1.45 (1.26-1.66)], with general obesity [OR=4.50 (4.02-5.04), and OR=5.20 (4.70-5.75)] and with WHtR ≥0.5 [OR=2.94 (2.52-3.43), and OR=3.02 (2.66-3.42)] in men and women respectively, besides abdominal obesity in men only [OR=3.51 (3.18-3.88)]. Diabetes showed the strongest association with abdominal obesity in women [OR=3,86 (3,09-4,89). The prevalence of obesity in Spain was high. Overweight, suboptimal WC, general, abdominal obesity and WHtR ≥0.5 was significantly associated with diabetes, hypertension, hypercholesterolemia and coronary risk. The use of lower cut-off points for both BMI and particularly WC and could help to better identify the population at risk and therefore achieve more effective preventive measures.

Sleep abnormalities, including obstructive sleep apnea (OSA), have been associated with insulin resistance. Chapter 10, by Cizza and colleagues, aims to determine the relationship between sleep, including OSA, and glucose parameters in a prospectively assembled cohort of chronically sleep-deprived obese subjects. Sleep duration and quality were assessed by actigraphy, sleep diaries and questionnaires, OSA was determined by a portable device; glucose metabolism assessed by oral glucose tolerance test (oGTT), and HbA1c concentrations in 96 obese individuals reporting sleeping less than 6.5 h on a regular basis. Sixty % of subjects had an abnormal respiratory disturbance index (RDI≥5) and 44% of these subjects had abnormal oGTT results. Severity of OSA as assessed by RDI score was associated with fasting glucose ($R = 0.325$, $p = 0.001$) and fasting insulin levels ($\rho = 0.217$, $p = 0.033$). Subjects with moderate to severe OSA (RDI>15) had higher glucose concentrations at 120 min than those without OSA (RDI<5) ($p = 0.017$). Subjects with OSA also had significantly higher concentrations of plasma ACTH ($p = 0.009$). Several proinflammatory cytokines were higher in subjects with OSA ($p<0.050$). CRP levels were elevated in this sample, suggesting increased cardiovascular risk. OSA is associated with impaired glucose metabolism in obese, sleep deprived individuals. Since sleep apnea is common and frequently undiagnosed, health care providers should be aware of its occurrence and associated risks.

Asthma is a heterogeneous disease with variability among patients in characteristics such as lung function, symptoms and control, body weight, markers of inflammation, and responsiveness to glucocorticoids (GC).

Cluster analysis of well-characterized cohorts can advance understanding of disease subgroups in asthma and point to unsuspected disease mechanisms. Chapter 11, by Sutherland, utilized an hypothesis-free cluster analytical approach to define the contribution of obesity and related variables to asthma phenotype. In a cohort of clinical trial participants (n = 250), minimum-variance hierarchical clustering was used to identify clinical and inflammatory biomarkers important in determining disease cluster membership in mild and moderate persistent asthmatics. In a subset of participants, GC sensitivity was assessed via expression of GC receptor alpha (GCRα) and induction of MAP kinase phosphatase-1 (MKP-1) expression by dexamethasone. Four asthma clusters were identified, with body mass index (BMI, kg/m^2) and severity of asthma symptoms (AEQ score) the most significant determinants of cluster membership ($F = 57.1$, $p<0.0001$ and $F = 44.8$, $p<0.0001$, respectively). Two clusters were composed of predominantly obese individuals; these two obese asthma clusters differed from one another with regard to age of asthma onset, measures of asthma symptoms (AEQ) and control (ACQ), exhaled nitric oxide concentration (FENO) and airway hyperresponsiveness (methacholine PC20) but were similar with regard to measures of lung function (FEV1 (%) and FEV1/FVC), airway eosinophilia, IgE, leptin, adiponectin and C-reactive protein (hsCRP). Members of obese clusters demonstrated evidence of reduced expression of GCRα, a finding which was correlated with a reduced induction of MKP-1 expression by dexamethasone. Obesity is an important determinant of asthma phenotype in adults. There is heterogeneity in expression of clinical and inflammatory biomarkers of asthma across obese individuals. Reduced expression of the dominant functional isoform of the GCR may mediate GC insensitivity in obese asthmatics.

Health care workers comprise a high-risk workgroup with respect to deterioration and early retirement. There is high prevalence of obesity and many of the workers are overweight. Together, these factors play a significant role in the health-related problems within this sector. In chapter 12, Christensen and colleagues evaluate the effects of the first 3-months of a cluster randomized controlled lifestyle intervention among health care workers. The intervention addresses body weight, general health variables, physical capacity and musculoskeletal pain. Ninety-eight female, overweight health care workers were cluster-randomized to an intervention group or a reference group. The intervention consisted of an individually dietary plan with an energy deficit of 1200 kcal/day (15 min/hour), strengthening exercises (15 min/hour) and cognitive behavioral training (30 min/hour) during working hours 1 hour/week. Leisure time aerobic fitness was planned for 2 hour/week. The reference group was offered monthly oral presentations. Body weight, BMI, body fat percentage (bio-impedance), waist circumference, blood pressure, musculoskeletal pain, maximal oxygen uptake (maximal bicycle test), and isometric maximal muscle strength of 3 body regions were measured before and after the intervention period. In an intention-to-treat analysis from pre to post tests, the intervention group significantly reduced body weight with 3.6 kg ($p < 0.001$), BMI from 30.5 to 29.2 ($p < 0.001$), body fat percentage from 40.9 to 39.3 ($p < 0.001$), waist circumference from 99.7 to 95.5 cm ($p < 0.001$) and blood pressure from 134/85 to 127/80 mmHg ($p < 0.001$), with significant difference between the intervention and control group ($p < 0.001$) on all measures. No effect of intervention was found in musculoskeletal pain, maximal oxygen uptake and muscle strength, but on aerobic fitness. The significantly reduced body weight, body fat, waist circumference and blood pressure as well as increased aerobic fitness in the intervention group show the great potential of workplace health promotion among this high-risk workgroup. Long-term effects of the intervention remain to be investigated.

A reduction in adiposity may be associated with an improvement in insulin sensitivity and β-cell function as well as cardiovascular disease (CVD) risk factors; however, few studies have investigated these associations in a longitudinal setting. To investigate these associations over a 1-year period, chapter 13, by Goto and colleagues conducted an observational analysis of 196 Japanese subjects with obesity in the Saku Control Obesity Program. The authors investigated the relations between changes in adiposity (body mass index [BMI], waist circumference, subcutaneous fat area [SFAT], and visceral fat area [VFAT]) and changes in HbA1c, fasting plasma glucose (FPG), insulin sensitivity index (ISI), the homeostasis model assessment β cell function (HOMA-β), lipids, and blood pressure. All adiposity changes were positively associated with HbA1c and FPG changes. Reductions in BMI and VFAT were associated with HOMA-β reduction. Reductions in all adiposity measures were associated with an improvement in the ISI. Changes in most adiposity measures were positively associated with changes in blood pressure and lipid levels, except for LDL. The present findings provide additional supportive evidence indicating that a reduction in adiposity may lead to an improvement in insulin sensitivity and the reduction of CVD risk factors in obese individuals.

Obesity is recognized as a global health crisis. Bariatric surgery offers a treatment that can reduce weight, induce remission of obesity-related diseases, and improve the quality of life. In chapter 14, Neff and colleagues outline the different options in bariatric surgery and summarize the recommendations for selecting and assessing potential candidates before proceeding to surgery. The authors present current data on post-surgical outcomes and evaluate the psychosocial and economic effects of bariatric surgery. Finally, they evaluate the complication rates and present recommendations for post-operative care.

REFERENCES

1. WHO Web site http://www.who.int/gho/ncd/risk_factors/obesity_text/en/. Accessed October 29, 2013.
2. Flegal KM, Carroll MD, Ogden CL, Curtin LR. Prevalence and trends in obesity among US adults, 1999–2008. JAMA. 2010;303(3):235–241.
3. Stommel M, Schoenborn CA. Variations in BMI and prevalence of health risks in diverse racial and ethnic populations. Obesity (Silver Spring). 2010;18(9):1821–1816.
4. Finucane MM, et al. Global Burden of Metabolic Risk Factors of Chronic Diseases Collaborating Group (Body Mass Index). National, regional, and global trends in body-mass index since 1980: systematic analysis of health examination surveys and epidemiological studies with 960 country-years and 9.1 million participants. Lancet. 2011;377(9765):557–567.
5. Guerrero RT, Paulino YC, Novotny R, Murphy SP. Diet and obesity among Chamorro and Filipino adults on Guam. Asia Pac J Clin Nutr. 2008;17(2):216–222.
6. El Rhazi K, Nejjari C, Zidouh A, Bakkali R, Berraho M, Gateau PB. Prevalence of obesity and associated sociodemographic and lifestyle factors in Morocco. Public Health Nutr. 2011;14(1):160–167.
7. Márquez-Sandoval F, Macedo-Ojeda G, Viramontes-Hörner D, Fernández Ballart J, Salas Salvadó J, Vizmanos B. The prevalence of metabolic syndrome in Latin America: a systematic review. Public Health Nutr. 2011;14(10):1702-1713.
8. Leibel RL. Molecular physiology of weight regulation in mice and humans. Int J Obes (Lond). 2008;32(suppl 7):S98–S108.

9. Ramachandrappa S, Farooqi IS. Genetic approaches to understanding human obesity. J Clin Invest. 2011;121(6):2080–2086.
10. WHO website http://www.who.int/gho/ncd/risk_factors/unhealthy_diet_text/en/. Accessed October 29, 2013.
11. Gross LS, Li L, Ford ES, Liu S. Increased consumption of refined carbohydrates and the epidemic of type 2 diabetes in the United States: an ecologic assessment. Am J Clin Nutr. 2004;79(5):774–779.
12. Mavoa HM, McCabe M. Sociocultural factors relating to Tongans' and Indigenous Fijians' patterns of eating, physical activity and body size. Asia Pac J Clin Nutr. 2008;17(3):375–384.
13. Mehio Sibai A, Nasreddine L, Mokdad AH, Adra N, Tabet M, Hwalla N. Nutrition transition and cardiovascular disease risk factors in Middle East and North Africa countries: reviewing the evidence. Ann Nutr Metab. 2010;57(3-4):193–203.
14. Malik VS, Popkin BM, Bray GA, Després JP, Hu FB. Sugar-sweetened beverages, obesity, type 2 diabetes mellitus, and cardiovascular disease risk. Circulation. 2010;121(11):1356–1364.
15. de Onis M, Blössner M, Borghi E. Global prevalence and trends of overweight and obesity among preschool children. Am J Clin Nutr. 2010;92(5):1257–1264.
16. WHO Web site http://www.who.int/gho/ncd/risk_factors/physical_activity_text/en/. Accessed October 29, 2013.
17. Williamson DF, Madans J, Anda RF, Kleinman JC, Kahn HS, Byers T. Recreational physical activity and ten-year weight change in a US national cohort. Int J Obes Relat Metab Disord. 1993;17(5):279–286.
18. Hu FB, Li TY, Colditz GA, Willett WC, Manson JE. Television watching and other sedentary behaviors in relation to risk of obesity and type 2 diabetes mellitus in women. JAMA. 2003;289(14):1785–1791.
19. Robinson TN. Reducing children's television viewing to prevent obesity: a randomized controlled trial. JAMA. 1999;282(16):1561–1567.
20. Bhargava SK, et al. Relation of serial changes in childhood body-mass index to impaired glucose tolerance in young adulthood. N Engl J Med. 2004;350(9):865–875.
21. Tirosh A, et al. Adolescent BMI trajectory and risk of diabetes versus coronary disease. N Engl J Med. 2011;364(14):1315–1325.
22. Berrington de Gonzalez A, et al. Body-mass index and mortality among 1.46 million white adults. N Engl J Med. 2010;363(23):2211–2219.
23. Flegal KM, Graubard BI, Williamson DF, Gail MH. Cause-specific excess deaths associated with underweight, overweight, and obesity. JAMA. 2007;298(17):2028–2037.
24. Zheng W, et al. Association between body-mass index and risk of death in more than 1 million Asians. N Engl J Med. 2011;364(8):719–729.

CHAPTER 1

POPULATION TRENDS AND VARIATION IN BODY MASS INDEX FROM 1971 TO 2008 IN THE FRAMINGHAM HEART STUDY OFFSPRING COHORT

JASON P. BLOCK, S. V. SUBRAMANIAN,
NICHOLAS A. CHRISTAKIS, and A. JAMES O'MALLEY

1.1 INTRODUCTION

The obesity epidemic has progressed rapidly in the United States over the last several decades. The mean body mass index (BMI) of US adults has increased from 25.7 kg/m^2 to 28.7 for men and 25.1 kg/m^2 to 28.7 for women from the 1960s to 2000s [1], [2], [3]. The prevalence of obesity (BMI $\geq$30 kg/m^2) among adults 20 to 74 years of age has increased nearly threefold [2], [4], [5]. These average trends, however, fail to capture potential heterogeneous patterns in body weight over time. For example, studies have found a prominent rightward skewing of the BMI distribution over time, contributing to a larger rise in mean BMI than might be seen if the mean was the only component of the BMI distribution to change over time [2], [6], [7]. Other studies have demonstrated variability in

This chapter was originally published under the Creative Commons Attribution License. Block JP, Subramanian SV, Christakis NA, and O'Malley AJ. Population Trends and Variation in Body Mass Index from 1971 to 2008 in the Framingham Heart Study Offspring Cohort. PLoS ONE ***8****,5 (2013), doi:10.1371/journal.pone.0063217.*

the prevalence of overweight and obese individuals by neighborhood of residence, with greater increases in those neighborhoods with lower socio-economic status [8], [9], [10], [11], [12].

Properly accounting for heterogeneity at both the individual and neighborhood levels using longitudinal data may determine true underlying patterns of population weight change over time with possible implications for interventions [13], [14], [15], [16]. The use of longitudinal data provides the unique opportunity to examine trajectories in BMI means and standard deviations over time and by baseline weight classification to determine what groups are at greatest risk for weight gain or have greater variability in weight gain over time.

Here, using data from the Framingham Heart Study (FHS) Offspring Cohort over 37 years, including a large number of individuals who moved great distances, we examined longitudinal trends in BMI between individuals and neighborhoods. The use of this cohort, linked together by common characteristics of their parents (or in-laws), enabled us to more confidently examine complex associations between BMI and social and geographic factors prone to endogeneity.

1.2 METHODS

1.2.1 ETHICS STATEMENT

The Institutional Review Board of Harvard Medical School approved this study. The Framingham Heart Study undertook a detailed written consent process for all aspects of data collection [17].

1.2.2 SAMPLE

Our sample came from the Framingham Heart Study (FHS) Offspring Cohort, which started in 1971 and enrolled 5124 subjects who were either the children of subjects enrolled in the FHS Original Cohort or their spouses.

The FHS Original Cohort included a random sample of residents of Framingham, Massachusetts, in the 1940s. Offspring Cohort subjects have been examined and surveyed up to eight times from enrollment through 2008, roughly every four years. Our final sample included all FHS Offspring Cohort subjects excluding observations with missing BMI, smoking status, alcohol intake, or census tract of residence; we also excluded subjects at any time points if they were living in a nursing home or were less than 21 years old.

For analyses, we intended to use three-level multi-level random effects models to account for BMI clustering by neighborhood and individual with an additional pure error variance term. However, contrary to our a priori hypothesis that we would find notable variance at the neighborhood level, we found that the neighborhood level contributed near zero variance in cross-sectional models for most of the eight waves (Table S1 in Appendix S1). Among women, the proportion of the variance contributed by the neigborhood level, calculated as the intra-class correlation coefficient (ICC) [neigborhood-level variance/(neighborhood-level variance+individual-level variance)], was less than 0.6% for five waves, and 1.5%, 1.1%, and 3.3% in Waves 5, 6 and 7, respectively. Among men, the ICC at the neighborhood level was less than 0.7% at each wave. To create the most parsimonious final models, we used only two-level multilevel models accounting for the individual-level variance and pure error variance. We included a random intercept at the individual level as well as random slopes for both time and the natural log of time. Including both fixed effects and random slopes for linear time and the natural log of time accounted for non-linearity in population-average and individual-specific BMI growth trajectories and allowed different amounts of heterogeneity between the linear and nonlinear components of individuals' trajectories. We required subjects to have at least two observations so that each individual contributed direct information about intra-individual change in BMI across time (Figure 1). Our final sample size was 4569 subjects with 28,625 observations.

1.2.3 VARIABLES

Time-varying individual-level BMI was the outcome variable, objectively calculated using in person measured weight and standing height at each

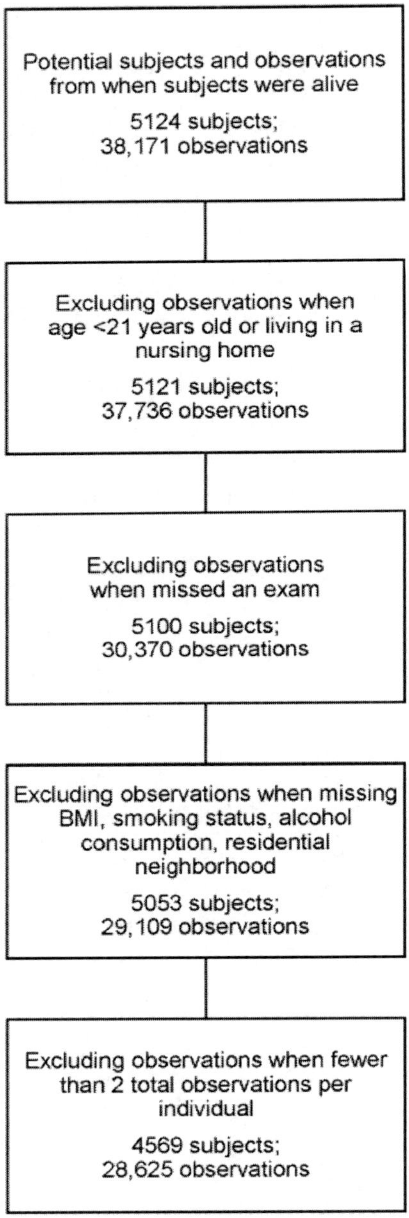

FIGURE 1: Flow Diagram for Framingham Heart Study Offspring Cohort Subjects and Observations Included in Analyses. The final sample size for this study included 4569 subjects with 28,625 observations over a nearly 40 year period.

wave [18]. Individual-level covariates included the time-varying variables age, marital status, employment status, smoking status, and alcohol consumption, and also the time-invariant education (only available in Waves 2 and 3). Despite not allowing neighborhood-level variance in the final model, we did include a covariate for census tract poverty. This measure is the percent of census tract residents with family incomes below the US poverty line, and we obtained the measure from the US Census for 1970, 1980, 1990, and 2000. Its effect represents the extent to which the average neighborhood BMI covaries with the poverty level of the neighborhood after adjusting for the other characteristics of the individuals in the neighborhood. Because of changing census tract borders over time, we used data from the commercial vendor Geolytics which adjusted all census data to the 2000 tract boundaries. We assigned census data to subjects by waves according to their census tract of residence and the date of their study examination, selecting the Census closest to the examination date. Residential addresses for subjects were collected at each of the eight waves of follow-up and were subsequently geocoded using ArcGIS, Version 9.3 (Redlands, CA).

1.2.4 MODEL BUILDING AND ANALYSIS

Our models were two-level multilevel models accounting for between-individual and within-individual (or pure "error") variance. When determining how best to account for individual-level variance, we explored several modeling strategies. In our data, the longitudinal trajectory in BMI appeared nonlinear with some evidence of nonlinear changes in the variance over time (Figure S1 in Appendix S1; Table S2 in Appendix S1); therefore, we chose models that included fixed effects and random slopes for both linear time and the natural log of time (see Figure S2 in Appendix S1 for model specification) to account for non-linearity. The variable time represented the wave of follow-up, with values from 1 to 8.

We first generated descriptive results using SAS statistical software, Version 9.1 (Cary, North Carolina). Using MLWin Version 2.24 (Bristol, United Kingdom) [19], we then examined the population means and the individual-level and pure error variation in BMI, controlling for individual- and neighborhood-level covariates (Methods Note S1 in Appendix S1 for details). Because of prior studies showing differential variation in BMI by gender, we ran sex-stratified models [8], [10], [12].

To determine how much of the unexplained individual-level variation in BMI was accounted for by baseline BMI, we subsequently fit separate models for Waves 2 through 8 with each model fit two ways: with Wave 1 BMI as a predictor and without. These models included all of the same covariates previously specified but had smaller sample sizes because we included outcomes only for Waves 2 through 8 (4569 subjects, 24,467 observations). We also included wave by age interactions to help differentiate temporal trends in BMI from aging trends.

Further, to determine whether BMI mean and standard deviation trajectories differed by baseline weight classification, we fit four models for each gender corresponding to the four categories of baseline BMI: underweight (BMI <18.5 kg/m^2), normal weight (BMI 18.5 to 24.9 kg/m^2), overweight (BMI 25 to 29.9 kg/m^2), and obese (BMI ≥ 30 kg/m^2). Our a priori hypothesis was that mean BMI increased more rapidly for overweight and obese participants [2]. In each case, a single longitudinal model was fit to BMI in Waves 2 through 8 with the same covariates, including Wave 1 BMI and wave by age interactions.

For all models, we used Markov Chain Monte Carlo (MCMC) analyses to generate multiple iterative samples from the joint posterior distribution of the parameters, from which parameter estimates could be constructed [20]. We used 10,000 iterative samples as a burn-in with 100,000 samples to generate final parameter estimates. We report posterior means and associated 95% credible intervals as point and interval estimates of the true model parameters. Significant findings are adjudicated to those predictors with estimated parameters whose 95% credible intervals excluded 0.

1.3 RESULTS

The mean number of observations per subject was 6.3 with a range of 2 to 8 observations (by construction, the lower limit was 2 not 1). The mean BMI increased from 24.0 kg/m^2 at Wave 1 to 27.7 at Wave 8 for women and from 26.6 kg/m^2 to 29.0 for men (Table 1, Figure S1 in Appendix S1).

TABLE 1: Characteristics of Sample, Framingham Heart Study Offspring Cohort, 1971 to 2008.

		Mean Across Waves	Wave 1 Mean, Wave 8 Mean	Mean Across Waves	Wave 1 Mean, Wave 8 Mean
		Female N = 2366* Observations = 15,016		Male N = 2203* Observations = 13,609	
BMI (kg/m^2)		26.1	24.0, 27.7	27.7	26.6, 29.0
Age (yr)		52.4	37.3, 66.9	52,6	38.4, 67.0
Education (%)	≤ High school	44.1	45.6, 35.3	37,4	39.0, 26.5
	> High school	51.8	46.9, 65.7	58.4	53.4, 73.4
	Missing Education	4.1	7.5, 0	4.3	7.6, 0.1
Married (%)		75.4	86.2, 65.0	85.4	88.6, 84.0
Employed (%)		60.0	53.3, 39.4	77.3	95.6, 46.1
Current Smoker (%)		24.8	43.0, 8.2	24.8	45.0, 7.5
Alcohol Intake (%)	0 drinks/day	35.8	16.6, 52.0	23.8	8.8, 38.0
	1-2 drinks/ day	59.0	77.4, 44.9	55.2	63.9, 48.4
	>2 drinks/day	5.2	6.0, 3.0	21.0	27.3, 13.6
Neighbor-hood Poverty		5.4	6.0, 5.6	5.3	6.1, 5.4

**The number of female subjects was 2148 in Wave 1 and 1518 in Wave 8. The number of male subjects was 2010 in Wave 1 and 1261 in Wave 8. The total number of subjects is greater than subjects in Wave 1 because some observations did not meet inclusion criteria (e.g. a subject had missing BMI in Wave 1 but available BMI in subsequent waves).*

In addition to the increase in mean BMI, the variation in BMI increased substantially over time (Table S2 in Appendix S1, Figure S3 in Appendix S1), with higher variability at each wave for women than for men. For women, the unadjusted standard deviation increased from 4.55 kg/m^2 in Wave 1 to 5.86 in Wave 8, and for men from 3.55 kg/m^2 to 4.67; the values of the coefficient of variation confirm the increase in BMI variability over time and the greater variability for women. Thus, the weight diversity of the population grew across time compared to a system where the standard deviation was proportional to the mean.

The pattern of BMI distribution also changed over time, with less skewness for both women (0.04 to 0.01) and no change for men (0.02 to 0.02), indicating a more normal distribution of BMI by Wave 8 for women. Consistent with the foregoing, kurtosis, a measure of the presence of outliers, declined quite substantially over time for women (5.62 to 1.52) with a slight increase for men (1.12 to 1.76). Overall, the distribution of BMI over time maintained a similar shape for men (slightly skewed and with thicker tails than the normal distribution) but became substantially more normal for women.

TABLE 2: Parameter Estimates from Final Models, Framingham Heart Study Offspring Cohort, 1971 to 2008.

		Female N = 2366 Obs = 15,016		Male N = 2203 Obs = 13,609	
Variable		β	95% Credible Interval	β	95% Credible Interval
Intercept		24.4	24.0, 24.9*	26.4	26.0, 26.8*
Time/Wave of Observation (1 to 8)		0.26	0.17, 0.34*	0.31	0.24, 0.38*
Natural Log of Time		0.61	0.38, 0.84*	0.02	-0.16, 0.21
Age		0.04	0.03-0.06*	0.02	0.003, 0.03*
Education	≤ high school	Ref		Ref	
	> high school	-0.61	-0.85, -0.36*	-0.48	-0.69, -0.27*
	Missing education	0.37	-0.06, 0.79	0.25	-0.10, 0.60
Married		0.47	0.34, 0.60*	0.26	0.14, 0.37*
Employed		0.12	0.03, 0.20	0.19	0.10, 0.28*
Smoker		-0.90	-1.0, -0.77*	-0.73	-0.84, -0.62*
Alcohol Consumption	0 drinks/day	Ref		Ref	
	1-2 drinks/day	0.19	0.10, 0.27*	0.22	0.13, 0.31*
	>2 drinks/day	0.29	0.10, 0.48*	0.32	0.20, 0.44*
Neighborhood poverty[+]		0.002	-0.01, 0.02	-0.006	-0.02, 0.004

TABLE 2: *Cont.*

		Female N = 2366 Obs = 15,016		Male N = 2203 Obs = 13,609	
Variance Components					
Level		Standard Deviation	95% Credible Interval	Standard Deviation	95% Credible Interval
Individual Level	Random Intercept	4.61	4.46, 4.75*	3.41	3.30, 3.52*
	Random Slope for Time	1.18	1.12, 1.24*	0.87	0.81, 0.93*
	Random Slope for Natural Log of Time	3.42	3.22, 3.62*	2.42	2.24, 2.61*
Pure Error Variance		1.49	1.46, 1.51*	1,25	1.23, 1.27*
Deviance Information Criteria (DIC) for model fit		59,538		49,167	

**95% credible interval does not cross 0.*

+Census tract information was unavailable for some tracts. Almost all of this missing data was from 1970 when some land areas were not yet assigned a census tract. For this analysis, we had census tract poverty data for 14,355 of the 15,016 observations among women and 12,989 of the 13,609 included observations among men. To ensure comparability across models, we included a dummy variable accounting for the availability of census tract poverty data along with a modified poverty variable (missing poverty data set to 0 rather than missing) in the final model. This did not change results for census tract poverty but did allow us to include all observations in the analyses that included this variable.

The final models included all individual-level covariates as well as neighborhood poverty (Table 2). For women and men, as expected, the covariates that were positively associated with BMI were time, increasing age, increasing alcohol consumption, and being married. Mean BMI increased in a non-linear pattern for women but not for men; the natural log of time for women was significantly positively associated with BMI. Smoking and higher education (> high school vs. ≤ high school) were negatively associated with BMI for both women and men. Neighborhood poverty was not associated with BMI. For men, being employed was positively associated with BMI. Model fit did not improve with the addition of demographic variables (age, marital status, employment status, education) or with the addition of census tract poverty; however, model fit did improve with the addition of behavioral variables (alcohol consumption and smoking status) (Table S3 in Appendix S1).

As we found for the unadjusted BMI variance, the individual-level random slopes for time and the natural log of time in fully-adjusted models revealed increasing heterogeneity in BMI across time for women and men (Table 2, Figure 2). The adjusted standard deviation in BMI increased more than the unadjusted, from 4.18 kg/m^2 at Wave 1 to 6.15 at Wave 8 for women and from 3.31 kg/m^2 to 4.73 for men (Figure 2). Thus, similar to unadjusted BMI, we found a greater increase in the BMI variance than the BMI mean after controlling for covariates and clustering.

To determine how much of the between-individual variation in BMI was accounted for by baseline BMI at Wave 1, we ran two sets of models restricted to observations from Waves 2 to 8, with baseline BMI and without, including all of the same covariates as for the prior models. In models without baseline BMI, the standard deviation in BMI at Wave 2 was 4.63 kg/m^2 for women and 3.46 for men (variance 21.5 kg/m^2 and 12.0). The addition of baseline BMI decreased standard deviations at Wave 2 to 1.95 kg/m^2 for women and 1.42 for men (variance 3.80 kg/m^2 and 2.01). The baseline BMI, thus, accounted for 82% and 83% of the between-individual variance in BMI, respectively, for women and men (data not shown in tables).

To assess the impact of baseline weight on the trajectories of BMI mean and variance, we then fit four models for each sex, stratified by baseline BMI classification—underweight, normal weight, overweight, obese—including BMI in Waves 2 to 8 as the outcome. These models also included wave by age interactions and Wave 1 BMI as predictors (Table S4 in Appendix S1, Table S5 in Appendix S1, Table S6 in Appendix S1, Table S7 in Appendix S1). In these models, being married was associated with higher BMI for normal weight and overweight women and men as well as obese women. Smoking was negatively associated with BMI in nearly all models, showing its strong negative effect on weight gain over time. Alcohol consumption was associated with higher weight only among overweight women and men and normal weight men. Higher baseline BMI was associated with higher subsequent BMI except among underweight women and men. The interaction effects between age and wave were negative and significant in nearly all models, suggesting that age became an increasingly

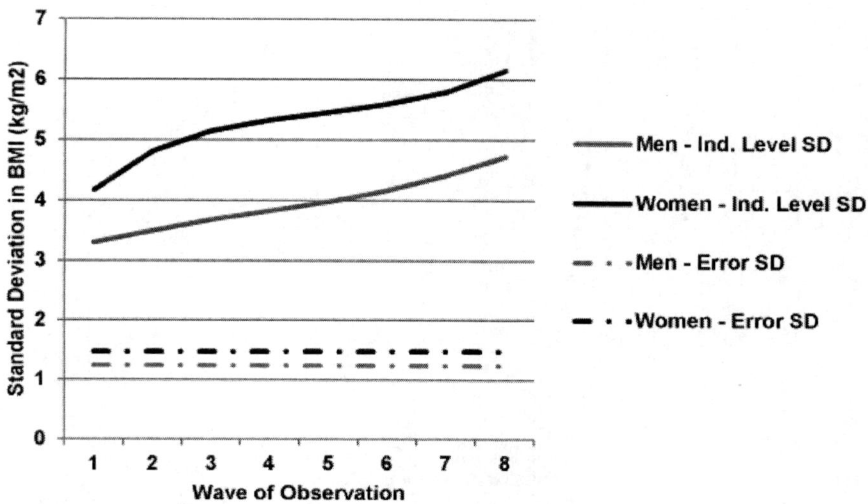

FIGURE 2: Adjusted Standard Deviation in Body Mass Index, Framingham Heart Study Offspring Cohort, 1971–2008. In the fully adjusted models, the total unexplained variation in BMI attributed to individuals across time (individual-level standard deviation) steadily increased from 1971 to 2008 for both women and men. The error standard deviation represents the idiosyncratic pure error variance. We accounted for non-linear increases in between-individual BMI standard deviation by including a random intercept at the individual level and random slopes for time and the natural log of time.

protective factor against weight gain over time. This trend likely represents the transition from being young adults (when metabolic rate and exercise levels may decline with age) to elderly (when reduced muscle mass and frailty may overpower reductions in metabolic rate).

In these models, mean BMI among men had parallel increases across baseline weight classifications with a plateau in BMI evident by Wave 8 (Figure 3B). Women had similar patterns except for obese women, who demonstrated somewhat more rapid weight gain in initial waves, followed by a partial reversal by Wave 8 (Figure 3A). Among women, standard deviation was proportion to baseline weight, with highest standard deviations for obese women over time and lowest for underweight women (Figure 4A). For men, underweight, normal weight, and overweight subjects at baseline had very similar standard deviations over time (Figure 4B).

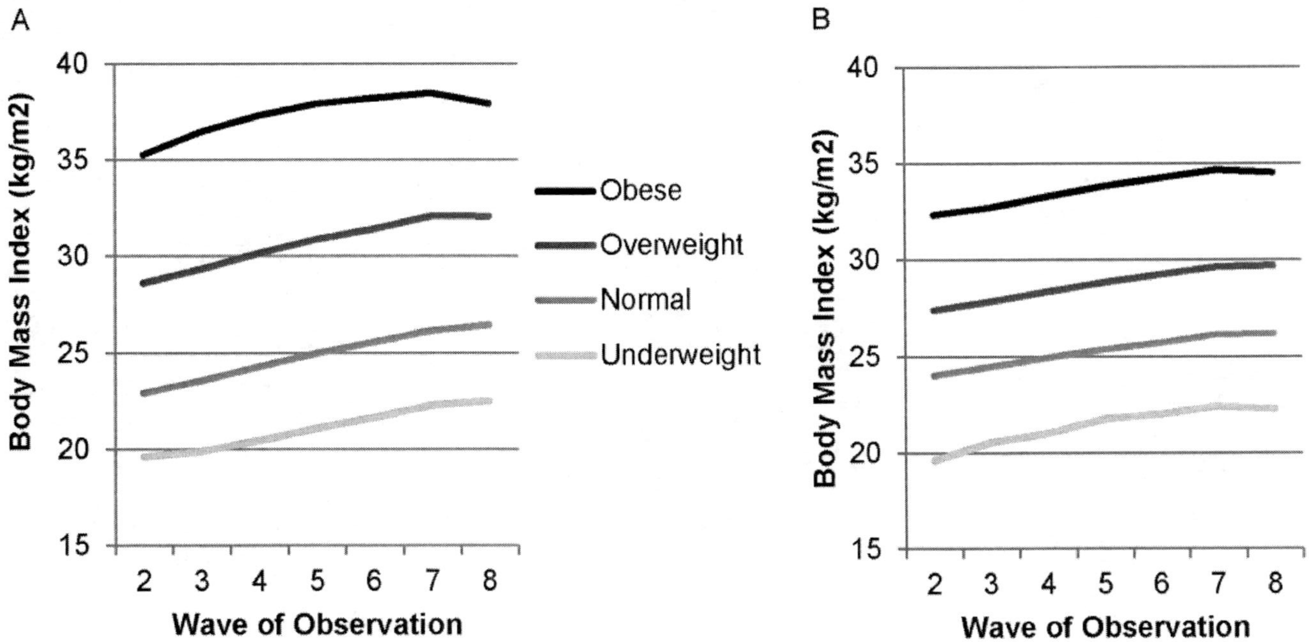

FIGURE 3: Body Mass Index Trajectories by Baseline Weight Classification, Framingham Heart Study Offspring Cohort, 1979–2008. Using results from the fully-adjusted models, we plotted the BMI trajectory for women (A) and men (B) based on their weight classification at baseline (during Wave 1, 1971–1975), controlling for covariates including baseline BMI. Weight classifications were underweight (BMI <18.5 kg/m2), normal weight (18.5 to 24.9), overweight (25 to 29.9), and obese (≥30). Lines represent trajectories for the typical male or female (mean age at each wave, married, employed,>high school education, non-smoker, consuming 1–2 alcoholic drinks daily, living in a census tract at mean poverty level, with mean baseline BMI for that weight classification).

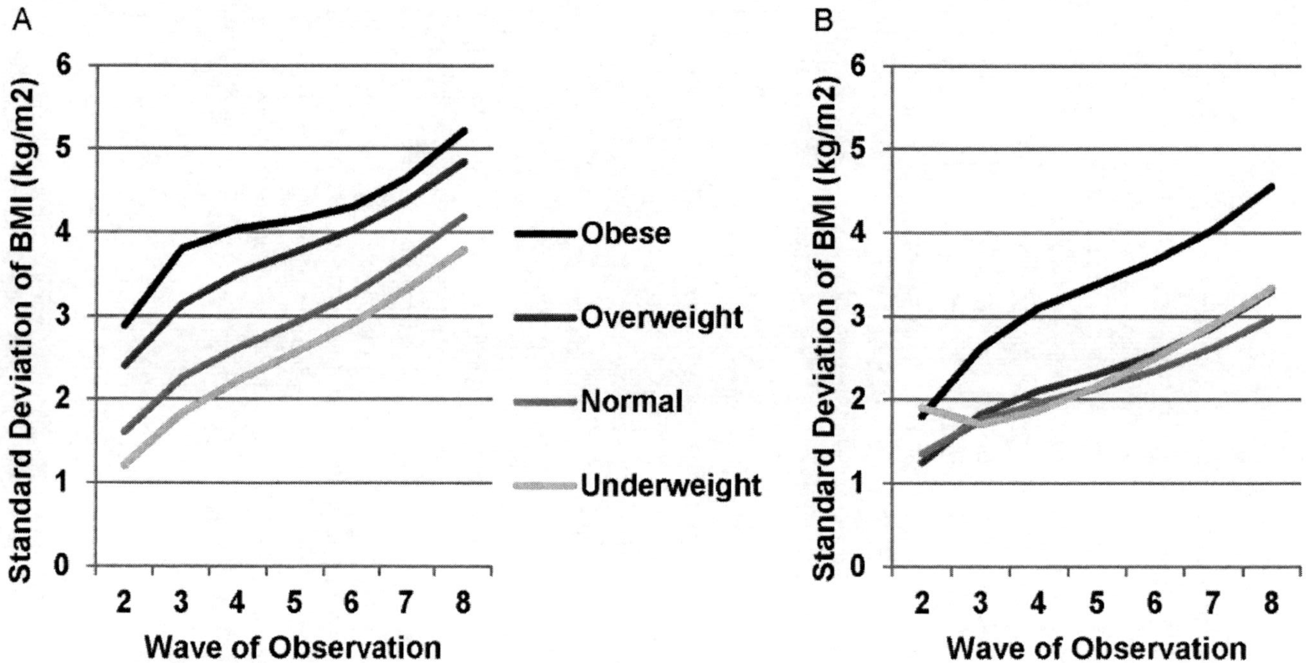

FIGURE 4: Individual-Level Standard Deviation in Body Mass Index by Baseline Weight Classification, Framingham Heart Study Offspring Cohort, 1979–2008. In the fully adjusted models, the individual-level standard deviation of BMI steadily increased from 1971 to 2008 for both women (A) and men (B) in all baseline weight classifications. Standard deviation increases were similar across most weight classifications with larger standard deviations for both obese women and men, and larger increases across time for obese men. We accounted for non-linear increases in between-individual BMI standard deviation by including a random intercept at the individual level and random slopes for time and the natural log of time.

Obese men had substantially higher standard deviations with continued divergence of these values from other weight classes over time.

1.4 DISCUSSION

Using data from the Framingham Heart Study Offspring Cohort over a nearly 40 year period, we show that factors intrinsic to individuals accounted for the overwhelming proportion of the variation in BMI over time. We also found increasing population means and variation for BMI over time. For both men and women, baseline BMI accounted for most of the unexplained individual-level variation in BMI, demonstrating that BMI reached by the late 30s (mean age at Wave 1 was 38 years for men, 37 for women), determined BMI until their late 60s (mean age at Wave 8 was 67 years for both men and women). The rapidity of weight gain was similar across all baseline weight classifications except for women who were obese at baseline. Obese women gained weight somewhat more rapidly than women with lower baseline BMIs until they were in their early 50s with an abatement of this trend thereafter. BMI variation increased over time for participants in all baseline weight categories. Variation was greatest for obese female and male subjects, demonstrating a more heterogeneous population across time.

The parallel increases in weight gain across baseline weight classifications calls for a relatively uniform population-targeted strategy to decrease risk for weight gain. Further, because weight trajectories appear to be set by the late 30s, strategies focused on children and young adults might be most effective [21]. The more rapid increases in BMI through middle age among obese women call for somewhat varied strategies to address risk for weight gain by age. Obese women may benefit from more aggressive interventions to counter risk for weight gain during middle age, with less need for interventions in the mid-to-late 60s due to a typical regression of weight gain by that point. Men have similar BMI increases across time irrespective of baseline BMI; however, the more rapid increase in variance among obese men also calls for somewhat more targeted approaches for this group.

These results, showing increasing variation in BMI but a more uniform distribution over time, contrasts somewhat with recent data from Flegal, et al. [2]. That study used data from the National Health and Nutrition Examination Survey (NHANES), a repeated cross-sectional survey of a representative sample of US adults, and found an increase in BMI mean and variation as well as a rightward skewing of the distribution of BMI over time for both women and men. Using our large longitudinal database, and accounting for both aging and secular trends, we find an increase in BMI mean and variation, with a more normal distribution of BMI emerging across time, especially for women.

Finally, our analyses shed light on the possible role of neighborhood of residence in the growth of obesity over the past four decades. In contrast to prior longitudinal studies, in our study, neighborhood of residence accounted for a very small proportion of BMI variance, and neighborhood poverty was unrelated to BMI [11], [22]. Because of the very small variance contributed by the neighborhood level in cross sectional models in most waves, we did not include neighborhood as a level in final models. We did find that census tracts accounted for 1% or more of the total variation in BMI for women during three waves; however, in the other five waves, neighborhoods accounted for less than 0.6% of the total BMI variation. Finding these differences across time highlights the importance of having longitudinal data for a cohort over a long period of time. Our study may differ from prior studies because of the characteristics of our sample, which included racially homogeneous subjects mostly living in smaller towns where public transportation is limited, typically requiring use of cars for transportation.

Our study has limitations. First, we could not measure characteristics of neighborhoods where subjects work, a possible source of unmeasured confounding between BMI and neighborhood characteristics. Second, we could more effectively determine the age at which BMI trajectories are established if we had measurements prior to the 1970s. Third, our sample lacks racial diversity, an unavoidable limitation of research with the FHS Offspring Cohort. However, this limitation in generalizability also could strengthen the plausibility of our findings. All subjects had some similar characteristics because they are the offspring (or an offspring's spouse) of the FHS Original Cohort, a random sampling of Framingham, Massachusetts, in the 1940s. One could argue that with fewer differences between individuals on observables, such as race, that it is reasonable to assume there are also fewer differences on unobservables and thus less impact from unmeasured confounding. Further, subjects were socioeconomically quite diverse. For example, in Wave 8, the mean census tract poverty for male subjects was 5.4% (SD 4.3%, Range 0.3% –31.0%). Fourth, we had a large number of census tracts in our sample, frequently with a small number of observations per tract. Our sample included participants from 2095 different census tracts over time, with a mean of 13.7 observations per tract (SD 79.8, range 1 to 1638). Multilevel models, by design, shrink the variance estimates toward the null for higher level units (tracts) with few observations and, therefore, may underestimate the ICC at the tract level in the cross-sectional models that we ran. Yet, shrunken residuals have the benefit of helping to avoid over-interpretation of random variation in the data as true neighborhood-level variation.

In sum, over nearly 40 years, BMI mean and variation increased in parallel across most baseline weight classifications in our sample. Individual-level characteristics, especially baseline BMI, were the primary factors in rising BMI. These findings have important implications not only for understanding the sources of the obesity epidemic in the United States but also for the targeting of interventions to address the epidemic.

REFERENCES

1. Ogden C, Fryar C, Carroll M, Flegal K (2004) Mean body weight, height, and body mass index, United States, 1960–2002. Advance Data From Vital and Health Statistics; no. 347. Hyattsville, MD: National Center for Health Statistics.
2. Flegal KM, Carroll MD, Kit BK, Ogden CL (2012) Prevalence of obesity and trends in the distribution of body mass index among US adults, 1999–2010. JAMA 307: 491–497. doi: 10.1001/jama.2012.39.
3. Malhotra R, Trulsostbye, Riley CM, Finkelstein E (2013) Young adult weight trajectories through midlife by body mass category. Obesity (Silver Spring) Epub ahead of print.
4. Ogden CL, Carroll MD (2010) Health E-stats: Prevalence of overweight, obesity and extreme obesity among adults: United States, trends 1960–1962 through 2007–2008. Hyattsville, MD: National Center for Health Statistics.

5. Flegal KM, Carroll MD, Ogden CL, Curtin LR (2010) Prevalence and trends in obesity among US adults, 1999–2008. JAMA 303: 235–241. doi: 10.1001/jama.2009.2014.
6. Sturm R, Hattori A (1038) Morbid obesity rates continue to rise rapidly in the United States. Int J Obes (Lond) 2012: 159. doi: 10.1038/ijo.2012.159.
7. Razak F, Corsi DJ, Subramanian SV (2013) Change in the body mass index distribution for women: analysis of surveys from 37 low- and middle-income countries. PLoS Med 10: e1001367. doi: 10.1371/journal.pmed.1001367.
8. King T, Kavanagh AM, Jolley D, Turrell G, Crawford D (2006) Weight and place: a multilevel cross-sectional survey of area-level social disadvantage and overweight/obesity in Australia. Int J Obes (Lond) 30: 281–287. doi: 10.1038/sj.ijo.0803176.
9. Regidor E, Gutierrez-Fisac JL, Ronda E, Calle ME, Martinez D, et al. (2008) Impact of cumulative area-based adverse socioeconomic environment on body mass index and overweight. J Epidemiol Community Health 62: 231–238. doi: 10.1136/jech.2006.059360.
10. Robert SA, Reither EN (2004) A multilevel analysis of race, community disadvantage, and body mass index among adults in the US. Soc Sci Med 59: 2421–2434. doi: 10.1016/j.socscimed.2004.03.034.
11. Sund ER, Jones A, Midthjell K (2010) Individual, family, and area predictors of BMI and BMI change in an adult Norwegian population: findings from the HUNT study. Soc Sci Med 70: 1194–1202. doi: 10.1016/j.socscimed.2010.01.007.
12. Harrington DW, Elliott SJ (2009) Weighing the importance of neighbourhood: a multilevel exploration of the determinants of overweight and obesity. Soc Sci Med 68: 593–600. doi: 10.1016/j.socscimed.2008.11.021.
13. Downs GW, Roche DM (1979) Interpreting heteroscedasticity. Am J Political Sci 23: 816–828. doi: 10.2307/2110809.
14. Davidoff F (2009) Heterogeneity is not always noise: lessons from improvement. JAMA 302: 2580–2586. doi: 10.1001/jama.2009.1845.
15. Merlo J, Ohlsson H, Lynch KF, Chaix B, Subramanian SV (2009) Individual and collective bodies: using measures of variance and association in contextual epidemiology. J Epidemiol Community Health 63: 1043–1048. doi: 10.1136/jech.2009.088310.
16. Braumoeller B (2006) Explaining variance; or, stuck in a moment we can't get out of. Political Analysis 14: 268–290. doi: 10.1093/pan/mpj009.
17. Framingham Heart Study Consent Forms website. Available: http://www.framinghamheartstudy.org/research/consentfms.html. Accessed 2013 Apr 16.
18. Davis N, Murabito J, Rich S, Wartofsky MJ (1994) Framingham Heart Study. Clinic protocol manual. Available: http://www.framinghamheartstudy.org/share/protocols/offspring_exam_5.pdf. Accessed 2013 Apr 16.
19. Rasbash J, Steele F, Browne WJ, Goldstein H (2009) A User's Guide to MLWin: Version 2.10. Bristol, United Kingdom: Centre for Multilevel Modeling. Available: http://www.bristol.ac.uk/cmm/software/mlwin/download/mlwin-userman-09.pdf. Accessed 2013 Apr 16.
20. Browne WJ (2012) MCMC estimation in MLWin: Version 2.26. Bristol, United Kingdom: Centre for Multilevel Modeling. Available: http://www.bristol.ac.uk/cmm/software/mlwin/download/2-26/mcmc-print.pdf. Accessed 2013 Apr 16.

21. de Kroon ML, Renders CM, van Wouwe JP, van Buuren S, Hirasing RA (2010) The Terneuzen Birth Cohort: BMI change between 2 and 6 years is most predictive of adult cardiometabolic risk. PLoS One 5: e13966. doi: 10.1371/journal.pone.0013966.
22. Stafford M, Brunner EJ, Head J, Ross NA (2010) Deprivation and the development of obesity: a multilevel, longitudinal study in England. Am J Prev Med 39: 130–139.

There is some online supporting information that is not included in this version of the article. To see these additional files, please use the citation in the beginning of the chapter to view the original article.

CHAPTER 2

COMMUNITY ENERGY BALANCE: A FRAMEWORK FOR CONTEXTUALIZING CULTURAL INFLUENCES ON HIGH RISK OF OBESITY IN ETHNIC MINORITY POPULATIONS

SHIRIKI KUMANYIKA, WENDELL C. TAYLOR, SONYA A. GRIER, VIKKI LASSITER, KRISTIE J. LANCASTER, CHRISTIAAN B. MORSSINK, and ANDRÉ M. N. RENZAHO

2.1 INTRODUCTION

Obesity is a major risk factor for the development of diabetes, cardiovascular diseases, certain cancers and other chronic conditions that cause disability and premature death and increase costs for health care systems (World Health Organization, 2000 and World Health Organization, 2003). It has taken a place alongside hunger and food insecurity as a major global nutrition concern (Food and Agricultural Organization of the United Nations, 2006). Levels of obesity worldwide show steep trajectories in recent decades (Al-Lawati and Jousilahti, 2004, Barr et al., 2006, Fezeu et al., 2007, Flegal et al., 2010, Katzmarzyk and Mason, 2006, Mbanya et al., 1997, New Zealand Ministry of Health, 2004, Ogden et al., 2010, Organisation for

---

Reprinted from Preventative Medicine, *55(5), Kumanyika S, Taylor WC, Grier SA, Lassiter V, Lancaster KJ, Morssink CB, Renzaho AM. Community Energy Balance: A Framework for Contextualizing Cultural Influences on High Risk of Obesity in Ethnic Minority Populations, Pages 371–381, 2012, with permission from Elsevier.*

Economic Co-operation and Development, 2010, Tremblay and Willms, 2000, Wang et al., 2002, World Health Organisation, 2005 and Wu, 2006). These population trends emanate from changes in environmental influences on eating and physical activity: underlying genetic or behavioral predispositions to obesity are more likely to be expressed under environmental conditions characterized by high availability of inexpensively-priced and heavily promoted high-calorie foods, combined with limited demand or opportunity for daily physical activity (Kumanyika et al., 2002 and World Health Organization, 2000). Conditions that predispose individuals to excess caloric consumption are now typical in high-income countries as well as many low- and middle-income countries. Humans are physiologically, socio-culturally, and psychologically geared to eat when food is available, store excess calories as fat, and have poorly developed systems of appetite regulation to prevent overconsumption of calories (World Health Organization, 2000). Hence, weight gain to obese levels reflects normal responses to an abnormal environment.

Within this overall picture, the higher obesity prevalence reported for many ethnic minority populations in high-income, plural societies demand attention to the specific environmental circumstances that could be responsible. Note that although current usage refers to "racial" or ethnic minorities, here the term 'ethnic' minority encompasses both, given our emphasis on cultural and contextual influences and recognizing that racial classifications, although socially meaningful, do not reflect biological "races" (Race Ethnicity and Genetics Working Group, 2005). Data on obesity prevalence differences in high income countries by ethnicity are in Table 1 and Table 2 for adults and children. Only data permitting the comparison of ethnic minority and majority reference populations are shown. The type of data presented and the ability to identify statistically significant differences were not consistent across sources but the data in the tables are illustrative. Higher obesity prevalence has been observed in non-Hispanic Black, Hispanic, and Native American populations in the United States (Anderson and Whitaker, 2009, Flegal et al., 2010, Ogden et al., 2012 and Schoenborn and Adams, 2010) and aboriginal populations in Canada, Australia, and New Zealand (Australian National Institute of Health and Welfare, 2007, New Zealand Ministry of Health, 2008 and Tjepkema, 2005) (see Table 1 and Table 2). In other cases, attention is focused on obesity in first or subsequent generations of immigrant populations, especially those from non-English speaking backgrounds, e.g. African and Middle Eastern migrants to Australia (Booth et al., 2006 and Saleh et al., 2002), Afro-Caribbean, Indian and Pakistani populations in the United Kingdom (Rennie and Jebb, 2005 and Saxena et al., 2004), Turkish and Moroccan immigrants in The Netherlands (de Wilde et al., 2009 and Dijkshoorn et al., 2011), Mexican American immigrants to the United States (Van Hook et al., 2012) and Asian Indian immigrants to several countries (Fernandez et al., 2011). Data for some of these populations are also shown in Table 1 and Table 2. In addition, although there is recent evidence of stabilization or decreases in obesity in some countries or localities, such findings are less likely to apply to their ethnic minorities (Centers for Disease Control, Prevention, 2011, de Wilde et al., 2009, Flegal et al., 2012 and Madsen et al., 2010). Also evident in Table 1 and Table 2 (although not addressed in this review), data for some Asian populations indicate lower than average prevalence of obesity. This may partly reflect underestimation of body fatness and related health risks in populations of Asian descent with standard body mass index cut offs (WHO Expert Panel, 2004). Overall, however, the data suggest that obesity-promoting environmental influences are somehow more prevalent or more potent in several ethnic minority populations, across diverse societal contexts. This review focuses on ways to improve understanding of the underlying nature of this excess risk and related implications for planning and evaluating interventions.

The commonly used ecological framework for understanding obesity in populations recognizes the interwoven relationships that exist between individuals and their physical, economic, political, and socio-cultural environments (Swinburn et al., 1999). However, ecological frameworks developed for specific application to socio-culturally distinctive and often socially disadvantaged population groups are relatively scarce, especially frameworks that define cultural contexts in ways that include structural variables (Krieger, 2001 and Kumanyika et al., 2007). The tendency is to focus on culturally influenced attitudes, values, and norms related to eating, physical, and body image that might predispose individuals to obesity, to be addressed in specially-designed, "culturally adapted" interventions (Caballero et al., 2003, Flynn et al., 2006, Klesges et al., 2010, Kumanyika, 2010a, Kumanyika, 2010b, Kumanyika et al., 2003, Lindberg and Stevens, 2007, Osei-Assibey et al., 2010, Paradis et al., 2005, Renzaho et al., 2010, Teufel-Shone, 2006, Thomas, 2002 and Whitt-Glover and Kumanyika, 2009).

TABLE 1: Examples of ethnic group differences in obesity prevalence in high income countries: adultsa.

Population and Data source[b and c] and year(s)	Ethnic group	Gender	
		Males	Females
USA (Flegal et al., 2010)	Total Population	32.2 (29.5–35.0)	35.5 (33.2–37.7)
National Health and Nutrition Examination Survey (NHANES), 2007–2008; age-adjusted % (95% CI) of adults ages 20 years and older with BMI ≥ 30 kg/m^2	Non-Hispanic White[d]	31.9 (28.1–35.7)	33.0 (29.3–36.6)
	Non-Hispanic Black	37.3 (32.3–42.4)	49.6 (45.5–53.7)
	Mexican American	35.9 (28.9–43.0)	45.1 (38.9–51.2)
USA (Schoenborn and Adams, 2010)	Total Population	25.7 (0.30)	25.0 (0.29)
National Health Interview Survey (NHIS), 2005–2007; age-adjusted % (SE) of adults ages 18 years and older with BMI ≥ 30 kg/m^2 based on self-reported weight and height	Non-Hispanic White[d]	25.6 (0.37)	22.9 (0.35)
	Non-Hispanic Black	29.4 (0.85)	38.8 (074)
	Mexican American	26.7 (0.93)	32.9 (0.96)
	American Indian or Alaska Native	33.9 (4.01)	33.4 (3.42)
	Asian	9.9 (0.84)	7.1 (0.70)
	Native Hawaiian/ Pacific Islander	35.5 (7.16)	21.8 (5.42)
Canada (Tjepkema, 2005)[e]	Total population[d]	22.9 (20.7–25.2)	23.2 (21.3–25.1)
Canadian Community Health Survey, 2004; % (95% CI) of adults ages 18 years and older with BMI ≥ 30 kg/m^2	White	25.5 (23.0–28.0)	24.8 (22.7–26.9)
	Aboriginal (off-reserve)	33.6 (19.2–48.0)	40.0 (27.9–52.0)

TABLE 1: *Cont.*

Population and Data source[b and c] and year(s)	Ethnic group	Gender	
		Males	Females
England (Rennie and Jebb, 2005)	General population[d]	18.9	20.9
Health Survey for England, 1999; % of adults ages 16 to 55 + years with BMI ≥ 30 kg/m²	Black Caribbean	18.3	31.0
	Indian	11.9	19.6
	Pakistani	12.6	25.6
	Bangladeshi	5.4	9.5
	Chinese	6.2	4.5
Amsterdam, Netherlands (Dijkshoorn et al., 2011)	Dutch[d]	12.6	19.8
Amsterdam Health Monitor Survey, 2004; % of adults 18 to 69 years with BMI ≥ 30 kg/m²	Turkish	26.4	49.8
	Moroccan	20.7	47.5
Australia (Australian National Institute of Health and Welfare, 2007)	Non-Indigenous[d]	17.8	14.9
2004–2005 National Aboriginal and Torres Strait Islander Health Survey and National Health Survey; age-standardized % of adults ages 18 years and older with BMI ≥ 30 kg/m² based on self-reported or measured weight and height	Indigenous	27.4	29.4

TABLE 1: *Cont.*

Population and Data source[b and c] and year(s)	Ethnic group	Gender	
		Males	Females
New Zealand (New Zealand Ministry of Health, 2008)	Non-Māori[d]	22.6 (21.0–24.2)	23.7 (22.2–25.3)
2006–2007 New Zealand Health Survey; age-adjusted % (95% CI) of adults ages 15 years and older with BMI ≥ 30 kg/m^2	Māori	43.2 (39.6–46.9)	43.2 (41.2–45.2)
	Non-Pacific[d]	22.4 (20.9–23.9)	23.8 (22.3–25.3)
	Pacific	63.9 (58.6–69.3)	66.3 (61.2–71.5)
	Non-Asian[d]	26.2 (24.6–27.7)	27.6 (26.0–29.2)
	Asian	10.0 (7.2–12.8)	13.6 (11.0–16.3)

[a] *Ethnic classifications are as reported in the source.*

[b] *Data for total population are reported if available and include other ethnic groups; whether prevalence is age-adjusted is reported if noted in the source; 95% confidence intervals (CI) or standard errors (SE) are provided where available, to assist with evaluation of group differences; bold type indicates significantly higher gender-specific obesity prevalence in the ethnic minority group relative to the indicated reference group when reported as such in the source.*

[c] *Based on measured weight and height unless otherwise noted.*

[d] *Reference group for comparison within source.*

[e] *Estimates for Canadian Blacks and South Asians were statistically unreliable and, therefore not reported.*

TABLE 2: Examples of ethnic group differences in overweight and obesity prevalence in high income countries: childrena.

Population and data source[b, c] and year (s)	Ethnic group	Age group (years) and gender	
USA (Ogden et al., 2012)		Males, ages 2 to 19	Females, ages 2 to 19
		Obese	Obese
National Health and Nutrition Examination Survey (NHANES), 2009–2010; % (95% CI) of children with obesity (CDC reference)[e]	Total population	18.6 (16.4–21.0)	15.0 (13.3–16.8)
	Non-Hispanic White[d]	16.1 (12.6–20.3)	11.7 (9.5–14.2)
	Non-Hispanic Black	24.3 (18.7–30.8)	24.3 (19.2–30.3)
	Hispanic	23.4 (20.5–26.6)	18.9 (15.4–22.9)
USA (Anderson and Whitaker, 2009)		Males, age 4	Females, age 4
Early Childhood Longitudinal Study, 2005; % (95% CI) of children with obesity (CDC reference)[e]		Obese	Obese
	Total population	19.8 (18.1–21.5)	17.0 (15.1–18.9)
	White, non-Hispanic[d]	17.4 (15.1–19.8)	14.3 (12.0–16.5)
	Black, non-Hispanic	22.5 (18.4–26.6)	19.0 (14.9–23.0)
	Hispanic	22.2 (19.2–25.3)	21.8 (17.9–25.7)
	American Indian/ Native Alaskan	37.0 (27.0–47.0)	25.8 (16.2–35.4)
	Asian	15.8 (11.5–20.2)	10.0 (5.9–14.0)

TABLE 2: *Cont.*

Population and data source[b, c] and year (s)	Ethnic group	Age group (years) and gender			
England (Saxena et al., 2004)		Males, ages 2 to 20		Females, ages 2 to 20	
Health Survey for England, 1999; % of children with overweight or obesity (IOTF Reference)[f]		Overweight	Obese	Overweight	Obese
	General population[d]	21.7	5.8	22.3	5.8
	Afro-Caribbean	22.6	5.1	33.3	13.0
	Indian	29.6	7.9	24.0	2.1
	Pakistani	26.2	9.0	25.7	8.0
	Bangladeshi	14.2	2.8	20.7	5.8
	Chinese	14.4	4.7	13.0	1.2
	Irish	17.3	3.3	25.6	8.3
The Hague, Netherlands (de Wilde et al., 2009)		Males, ages 3 to 16		Females, ages 3 to 16	
Electronic health records from nutrition surveillance, 2007; % of children with overweight or obesity (IOTF Reference)[f]		Overweight	Obese	Overweight	Obese
	Dutchd	8.9	2.3	10.9	3.3
	Turkish	21.4	13.1	23.2	10.7
	Moroccan	16.7	7.2	20.5	6.6
	Surinamese South Asian	14.5	5.4	12.6	4.5

TABLE 2: *Cont.*

Population and data source[b, c] and year (s)	Ethnic group	Age group (years) and gender	
New South Wales (NSW), Australia (Hardy et al., 2010)		Males, ages 5 to 16	Females, ages 5 to 16
NSW Schools Physical Activity and Nutrition Survey (SPANS), 2010; % of children with combined overweight and obesity (IOTF Reference)[f]		Combined overweight and obesity	
	English-speaking[d]	23.2	21.5
	European	34.6	12.5
	Middle-Eastern	37.3	24.6

TABLE 2: *Cont.*

Population and data source[b, c] and year (s)	Ethnic group	Age group (years) and gender			
	Asian	24.3		17.9	
New Zealand (New Zealand Ministry of Health, 2008)		Males, ages 2 to 14		Females, ages, 2 to 14	
2006–2007 New Zealand Health Survey; age-standardized % (95% CI) of children ages 2–14 years with overweight or obesity (IOTF Reference)f		Overweight	Obese	Overweight	Obese
	Non-Māori[d]	19.1 (16.4–21.8)	7.0 (5.4–8.5)	19.9 (17.2–22.6)	7.7 (5.8–9.6)
	Māori	25.3 (21.9–28.7)	11.4 (8.9–13.8)	26.4 (21.6–31.2)	12.3 (9.3–15.4)
	Non-Pacificd	19.2 (16.9–21.5)	6.3 (5.0–7.7)	19.9 (17.3–22.5)	6.5 (4.9–8.1)
	Pacific	30.6 (25.8–35.5)	21.0 (16.8–25.1)	32.0 (26.2–37.8)	26.0 (20.4–31.6)
	Non-Asiand	20.8 (18.5–23.1)	8.2 (6.9–9.5)	22.3 (19.7–24.8)	8.9 (7.3–10.6)
	Asian	16.9 (11.5–22.2)	5.2 (2.8–8.7)	12.2 (8.2–16.2)	6.7 (3.3–11.8)

[a] *Ethnic classifications are as reported in the source.*

[b] *Data for total population are reported if available and include other ethnic groups; whether prevalence is age-adjusted is reported if noted in the source; 95% confidence intervals (CI) or standard errors (SE) are provided, where available to assist with evaluation of group differences; bold type indicates significantly higher gender-specific, obesity prevalence in the ethnic minority group relative to the indicated reference group when reported as such in the source.*

[c] *Based on measured weight and height unless otherwise noted.*

[d] *Reference group for comparison within source.*

[e] *CDC = 85th to < 95 percentile (overweight) or ≥ 95th percentile (obese) of Centers for Disease Control and Prevention BMI reference curves.*

[f] *IOTF* = International Obesity Task Force standard equivalent to adult BMI 25.0–29.9 (overweight) or ≥ 30 (obese).

Table options

The Community Energy Balance (CEB) Framework introduced in this paper addresses the need for more comprehensive guidance. The objective was to develop a visual and narrative framework describing a broad range of relevant considerations for community-level interventions.

2.2 METHODS

Six of the (SK, WCT, SAG, VL, KJL, and AMNR) authors, a group of scholars comprising expertise in nutrition, obesity prevention and treatment, physical activity, marketing, cultural anthropology, public health, and social psychology, developed a preliminary framework at a two-day brainstorming session convened for this purpose by the African American Collaborative Obesity Research Network (Kumanyika et al., 2005 and Kumanyika et al., 2007) in collaboration with the African Migrant Capacity Building and Appraisal program, an Australian obesity prevention initiative among newly arrived migrants (Renzaho, 2009, Renzaho, 2011, Renzaho et al., 2008 and Renzaho et al., 2012). The initial framework, therefore, emerged from issues and concepts identified in studies and reviews, including our own work, that focused primarily on populations of African descent in the United States or Australia. Through multiple rounds of discussions and literature reviews over a period of approximately two years, the framework development was further informed by several theoretical articles and conceptual frameworks related to cultural and structural influences on food, physical activity, and obesity, and an additional author (CBM) with training in non-western sociology was added. Although our knowledge and experiences relate to African descent populations in English-speaking nations, we made an effort to create a more generalizable framework with potential applicability to ethnic minority populations in diverse countries. Hence, we expanded the scope of considerations and literature reviews to include some evidence related to other U.S. ethnic minority populations as well as those in New Zealand, Canada and Europe. Topics and references we explored were as follows:

- cultural influences, lifestyles, eating, immigration, acculturation, food habits, physical activity, and body size from the perspectives of multiple disciplines (Anderson, 2011, Axelson, 1986, Berry, 1997, Brown and Konner,

1987, Butterfoss, 2006, Cockerham, 2005, De Garine and Koppert, 1991, De Garine and Pollock, 1995, Harrison, 2005, Jelliffe, 1967, Mintz, 1996, Mintz and DuBois, 2002, Murcott, 2002, Nelson et al., 2010, Popenoe, 2005, Sallis et al., 2006, Scheffer, 2011 and Tharp, 2001);
- ecological and life course models for analyzing influences on obesity-related risks or outcomes (Booth et al., 2001, Castro et al., 2009, Daniel et al., 2011, Glass and McAtee, 2006, Kumanyika et al., 2002, Swinburn et al., 1999 and Wetter et al., 2001);
- frameworks for understanding and addressing health inequalities related to race/ethnicity or socioeconomic status (Adler and Newman, 2002, Adler and Stewart, 2009, Dressler, 2005, Gutmann, 2003, Krieger, 2005, Kumanyika and Morssink, 2006, LaVeist, 2005, Thomas, 1998 and Thomas et al., 2011);
- frameworks for addressing cultural influences in obesity and in behavior change and health promotion more broadly (Airhihenbuwa, 1995, Caperchione et al., 2009 and Castro et al., 2010; Corneille et al., 2005, Dressler, 2005, James, 2004 and Kreuter et al., 2003; Kumanyika and Morssink, 1997 and Williams et al., 2012; Kumanyika et al., 2003, Kumanyika et al., 2007, Mavoa and McCabe, 2008, Page, 2005, Resnicow et al., 1999, Robinson, 2005, Singer, 1990, Thomas, 2002 and Vrazel et al., 2008);
- empirical studies and reviews about cultural and contextual influences on eating, physical activity, and body size (Airhihenbuwa et al., 1995, Airhihenbuwa et al., 1996, Brewis et al., 1998, Casagrande et al., 2009, Craig et al., 1996, D'Alonzo and Fischetti, 2008, Diaz et al., 2007, Gray et al., 2005, James and Underwood, 1997, Nicolaou et al., 2008, Nicolaou et al., 2009, Nicolau et al., 2012, Parham and Scarinci, 2007, Renzaho, 2004, Renzaho, 2009, Renzaho, 2011, Renzaho and Mellor, 2010, Renzaho et al., 2008, Renzaho et al., 2009a, Renzaho et al., 2009b, Renzaho et al., 2011, Rucker and Cash, 1992, Taylor et al., 1994, Taylor et al., 1998, Taylor et al., 1999, Taylor et al., 2001, Taylor et al., 2006, Taylor et al., 2007a, Taylor et al., 2007b, Teufel-Shone, 2006, Vallianatos and Raine, 2008, Van Duyn et al., 2007, Whitt-Glover and Kumanyika, 2009 and Wilson et al., 2010).

Consensus was reached on the elements and graphical presentation shown in Fig. 1 as a useful way of organizing and highlighting important issues that might otherwise be overlooked or inadequately examined. We included key elements applicable to any public health or health promotion intervention on population-wide obesity but went considerably beyond these elements to emphasize factors of particular relevance to ethnically distinct communities living within larger, majority reference populations. We recognized the applicability of many factors to non-minority populations, particularly in the ancestral or home countries of the minority populations of interest (Finucane et al., 2011 and World Health Organization,

2000) but retained the focus on African descent and other ethnic minorities in high-income, plural societies to avoid undue complexity.

2.3 RESULTS

2.3.1 OVERVIEW

The framework depicts the public health/health promotion goal—achievement of energy balance and healthy weight status at the community level (bottom, center of Fig. 1)—and the dynamic societal contexts that affect eating and activity patterns (top). Intervention considerations relate to: settings and change agents for obesity prevention initiatives (middle); types of initiatives and action pathways (targets) that can contribute to goal achievement (right side); and cultural-contextual variables that influence change perspectives and processes (left side). Each of these elements is described below.

2.3.2 PUBLIC HEALTH GOAL

The scale showing a balance between food intake and physical activity represents the goal. Energy balance is a function of energy intake (calories in foods eaten) and energy expenditure (calories expended through physical activity). Although the excess of intake over expenditure that leads to excess weight gain and obesity is usually defined at the individual level, the CEB framework uses the concept of energy balance to refer to the balance of community level influences on energy intake to reflect collective, historical, and cultural constructs or drivers associated with both physical activity and food intake. In the text that follows, we will identify several of these constructs and discuss the ways social forces shape communities, the arenas of power and social interactions, as well as social systems and their impacts on the health and welfare of individuals as members of communities.

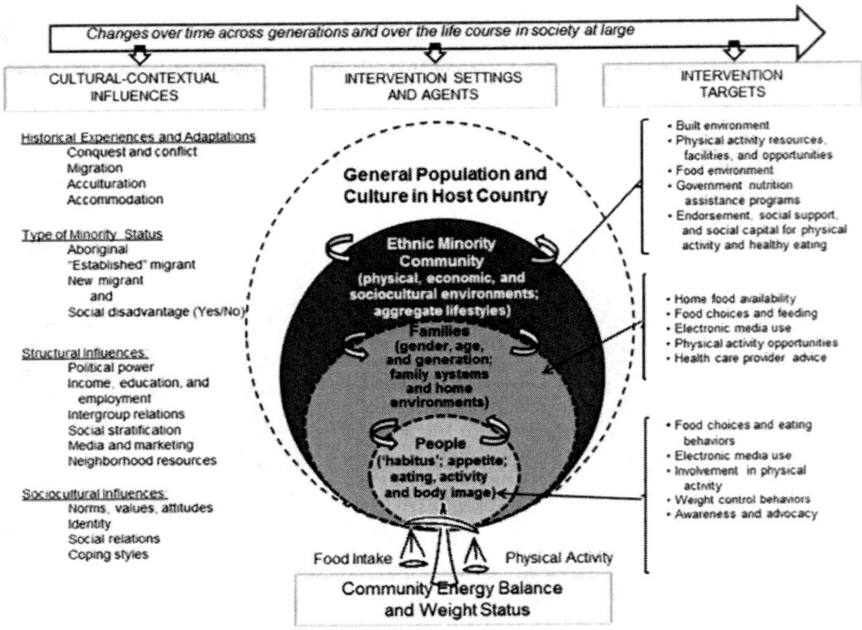

FIGURE 1: A "community energy balance" framework for identifying cultural and contextual influences predisposing to high risk of obesity in ethnic minority populations.

2.3.3 CHANGES OVER TIME, ACROSS GENERATIONS, AND OVER THE LIFE COURSE IN SOCIETY AT LARGE

The arrow at the top highlights the ever changing, societal contexts related to food intake and physical activity in whole populations across the life course (Kumanyika et al., 2002, World Health Organization, 2000 and World Health Organization, 2003) and refers to the availability and affordability of foods, socio-cultural meanings and health values, and opportunities and expectations related to utilitarian, recreational, and health-related physical activity behaviors. The marked increases in the availability and affordability of food energy, especially when experienced in terms of prolonged exposure to hunger and food insecurity, can lead to norms of overeating and seeking satiety that cannot easily be corrected by cognition and sheer knowledge. This part of the framework also captures advances in technology, population dynamics, political and social globalization, and economic development. Major societal changes also follow events such as wars, natural disasters, and changes in political boundaries, or in stratification systems.

2.3.4 INTERVENTION SETTINGS AND AGENTS

2.3.4.1 GENERAL POPULATION AND CULTURE IN HOST COUNTRY OR AREA

Referring to the circles in the middle, the unshaded layer contrasts the environments and aggregate lifestyles of the respective general population with those of the ethnic minority community of interest. The shading indicates that circumstances in the population at large are the background against which interventions happen (Swinburn et al., 1999 and World Health Organization, 2000) (Booth et al., 2001 and Kumanyika et al., 2002). The country characteristics are presumed to reflect dominant structures and perspectives, e.g., the nature and intensity of the obesity-promoting or protective forces in the physical, economic, and sociocultural environments in the general population and how they enhance or deter social forces in ethnic subpopulations.

2.3.4.2 COMMUNITIES

Communities are the key cultural and structural entities between members and the society at large. They are the settings within which social life occurs and in which people experience the stresses of daily living. Communities include physical and social settings, formal and informal institutions (e.g., businesses, schools, religious organizations, social and civic organizations), communication channels and legally-recognized or formal governance structures. Communities are the intervention settings most likely to be within the reach of change agents. Change agents may be community leaders, members or "outsiders" who provide services or have influence within a community. Community processes involve shared customs, traditions, rituals, perceptions (including self-identity) and expectations and dynamically blend historical and current experiences and exposures (Robinson, 2005). Minority communities then are contrasted, and contrast themselves, with the "general" population on these variables. Considering lifestyles in the aggregate acknowledges the reciprocal and social norming effects of a person's behavior in relation to the behavior of others in the group and society at large. However, each individual responds uniquely to exposures and experiences.

2.4.3.3 FAMILIES

Family systems and homes include both nuclear and extended kinship networks that describe an array of circumstances and influence pathways: communication styles; inter- and intra-generational relationships among family members; family cohesion and family support; role modeling; gender role differentiation; status hierarchies; and intergenerational influences. Also, family systems reflect material resources and their distribution as they affect feeding, food provision, and food and activity-related roles, obligations, choices, motivations, and preferences. Families are major sources and channels for transmission of cultural perspectives and mediators of interactions with the surrounding contexts. The quality of family life, and factors such as gender, rank, generation, and opportunities (education, income, social support) as aspects of family dynamics impact directly the agency of its individual members, as well as whole families in relation to community.

2.4.3.4 PEOPLE

Individuals and communities incorporate into their outlook and behaviors the learned and daily (re)-negotiated responses that reflect the settings (Super and Harkness, 2002) fields or social arenas (Bourdieu, 1984), in which they live. In these social arenas ethnicity and minority labels are extra structuring forces that influence the negotiation and the eventual behaviors. The resulting individual behaviors are often referred to as "lifestyles", although in sociology this term is more appropriately applied to aggregate than individual behavior (Cockerham, 2005 and Korp, 2010). The concept of habitus is better suited to express the way people use, wittingly or unwittingly, their agency, or lack thereof, in the daily course of living. '…Habitus is neither a result of free will, nor determined by structures, but created by a kind of interplay between the two over time: dispositions that are both shaped by past events and structures, and that shape current practices and structures and also, importantly, that condition our very perceptions of these' ((Bourdieu, 1984), page 170). In this sense habitus is created and reproduced unconsciously, 'without any deliberate pursuit of coherence… without any conscious concentration' (Bourdieu, 1984, p 170). Building on Bourdieu's work, using specifically the power dynamics of the social arenas, we propose that in the plural society, the habitus of majority and the habitus of minority peoples differ, yet interlink. Power dynamics in turn are influenced by the availability of capital. Bourdieu argues that 'capital' extends beyond the notion of material assets to capital that may be social, cultural or symbolic (Bourdieu, 1986). This construct of capital, in association with habitus, provides the core "modus operandi" that the minority member uses to be a minority, to be "in place" to be "not the other". The state of being a minority constitutes social, cultural and symbolic capital, for better or for worse.

Habitus and capital with respect to eating, physical activity, and body size are critical given the fundamental nature of these aspects of life and are shaped by historical and current societal processes related to survival and day-to-day functioning. Living in a plural society as a member of an ethnic minority group generally means coming into daily contact with cultural perspectives that challenge one's ability to maintain day to day harmony. Depending on the person and the circumstance, people may ignore or reject pressures (including behavior change messages) that are not consistent with their habitus. Or, they may change their ways of thinking and feeling about how to survive and assimilate, or negotiate compromises that fall somewhere in between. Rejecting pressure from the larger society may lead to marginalization or to an overemphasis on ethnic identity. With ethnicity in the mix, whether by race, language, or religion, social arenas become even more complex. In plural societies, majority and minority people also need to "co-exist" and participate together in the larger entity (Anderson, 2011 and Gutmann, 2003).

2.4.4 INTERVENTION TARGETS

Achieving a balance between energy intake and energy output and preventing excess weight gain require identifying ways to change obesity-promoting environments and the ways people react to them (Kumanyika et al., 2002 and Kumanyika et al., 2008). Policies and practices to foster healthy weight involve transportation, housing and urban development, social welfare, education, financial, agricultural, media and cultural sectors. Table 3 illustrates key targets and approaches for addressing them. In this ecological system, individually-focused interventions cannot be successful without also attending to the contextual factors influencing the individual's behavior (Adler and Stewart, 2009). The goal is to intervene in the environment to enable individuals to achieve energy balance and facilitate favorable individual responses to changes. Community-level approaches focus on specific policies and practices to counteract the pervasive availability of inexpensive, high-calorie food, the promotion of these foods, and decreased demands and opportunities for physical activity, based on mandates and guidelines from government agencies, advisory bodies, and non-governmental organizations (Commonwealth of Australia, 2009, Institute of Medicine, 2006, Institute of Medicine, 2009, Institute of Medicine, 2011, Koplan et al., 2005, Koplan et al., 2007, Kumanyika et al., 2008, McLean et al., 2009, Organisation for Economic Co-operation and Development, 2010 and World Health Organization, 2003). Family-level and individual-level interventions target awareness, availability, access, motivation, and utilization with respect to environments or resources for improving energy balance. Dietary targets include considerations of dietary quality in addition to the amount of calories consumed.

TABLE 3: Obesity prevention policy and environmental change targets and potential intervention approaches at community, family/household, and individual levels.

Level of intervention	Intervention target	Examples of intervention approaches or content
Communities	Built environment	• Neighborhood renewal programs to upgrade parks and nature reserves in order to address crime, increase cleanliness and esthetic appeal of the neighborhood (e.g., address vandalism), to increase a sense of community or cohesion and facilitate social events
		• Public–private partnerships to provide financial incentives and mobilize community support for locating supermarkets and other food retail outlets that offer healthy foods in neighborhoods with limited availability of healthy foods at affordable prices
		• More socially and culturally-centered urban design, land use patterns, and transportation systems that promote walking or bicycling as strategies to create active, healthier, and more livable communities
		• Raising fees associated with automobile use (bridge tolls, parking fees) combined with improving the availability and affordability of public transportation
	Physical activity resources, facilities, and opportunities	• Advocacy for fair distribution of parks, resources, and recreational facilities
		• Establishing linkages between neighborhoods and schools for joint use of local facilities and school playgrounds/parks for community use to promote physical activity
		• Promotion of physical activity by community organizations and institutions (e.g., schools, faith organizations, worksites), including the incorporation of short physical activity breaks into meetings or classroom activities
	Food environment (products, distribution, advertising and promotion, and price)	• Improving food options in small neighborhood stores (e.g. "corner stores" or "bodegas" in the US) in neighborhoods with limited access to affordable, healthy foods
		• Fiscal policies and local ordinances to discourage the consumption of nutrient-poor foods and beverages (e.g., taxes of unhealthy foods, incentives, land use and zoning regulations related to the mix of retail food outlets)
		• Special initiatives to encourage mobile vendors with healthy food options in local neighborhoods
		• Food policy councils and consumer coalitions formed to improve healthy food availability and access in local areas

TABLE 3: *Cont.*

Level of intervention	Intervention target	Examples of intervention approaches or content
		• Consumer education and counter-marketing activities to decrease exposure of children to marketing of high calorie low nutrition foods and beverages (e.g., "The Parents Jury" http://www.parentsjury.org.au/food-marketing-to-kids, "Change 4 Life" in the UK http://www.nhs.uk/change4life/Pages/change-for-life.aspx, and the "Life's Sweeter with Fewer Sugary Drinks" campaign in the USA http://fewersugarydrinks.org/)
		• Encouraging food outlets or groceries that serve culturally diverse communities to create culturally appropriate "healthy food baskets" to minimize the effect of dietary acculturation and improve affordability
		• Health-oriented food procurement guidelines for government run facilities
		• Regulations requiring employers to provide breastfeeding facilities and opportunities
	Government nutrition assistance programs	• Monitoring and advocating for healthy changes in school food menus and other government sponsored nutrition assistance programs
		• Making provisions for use of government nutrition program benefits at local farmers' markets
		• Advocacy and initiatives to increase participation in government programs that provide money to purchase foods, both general programs (e.g., food stamps) and specially targeted programs (such as the Supplemental Nutrition Program for Women, Infants, and Children in the USA)
		• Regulations that require adherence to health-oriented nutrition standards for foods served in school cafeterias and snack bars or canteens
	Endorsement, social support, and social capital for physical activity and healthy eating	• Concerned citizens and community leaders (from faith-based and other organizations) advocating for initiatives to increase community trust and solidarity and prevent crime and violence
		• Community walking or cycling clubs
		• Community garden and school kitchen and garden programs
		• Intergenerational nutrition and physical activity programs
Families and households	Home food availability	• Providing nutrition program recipients with discounts for purchases of fruits and vegetables
		• Facilitating enrollment in government funded programs that provide money for food purchase
	Food choices and feeding	• Contextually and culturally appropriate nutrition and physical activity counseling incorporated into parent-education or other home visiting programs

TABLE 3: *Cont.*

Level of intervention	Intervention target	Examples of intervention approaches or content
		• General social marketing and health literacy programs
		• Breastfeeding support
		• Food and nutrition education in schools, faith organizations, and other community settings
		• Worksite wellness programs
	Electronic media use	TV turnoff days and other initiatives to encourage parents to limit children's screen time
		• Advice to parents against putting televisions in a child's bedroom
	Physical activity opportunities	• Social marketing programs (e.g., the VERB campaign in the USA; see http://www.cdc.gov/youthcampaign/)
		• Resource guides and assistance to help families identify convenient and affordable opportunities for physical activity
		• Games, DVDs and cable TV shows that require or promote physical activity
		• Physical education in schools and child care centers
		• Promotion of opportunities for all types of physical activity congruent with cultural norms and expectations
	Health care provider advice	• Assessment and counseling about obesity prevention
Individuals	Food choices and eating behaviors	• Contextually and culturally appropriate counseling and skills training for acquisition and preparation of foods and meals meeting dietary guidelines for quality and quantity of foods consumed
	Electronic media use	• Limit screen time for children to no more than 2 h per day outside of schoolwork
		• Encourage the use of media in ways that require or promote physical activity
	Involvement in physical activity	• Encouragement to engage in utilitarian physical activity such as walking and gardening
		• Contextually and culturally appropriate counseling and skills training for engagement in leisure time physical activity and sports at levels sufficient to meet guidelines
	Weight control behaviors	• Contextually and culturally appropriate counseling to promote a positive body image and avoid potentially harmful or counterproductive dietary restriction
	Citizen advocacy	• Link to opportunities for engagement in community activities to promote healthier environments
		• Training for effective advocacy
		• On-line advocacy networks

2.4.5 CULTURAL-CONTEXTUAL INFLUENCES

2.4.5.1 HISTORICAL EXPERIENCES, STRUGGLES, AND ACCOMMODATIONS

The environments of ethnic minority populations may reflect adaptations to circumstances created by conquest or migration. The subsequent population contexts reflect interrelated factors such as political relationships and economic variables, reasons for migration (e.g., forced migration or enslavement, asylum seeking, labor migration, or voluntary migration), the geographical and cultural distance between the home country and the host country, and the duration of residence in the host country. People and whole populations adjust over time, through acculturation, assimilation, or negotiated segregation. These contextual adjustments lead to changes in perspectives related to food, physical activity, and a variety of other aspects of lifestyle (e.g., appropriate and/or preferred recreational pursuits, health-related values). Perceptions of physical activity and body size related to health, wealth, and social status or acceptance are influenced by these historical experiences and the paths followed.

From an obesity prevention or health perspective, people's adoption of strategies of survival as a minority may be health promoting, health adverse, or a mixture of both. This depends on structural variables (see below), the direction of the gradient of change (e.g., whether acculturation results in more healthful or less healthful eating practices and physical activity behaviors relative to those in the reference culture), generation and life stage. Together with the aforementioned differences in the effects of broad societal influences across generations and developmental stages, differences in acculturation and the obstacles endured across generations may become manifest in sometimes conflicting responses of youth vs. their elders to the surrounding social context and structures (Renzaho et al., 2012). Also, the nature and extent of acculturation and adaptation will vary within the same population and over time. Assessing the specifics of survival strategies, cultural and symbolic capital, agency empowerment, and acculturation within the population targeted for intervention is, therefore, critical.

2.4.5.2 TYPE OF MINORITY STATUS

Classification of ethnic minority populations along the lines shown in Table 4 (Kumanyika, 2006 and Mavoa et al., 2010) prompts for differentiation of challenges in the relevant structural and sociocultural contexts. For example, with respect to indigenous populations or formerly enslaved populations, one might explore ways in which the major cultural trauma associated with conquest or enslavement has disrupted or distorted original, traditional dietary patterns and current perceptions of traditional or preferred diets. What have been the more health adverse adaptations? What positive eating and physical activity traditions have been maintained? How do social disadvantages influence the nature of adaptations made? Compared to populations whose minority status is associated with cultural disruption and explicit subjugation, these questions may elicit different responses when asked of established migrants for whom aspects of a relatively healthful, traditional dietary pattern are still dominant or where systematic social disadvantage based on ethnicity is not observed. With respect to new migrant populations, one might ask whether an adequate and relatively healthful dietary pattern was intact before migration and what types of dietary adaptations are being made post migration and why. Answers would differ for refugee populations and for migrant workers (e.g., Turkish migrants in Northern Europe) compared to relatively advantaged, voluntary migrants, (e.g., professionals who migrate from low and middle income to high income countries) and also according to post migration social and economic circumstances. Comparable questions can be asked about attitudes, values, and patterns related to physical activity. What were the physical activity opportunities and patterns in the home country? What accommodations have been made as a response to the culture in the host country? Are these favorable or unfavorable to engagement in physical activity? Do they differ by gender or age?

TABLE 4: Cultural-contextual classification of ethnic minority populations in high income countries.

Type of minority group	Examples	Social disadvantage/ disparities[a]
"Aboriginal" populations	Indigenous populations in Australia, New Zealand, the United States and Canada	Yes
"Established" migrant populations	People of African, Hispanic, and Asian descent who have lived in countries such as the United States or United Kingdom for many generations	In many cases, but varies by population and country
"New migrants"	First or second generation refugee and other immigrant non-European populations	Varies with circumstances in home country and reasons for migration

[a] *May refer to any of the above populations for whom historical or current political contexts are associated with disparities in income, education, and health status relative to the respective general population.*

2.4.5.3 STRUCTURAL INFLUENCES

Attention to structural influences on obesity development is crucial, particularly for socially disadvantaged minority populations. Negotiating environments that are not aligned with one's sociocultural perspectives requires effort, agency and stress. Lack of political power, prejudice and discrimination, and negative social stratification combine to place many ethnic minority populations at the bottom or lower rungs of the social hierarchy, resulting in poverty, low educational attainment, underemployment, and limited agency (Braveman et al., 2011 and Friel and Marmot, 2011). Neighborhood segregation, whether voluntary or enforced, may worsen circumstances if services and resources are substandard or lacking. Within the food and physical activity sphere specifically, socially disadvantaged ethnic minority populations may be less likely to have neighborhood access to affordable healthy foods or safe and affordable opportunities for physical activity (Grier and Kumanyika, 2008 and Taylor et al., 2006). In addition, media targeted toward ethnic minority populations may include heavier than average promotion of foods and beverages which, even if apparently justified by ethnic consumer demand, are less healthful than foods promoted to other communities (Grier and Kumanyika, 2008 and

Yancey et al., 2009). Intervention approaches should recognize the potential health implications of these structural influences.

2.4.5.4 SOCIO-CULTURAL INFLUENCES

The use of food to create ethnic identity, express caring, cope with stress, reward children, and define celebrations and other social interactions establishes cultural anchors for eating behaviors that are unrelated to the nutritional or health values in current food guidance (Axelson, 1986, Beagan and Chapman, 2012, Counihan and Van Esterik, 1997, James, 2004, Mintz, 1996, Mintz and DuBois, 2002 and Murcott, 2002). Along with its value as sustenance, food is a symbol of hospitality, generosity, status, and goodwill (Nicolaou et al., 2009). Moreover, symbolic meanings and cultural uses of food may reflect health values relevant in prior eras.

Sociocultural influences can only be understood in association with contextual influences (Krieger, 2001). For example, traditions that encourage overeating (feasting) have their roots in attitudes that evolved during shortages of food or cash. Even when historical experiences of hunger are in the distant past, deeply embedded cultural memory of such food insecurity may persist even when food is readily available in large quantities, leading to overeating and excess weight gain. Once expensive foods may be considered high-status and consumed preferentially. Caloric overconsumption emerges when changes in the global food supply make formerly scarce and costly but desirable foods or food components (such as sugar and fat) widely available at very low cost. Thus, structural changes (e.g. in the types of foods available and promoted) can combine with sociocultural influences to predispose ethnic minority populations toward obesity (Williams et al., 2012).

With respect to energy expenditure, physical work may be seen as something to avoid in both occupational and leisure settings. Sedentary entertainment and automobile use may be associated with upward mobility and high social status. Recreational and utilitarian physical activities may not be valued or emphasized for their health benefits (Airhihenbuwa et al., 1995 and Taylor et al., 1994), although in some communities, physical activity and exercise are associated with traditional sports involvement and economic advancement through sports (Teufel-Shone, 2006 and Yancey et al., 2006). In socially disadvantaged environments, outdoor physical activity may be constrained by fears for personal safety (Taylor et al., 2012).

Barring severe obesity, numerous studies demonstrate positive or relatively tolerant attitudes toward large body size among ethnic minority populations, i.e., a perception that being somewhat heavy means being fertile and attractive (women), robust, well off, and powerful (both sexes), accompanied by relatively negative attitudes toward thinness as being unhealthy, unattractive, uncared for, or weak (Brown and Konner, 1987, Popenoe, 2005, Renzaho, 2004 and Rguibi and Belahsen, 2006). Persistent high prevalence of obesity may render large body size socially normative, further reinforcing cultural attitudes (Brewis et al., 1998). However, traditional preferences for large body size may change over time and with exposure to European culture (Craig et al., 1996, Nicolau et al., 2012 and Popenoe, 2005). Understanding how strongly held cultural attitudes about body size might limit uptake of improved opportunities for healthy eating and physical activity is critical when planning obesity prevention initiatives.

2.5 CONCLUSION

The CEB Framework emphasizes cultural and contextual considerations relevant to obesity prevention interventions with a focus on influences that differentiate ethnic minority populations from their respective reference populations. These considerations can be incorporated into available intervention planning and evaluation systems using both qualitative and quantitative methods to explore and elucidate factors of greatest relevance to caloric consumption or being physically active. Recognizing that many of the identified variables are the subject of discourse in the humanities and social sciences, we acknowledge that this article only touches the surface. We recommend collaborations with scholars in fields such as history, anthropology, marketing, sociology, and family studies as well as scholars who work with other ethnic minorities to achieve a greater depth of understanding and to further develop the framework (Kumanyika et al.,

2007). For example, Hispanic or Latino Americans are now the largest U.S. ethnic minority, and comprise diverse populations with different regional, historical, and cultural origins and political histories (Saenz, 2010 and U.S. Census Bureau, 2012). Reflecting on CEB framework elements from the perspectives of these populations will undoubtedly reveal additional concepts and issues for consideration.

The CEB Framework underscores the reality among ethnic minorities that cultural-contextual interactions cause stresses that negatively influence eating and physical activity patterns, having long-term, adverse consequences (Thomas, 1998). The framework may inform the design of interventions that both acknowledge contextual stressors and reshape health adverse behaviors to more health promoting coping strategies. The framework elements reinforce the importance of community-based participatory research approaches and of leveraging supportive community assets. This suggests that professionals interested in working with ethnic minority populations need advocacy and policy/environmental change skills as much as or more than behavioral modification skills, which tend to assume a fixed environmental reality and place the entire burden of change on the individual. Furthermore, we believe that, following Bourdieu, scientists must at all times conduct their research with conscious attention to the effects of their own position, their own set of internalized structures, and how these are likely to distort or prejudice their worldview (Bourdieu, 1990).

In conclusion, this article presents a Community Energy Balance framework, an approach above and beyond traditional socio-ecologic models of obesity prevention, with the objective of stimulating others to creatively address obesity prevention needs in ethnic minorities, particularly socially disadvantaged groups. The ultimate value of this framework will be in its application by scholars in developing effective interventions to achieve equity in addressing the obesity epidemic plaguing all communities.

REFERENCES

1. N.E. Adler, K. Newman Socioeconomic disparities in health: pathways and policies Health Aff. (Millwood), 21 (2002), pp. 60–76

2. N.E. Adler, J. Stewart Reducing obesity: motivating action while not blaming the victim Milbank Q, 87 (2009), pp. 49–70
3. C.O. Airhihenbuwa Health and culture Beyond the Western paradigmSage Publications, Inc, Thousand Oaks, CA (1995)
4. C.O. Airhihenbuwa, S. Kumanyika, T.D. Agurs, A. Lowe Perceptions and beliefs about exercise, rest, and health among African-Americans Am. J. Health Promot., 9 (1995), pp. 426–429
5. C.O. Airhihenbuwa, S. Kumanyika, T.D. Agurs, A. Lowe, D. Saunders, C.B. Morssink Cultural aspects of African American eating patterns Ethn. Health, 1 (1996), pp. 245–260
6. J.A. Al-Lawati, P.J. Jousilahti Prevalence and 10-year secular trend of obesity in Oman Saudi Med. J., 25 (2004), pp. 346–351
7. E. Anderson The cosmopolitan canopy Race and Civility in Everyday LifeW.W. Norton and Company, New York, NY (2011)
8. S.E. Anderson, R.C. Whitaker Prevalence of obesity among US preschool children in different racial and ethnic groups Arch. Pediatr. Adolesc. Med., 163 (2009), pp. 344–348
9. Australian National Institute of Health and Welfare. Prevalence of overweight and obesity, Aboriginal and Torres Strait Islander Health Performance Framework 2006 report. Detailed analyses, Canberra, Australia (2007), pp. 810–816 pp. Section 2.24
10. M.L. Axelson. The impact of culture on food-related behavior. Annu. Rev. Nutr., 6 (1986), pp. 345–363
11. E. Barr, D.J. Magliano, P.Z. Zimmet et al. AusDiab 2005 the Australian Diabetes, Obesity and Lifestyle Survey. Tracking the accelerating epidemic: its causes and outcomes. International Diabetes Institute, Melbourne (2006)
12. B.L. Beagan, G.E. Chapman. Meanings of food, eating and health among African Nova Scotians: 'certain things aren't meant for Black folk'. Ethn. Health (2012) Feburary, (e-pub ahead of print)
13. J.W. Berry. Immigration, acculturation, and adaptation. Appl. Psychol., 46 (1997), pp. 5–68
14. Booth, S.L., Sallis, J.F., Ritenbaugh, C., Hill, J.O., Birch, L.L., Frank, L.D., Glanz, K., Himmelgreen, D.A., Mudd, M., et al., 2001. Environmental and societal factors affect food choice and physical activity: rationale, influences, and leverage points. Nutr Rev 59:S21-39; discussion S57-65.
15. M. Booth, A.D. Okely, E. Denney-Wilson, L. Hardy, B. Yang, T. Dobbins. NSW Schools Physical Activity and Nutrition Survey (SPANS) 2004: Summary Report. NSW Department of Health, Sydney (2006)
16. P. Bourdieu. Distinction: A Social Critique of the Judgement of Taste. Routledge, London (1984)
17. P. Bourdieu. The forms of capital. J.G. Richardson (Ed.), Handbook of Theory and Research for the Sociology of Capital, Greenwood Press, New York (1986), pp. 241–258
18. P. Bourdieu. In Other Words. Essays Towards a Reflexive Sociology (translated from French). Stanford University Press, Palo Alto, CA (1990)
19. B.P. Braveman, S. Kumanyika, J. Fielding et al. Health disparities and health equity: the issue is justice Am. J. Public Health, 101 (2011), pp. S149–S155

20. A.A. Brewis, S.T. McGarvey, J. Jones, B.A. Swinburn. Perceptions of body size in Pacific Islanders. Int. J. Obes. Relat. Metab. Disord., 22 (1998), pp. 185–189
21. P.J. Brown, M. Konner. An anthropological perspective on obesity. Ann. N. Y. Acad. Sci., 499 (1987), pp. 29–46
22. F.D. Butterfoss. Process evaluation for community participation. Annu. Rev. Public Health, 27 (2006), pp. 323–340
23. B. Caballero, T. Clay, S.M. Davis et al. Pathways: a school-based, randomized controlled trial for the prevention of obesity in American Indian schoolchildren. Am. J. Clin. Nutr., 78 (2003), pp. 1030–1038
24. C.M. Caperchione, G.S. Kolt, W.K. Mummery. Physical activity in culturally and linguistically diverse migrant groups to Western society: a review of barriers, enablers and experiences. Sports Med., 39 (2009), pp. 167–177
25. S.S. Casagrande, M.C. Whitt-Glover, K.J. Lancaster, A.M. Odoms-Young, T.L. Gary. Built environment and health behaviors among African Americans: a systematic review. Am. J. Prev. Med., 36 (2009), pp. 174–181
26. F.G. Castro, G.Q. Shaibi, E. Boehm-Smith. Ecodevelopmental contexts for preventing type 2 diabetes in Latino and other racial/ethnic minority populations. J. Behav. Med., 32 (2009), pp. 89–105
27. F.G. Castro, M. Barrera Jr., L.K. Holleran Steiker. Issues and challenges in the design of culturally adapted evidence-based interventions. Annu Rev Clin Psychol, 6 (2010), pp. 213–239
28. U.S. Census Bureau. USA Quick Facts. (2012)
29. Centers for Disease Control, Prevention. Obesity in K-8 students—New York City, 2006–07 to 2010–11 school years. MMWR Morb. Mortal Wkly. Rep., 60 (2011), pp. 1673–1678
30. W.C. Cockerham. Health lifestyle theory and the convergence of agency and structure. J. Heal. Soc. Behav., 46 (2005), pp. 51–67
31. Commonwealth of Australia. Australia: the healthiest country by 2020. Technical Report No 1. Obesity in Australia: a Need for Urgent Action. Including Addendum for October 2008 to June 2009 (2009) Retrieved from: http://www.health.gov.au/internet/preventativehealth/publishing.nsf/content/E233F8695823F16CCA2574DD00818E64/$File/obesity-jul09.pdf.
32. M.A. Corneille, A.M. Ashcroft, F.Z. Belgrave. What's culture got to do with it? Prevention programs for African American adolescent girls. J. Health Care Poor Underserved, 16 (2005), pp. 38–47
33. C. Counihan, P. Van Esterik. Food and culture: A Reader. Routledge, New York, NY (1997)
34. P.L. Craig, B.A. Swinburn, T. Matenga-Smith, H. Matangi, G. Vaughn. Do Polynesians still believe that big is beautiful? Comparison of body size perceptions and preferences of Cook Islands, Maori and Australians. N. Z. Med. J., 109 (1996), pp. 200–203
35. K.T. D'Alonzo, N. Fischetti. Cultural beliefs and attitudes of Black and Hispanic college-age women toward exercise. J. Transcult. Nurs., 19 (2008), pp. 175–183
36. M. Daniel, P. Lekkas, M. Cargo, I. Stankov, A. Brown. Environmental risk conditions and pathways to cardiometabolic diseases in indigenous populations. Annu. Rev. Public Health, 32 (2011), pp. 327–347

37. I. De Garine, G.J. Koppert. Guru fattening sessions among the Massa. Ecol. Food Nutr., 25 (1991), pp. 1–28
38. I. De Garine, N. Pollock. Social Aspects of Obesity. Overseas Publishers Association, Amsterdam BV (1995)
39. J.A. de Wilde, P. van Dommelen, B.J. Middelkoop, P.H. Verkerk. Trends in overweight and obesity prevalence in Dutch, Turkish, Moroccan and Surinamese South Asian children in the Netherlands. Arch. Dis. Child., 94 (2009), pp. 795–800
40. V.A. Diaz, A.G. Mainous III, C. Pope. Cultural conflicts in the weight loss experience of overweight Latinos. Int. J. Obes. (Lond), 31 (2007), pp. 328–333
41. H. Dijkshoorn, J.K. Ujcic-Voortman, L. Viet, A.P. Verhoeff, D.G. Uitenbroek. Ethnic variation in validity of the estimated obesity prevalence using self-reported weight and height measurements BMC Public Health, 11 (2011), p. 408
42. W.W. Dressler. Race and ethnicity in public health research. Models to explain health disparities. Annu. Rev. Anthropol., 34 (2005), pp. 231–252
43. R. Fernandez, C. Miranda, B. Everett. Prevalence of obesity among migrant Asian Indians: a systematic review and meta-analysis. Int. J. Evid. Based Healthc, 9 (2011), pp. 420–428
44. L. Fezeu, B. Balkau, A. Kengne, E. Sobngwi, J. Mbanya. Metabolic syndrome in a sub-Saharan African setting: central obesity may be the key determinant. Atherosclerosis, 193 (2007), pp. 70–76
45. M.M. Finucane, G.A. Stevens, M.J. Cowan et al.. National, regional, and global trends in body-mass index since 1980: systematic analysis of health examination surveys and epidemiological studies with 960 country-years and 9.1 million participants. Lancet, 377 (2011), pp. 557–567
46. K.M. Flegal, M.D. Carroll, C.L. Ogden, L.R. Curtin. Prevalence and trends in obesity among US adults, 1999–2008. JAMA, 303 (2010), pp. 235–241
47. K.M. Flegal, M.D. Carroll, B.K. Kit, C.L. Ogden. Prevalence of obesity and trends in the distribution of body mass index among US adults, 1999–2010. JAMA, 307 (2012), pp. 491–497
48. M.A. Flynn, D.A. McNeil, B. Maloff et al. Reducing obesity and related chronic disease risk in children and youth: a synthesis of evidence with 'best practice' recommendations. Obes. Rev., 7 (Suppl. 1) (2006), pp. 7–66
49. Food and Agricultural Organization of the United Nations. The double burden of malnutrition. Case Studies in Six Developing Countries, Rome, Italy (2006)
50. S. Friel, M.G. Marmot. Action on the social determinants of health and health inequities goes global. Annu. Rev. Public Health, 32 (2011), pp. 225–236
51. T.A. Glass, M.J. McAtee. Behavioral science at the crossroads in public health: extending horizons, envisioning the future. Soc. Sci. Med., 62 (2006), pp. 1650–1671
52. V.B. Gray, J.S. Cossman, W.L. Dodson, S.H. Byrd. Dietary acculturation of Hispanic immigrants in Mississippi. Salud Publica Mex., 47 (2005), pp. 351–360
53. S.A. Grier, S.K. Kumanyika. The context for choice: health implications of targeted food and beverage marketing to African Americans. Am. J. Public Health, 98 (2008), pp. 1616–1629
54. A. Gutmann. Chapter 1. The claims of cultural identity groups, pages 38–85, Identity in Democracy. Princeton University Press, Princeton, NJ (2003)
55. J. Harrison. Spam. D. Kulick, A. Meneley (Eds.), Fat. The Anthropology of an Obsession, Penguin Group, New York (2005), pp. 185–198

56. Institute of Medicine. Food marketing to children and youth. Threat or Opportunity, National Academies Press (2006), p. 516
57. Institute of Medicine. Local Government Actions to Prevent Obesity. National Academies Press, Washington, DC (2009)
58. Institute of Medicine. Early Childhood Obesity Prevention Policies. National Academies Press, Washington, DC (2011)
59. D.C. James. Factors influencing food choices, dietary intake, and nutrition-related attitudes among African Americans: application of a culturally sensitive model. Ethn. Health, 9 (2004), pp. 349–367
60. J. James, A. Underwood. Ethnic influences on weaning diet in the UK. Proc. Nutr. Soc., 56 (1997), pp. 121–130
61. D.B. Jelliffe. Parallel food classifications in developing and industrialized countries. Am. J. Clin. Nutr., 20 (1967), pp. 279–281
62. Katzmarzyk and Mason, 2006. P. Katzmarzyk, C. Mason. Prevalence of class I, II and III obesity in Canada. CMAJ, 174 (2006), pp. 156–157
63. R.C. Klesges, E. Obarzanek, S. Kumanyika, D.M. Murray, L.M. Klesges, G.E. Relyea, M.B. Stockton, J.Q. Lanctot, B.M. Beech et al.. The Memphis girls' health enrichment multi-site studies (GEMS): an evaluation of the efficacy of a 2-year obesity prevention program in African American girls. Arch Pediatr Adolesc Med, 164 (2010), pp. 1007–1014
64. J.P. Koplan, C.T. Liverman, V.I. Kraak (Eds.), Preventing Childhood Obesity, Health in the Balance, National Academies Press, Washington, DC (2005)
65. J.P. Koplan, C.T. Liverman, V.I. Kraak, S.L. Wisham (Eds.), Progress in Preventing Childhood Obesity, How Do We Measure Up?, National Academies Press, Washington, DC (2007)
66. P. Korp. Problems of the Healthy Lifestyle Discourse. Sociol. Compass, 4 (2010), pp. 800–810
67. M.W. Kreuter, S.N. Lukwago, R.D. Bucholtz, E.M. Clark, V. Sanders-Thompson. Achieving cultural appropriateness in health promotion programs: targeted and tailored approaches. Health Educ. Behav., 30 (2003), pp. 133–146
68. N. Krieger. A glossary for social epidemiology. J. Epidemiol Community Health, 55 (2001), pp. 693–700
69. N. Krieger. Embodiment: a conceptual glossary for epidemiology. J. Epidemiol Community Health, 59 (2005), pp. 350–355
70. S. Kumanyika. Nutrition and chronic disease prevention: priorities for US minority groups. Nutr. Rev., 64 (2006), pp. S9–S14
71. S. Kumanyika. Church- and other community-interventions to promote healthy lifestyle: tailoring to ethnicity and culture. L. Dubé, A. Bechara, A. Dagher, A. Drewnowski, J. Lebel, P. James, R.Y. Yada, M.-C. Laflamme-Sanders (Eds.), Obesity Prevention: The Role of Society and Brain on Individual Behavior. A Handbook for Integrative Science, Policy, and Action to Stop the Progression of the Obesity Pandemic, Elsevier, Amsterdam (2010), pp. 619–651
72. S. Kumanyika. Targeted approaches by culturally appropriate programs/ J.A. O'Dea, M. Eriksen, M. Eriksen (Eds.), Childhood Obesity Prevention—International Research, Controversies, and Interventions, Oxford Press, London (2010), pp. 348–362

73. S.K. Kumanyika, C.B. Morssink. Cultural appropriateness of weight management programs. S. Dalton (Ed.), Overweight and Weight Management, Aspen, Gaithersburg, MD (1997), pp. 69–106
74. S.K. Kumanyika, C.B. Morssink. Bridging domains in efforts to reduce disparities in health and health care. Health Educ. Behav., 33 (2006), pp. 440–458
75. S. Kumanyika, R.W. Jeffery, A. Morabia, C. Ritenbaugh, V.J. Antipatis. Obesity prevention. The case for action. Int. J. Obes. Relat. Metab. Disord., 26 (2002), pp. 425–436
76. S.K. Kumanyika, M. Story, B.M. Beech et al.. Collaborative planning for formative assessment and cultural appropriateness in the girls health enrichment multi-site studies (GEMS): a retrospection. Ethn. Dis., 13 (2003), pp. S15–S29
77. S.K. Kumanyika, T.L. Gary, K.J. Lancaster et al. Achieving healthy weight in African-American communities: research perspectives and priorities. Obes. Res., 13 (2005), pp. 2037–2047
78. S.K. Kumanyika, M.C. Whitt-Glover, T.L. Gary et al.. Expanding the obesity research paradigm to reach African American communities. Prev. Chronic Dis., 4 (2007), p. A112
79. S.K. Kumanyika, E. Obarzanek, N. Stettler et al. Population-based prevention of obesity: the need for comprehensive promotion of healthful eating, physical activity, and energy balance: a scientific statement from American Heart Association Council on Epidemiology and Prevention, Interdisciplinary Committee for Prevention (formerly the expert panel on population and prevention science). Circulation, 118 (2008), pp. 428–464
80. T.A. LaVeist. Disentangling race and socioeconomic status: a key to understanding health inequalities. J. Urban Health, 82 (2005), pp. iii26–iii34
81. N.M. Lindberg, V.J. Stevens. Review: weight-loss interventions with Hispanic populations. Ethn. Dis., 17 (2007), pp. 397–402
82. K.A. Madsen, A.E. Weedn, P.B. Crawford. Disparities in peaks, plateaus, and declines in prevalence of high BMI among adolescents. Pediatrics, 126 (2010), pp. 434–442
83. H.M. Mavoa, M. McCabe. Sociocultural factors relating to Tongans' and Indigenous Fijians' patterns of eating, physical activity and body size. Asia Pac. J. Clin. Nutr., 17 (2008), pp. 375–384
84. H. Mavoa, S. Kumanyika, A. Renzaho. Socio-cultural issues and body image. E. Waters, J. Seidell, B. Swinburn, R. Uauy (Eds.), Preventing Childhood Obesity, Wiley-Blackwell, Chichester, UK (2010), pp. 138–146
85. J. Mbanya, J. Ngogang, J. Salah, E. Minkoulou, B. Balkau. Prevalence of NIDDM and impaired glucose tolerance in a rural and an urban population in Cameroon. Diabetologia, 40 (1997), pp. 824–829
86. R.M. McLean, J.A. Hoek, S. Buckley et al.. "Healthy eating—healthy action": evaluating New Zealand's obesity prevention strategy. BMC Publ. Health, 9 (2009), p. 452
87. S.W. Mintz. Tasting food, tasting freedom. Excursions into Eating, Culture, and the PastBeacon Press, Boston, MA (1996)
88. S.W. Mintz, C.M. DuBois. The anthropology of food and eating. Annu. Rev. Anthropol., 31 (2002), pp. 99–119

89. A. Murcott. Nutrition and inequalities. A note on sociological approaches. Eur. J. Public Health, 12 (2002), pp. 203–207
90. A. Nelson, R. Abbott, D. Macdonald. Indigenous Austalians and physical activity: using a social-ecological model to review the literature. Health Educ. Res., 25 (2010), pp. 498–509
91. New Zealand Ministry of Health. A Portrait of Health: Key Results of the 2002/03 New Zealand Health Survey. NZ Ministry of Health, Wellington (2004)
92. New Zealand Ministry of Health. A portrait of health. Key Results of the 2006/07 New Zealand Health SurveyNZ Ministry of Health, Wellington (2008)
93. M. Nicolaou, C. Doak, R. Dam, K. Hosper, J. Seidell, K. Stronks. Body size preference and body weight perception among two migrant groups of non-Western origin. Public Health Nutr., 11 (2008), pp. 1332–1341
94. M. Nicolaou, C.M. Doak, R.M. van Dam, J. Brug, K. Stronks, J.C. Seidell. Cultural and social influences on food consumption in Dutch residents of Turkish and Moroccan origin: a qualitative study. J. Nutr. Educ. Behav., 41 (2009), pp. 232–241
95. M. Nicolaou, S. Benjelloun, K. Stronks, R.M. van Dam, J.C. Seidell, C.M. Doak. Influences on body weight of female Moroccan migrants in the Netherlands: A qualitative study. Health Place, 18 (2012), pp. 883–891
96. C.L. Ogden, M.D. Carroll, L.R. Curtin, M.M. Lamb, K.M. Flegal. Prevalence of high body mass index in US children and adolescents, 2007–2008. JAMA, 303 (2010), pp. 242–249
97. C.L. Ogden, M.D. Carroll, B.K. Kit, K.M. Flegal. Prevalence of obesity and trends in body mass index among US children and adolescents, 1999–2010. JAMA, 307 (2012), pp. 483–490
98. Organisation for Economic Co-operation and Development. Obesity and the Economics of Prevention. Fit not Fat, Paris (2010)
99. G. Osei-Assibey, I. Kyrou, Y. Adi, S. Kumar, K. Matyka. Dietary and lifestyle interventions for weight management in adults from minority ethnic/non-White groups: a systematic review. Obes Rev, 11 (2010) 769–76
100. J.B. Page. The concept of culture: a core issue in health disparities. J. Urban Health, 82 (2005), pp. iii35–iii43
101. G. Paradis, L. Levesque, A.C. Macaulay et al. Impact of a diabetes prevention program on body size, physical activity, and diet among Kanien'keha:ka (Mohawk) children 6 to 11 years old: 8-year results from the Kahnawake Schools Diabetes Prevention Project Pediatrics, 115 (2005), pp. 333–339
102. G.P. Parham, I.C. Scarinci. Strategies for achieving healthy energy balance among African Americans in the Mississippi Delta. Prev. Chronic Dis., 4 (2007), p. A97
103. R. Popenoe. Ideal. D. Kulick, A. Meneley (Eds.), Fat. The Anthropology of an Obsession, Penguin Group, New York (2005), pp. 9–28
104. Race Ethnicity and Genetics Working Group. The use of racial, ethnic, and ancestral categories in human genetics research. Am. J. Hum. Genet., 77 (2005), pp. 519–532
105. K.L. Rennie, S.A. Jebb. Prevalence of obesity in Great Britain. Obes. Rev., 6 (2005), pp. 11–12
106. A.M. Renzaho. Fat, rich and beautiful: changing socio-cultural paradigms associated with obesity risk, nutritional status and refugee children from sub-Saharan Africa Health Place, 10 (2004), pp. 105–113

107. A.M.N. Renzaho. Challenges of negotiating obesity-related findings with African migrants in Australia: lessons learnt from the African Migrant Capacity Building and Performance Appraisal Project. Nutr. Diet., 66 (2009), pp. 146–151
108. A.M.N. Renzaho. Parenting, family functioning and lifestyle in a new culture: the case of African migrants in Melbourne, Victoria, Australia. Child Fam. Soc. Work, 16 (2011), pp. 228–240
109. A. Renzaho, D. Mellor. Applying socio-cultural lenses to childhood obesity prevention among African migrants to high-income Western countries: the role of acculturation, parenting and family functioning. Int. J. Migrat. Health Soc. Care, 6 (2010), pp. 34–42
110. A.M. Renzaho, B. Swinburn, C. Burns. Maintenance of traditional cultural orientation is associated with lower rates of obesity and sedentary behaviours among African migrant children to Australia. Int. J. Obes. (Lond), 32 (2008), pp. 594–600
111. A. Renzaho, J. Oldroyd, C. Burns, E. Waters, E. Riggs, C. Renzaho. Over and undernutrition in the children of Australian immigrants: assessing the influence of birthplace of primary carer and English language use at home on the nutritional status of 4–5-year-olds. Int. J. Pediatr. Obes., 4 (2009), pp. 73–80
112. A.M.N. Renzaho, M. McCabe, W.J. Sainsbury. Immigration and social exclusion. examining health inequalities of immigrants through acculturation lenses. A. Taket, B. Crisp, A. Nevill, G. Lamaro, M. Graham, S. Barter-Godfrey (Eds.), Theorising Social Exclusion, Routledge, Oxon (2009), pp. 117–126
113. A.M. Renzaho, D. Mellor, K. Boulton, B. Swinburn. Effectiveness of prevention programmes for obesity and chronic diseases among immigrants to developed countries—a systematic review. Public Health Nutr., 13 (2010), pp. 438–450
114. A.M.N. Renzaho, M. McCabe, W.J. Sainsbury. Parenting, role reversals and the preservation of cultural values among Arabic speaking migrant families in Melbourne, Australia. Int. J. Intercul. Relations, 35 (2011), pp. 416–424
115. A.M. Renzaho, M. McCabe, B. Swinburn. Intergenerational differences in food, physical activity, and body size perceptions among African migrants. Qual. Health Res., 22 (2012), pp. 740–754
116. K. Resnicow, T. Baranowski, J.S. Ahluwalia, R.L. Braithwaite. Cultural sensitivity in public health: defined and demystified. Ethn. Dis., 9 (1999), pp. 10–21
117. M. Rguibi, R. Belahsen. Body size preferences and sociocultural influences on attitudes towards obesity among Moroccan Sahraoui women. Body Image, 3 (2006), pp. 395–400
118. R.G. Robinson. Community development model for public health applications: overview of a model to eliminate population disparities. Health Promot. Pract., 6 (2005), pp. 338–346
119. C.E. Rucker, T.F. Cash. Body images, body size perceptions and eating behaviors among African American and white college women. Int. J. Eat. Disord., 3 (1992), pp. 291–299
120. R. Saenz. Latinos in the United States 2010, population bulletin update. Population Reference Bureau (2010) Available at. http://www.prb.org/pdf10/latinos-update2010.pdf, Washington D.C.

121. A. Saleh, S. Amanatidis, S. Samman. The effect of migration on dietary intake, type 2 diabetes and obesity: the Ghanaian Health and Nutrition Analysis in Sydney, Australia (GHANAISA). Ecol. Food Nutr., 41 (2002), pp. 255–270
122. J.F. Sallis, R.B. Cervero, W. Ascher, K.A. Henderson, M.K. Kraft, J. Kerr. An ecological approach to creating active living communities. Annu. Rev. Public Health, 27 (2006), pp. 297–322
123. S. Saxena, G. Ambler, T.J. Cole, A. Majeed. Ethnic group differences in overweight and obese children and young people in England: cross sectional survey. Arch. Dis. Child., 89 (2004), pp. 30–36
124. P. Scheffer. Immigrant Nations. Wiley, Hoboken, NJ (2011)
125. C.A. Schoenborn, P.E. Adams. Health behaviors of adults: United States, 2005–2007. Vital Health Stat., 10 (2010), pp. 1–132
126. M. Singer. Reinventing medical anthropology: toward a critical realignment. Soc. Sci. Med., 30 (1990), pp. 179–187
127. C.M. Super, S. Harkness. Culture structures the environment for development. Hum. Dev., 45 (2002), pp. 270–274
128. B. Swinburn, G. Egger, F. Raza. Dissecting obesogenic environments: the development and application of a framework for identifying and prioritizing environmental interventions for obesity. Prev. Med., 29 (1999), pp. 563–570
129. W.C. Taylor, T. Baranowski, J.F. Sallis. Family determinants of childhood physical activity. A social cognitive model. R.K. Dishman (Ed.), Advances in Exercise Adherence, Human Kinetics, Champaign, IL (1994), pp. 319–342
130. W.C. Taylor, T. Baranowski, D.R. Young. Physical activity interventions in low-income, ethnic minority, and populations with disability. Am. J. Prev. Med., 15 (1998), pp. 334–343
131. W.C. Taylor, A.K. Yancey, J. Leslie et al.. Physical activity among African American and Latino middle school girls: consistent beliefs, expectations, and experiences across two sites. Women Health, 30 (1999), pp. 67–82
132. W.C. Taylor, A.K. Yancey, D. Rohm-Young, W.J. McCarthy. Physical activity. R.L. Braithwaite, S.L. Taylor (Eds.), Health Issues in the Black Community, Jossey-Bass, San Franscisco (2001), pp. 448–468
133. W.C. Taylor, W.S.C. Poston, L. Jones, M.K. Kraft. Environmental justice: obesity, physical activity, and healthy eating. J. Phys. Act. Heal., 3 (2006), pp. S30–S54
134. W.C. Taylor, M.F. Floyd, M.C. Whitt-Glover, J. Brooks. Environmental justice: a framework for collaboration between the public health and parks and recreation fields to study disparities in physical activity. J. Phys. Act. Health, 4 (Suppl. 1) (2007), pp. S50–S63
135. W.C. Taylor, J.F. Sallis, E. Lees et al.. Changing social and built environments to promote physical activity: recommendations from low income, urban women. J. Phys. Act. Health, 4 (2007), pp. 54–65
136. W.C. Taylor, L. Franzini, N. Olvera, W.S. Carlos Poston, G. Lin. Environmental audits of friendliness toward physical activity in three income levels. J Urban Health, 89 (2012), pp. 296–297
137. N.I. Teufel-Shone. Promising strategies for obesity prevention and treatment within American Indian communities. J. Transcult. Nurs., 17 (2006), pp. 224–229

138. M. Tharp (Ed.), Marketing and consumer identity in multicultural America, Sage Publications, Inc, Thousand Oaks, CA (2001)
139. R.B. Thomas. The evolution of human adaptability paradigms. Toward a biology of poverty. A.H. Goodman, T.L. Leatherman (Eds.), Building a New Biosynthesis, University of Michigan Press, Ann Arbor, MI (1998), pp. 43–73
140. J. Thomas. Nutrition intervention in ethnic minority groups. Proc. Nutr. Soc., 61 (2002), pp. 559–567
141. S.B. Thomas, S.C. Quinn, J. Butler, C.S. Fryer, M.A. Garza. Toward a fourth generation of disparities research to achieve health equity. Annu Rev Public Health, 32 (2011), pp. 399–416
142. M. Tjepkema. Measured obesity–adult obesity in Canada: measured height and weight. Nutrition: Findings from the Canadian Community Health Survey. OttawaStatistics Canada, Ontario (2005) Accessible at http://www.statcan.ca/english/research/82-620-MIE/2005001/articles/adults/aobesity.htm
143. M.S. Tremblay, J.D. Willms. Secular trends in the body mass index of Canadian children. CMAJ, 163 (2000), pp. 1429–1433 November
144. H. Vallianatos, K. Raine. Consuming food and constructing identities among Arabic and South Asian immigrant women. Food Culture Soc., 11 (2008), pp. 356–373
145. M.A. Van Duyn, T. McCrae, B.K. Wingrove et al.. Adapting evidence-based strategies to increase physical activity among African Americans, Hispanics, Hmong, and Native Hawaiians: a social marketing approach. Prev. Chronic Dis., 4 (2007), p. A102
146. J. Van Hook, E. Baker, C.E. Altman, M.L. Frisco. Canaries in a coalmine: immigration and overweight among Mexican-origin children in the US and Mexico. Soc. Sci. Med., 74 (2012), pp. 125–134
147. J. Vrazel, R.P. Saunders, S. Wilcox. An overview and proposed framework of social-environmental influences on the physical-activity behavior of women. Am. J. Health Promot., 23 (2008), pp. 2–12
148. Y. Wang, C. Monteiro, B.M. Popkin. Trends of obesity and underweight in older children and adolescents in the United States, Brazil, China and Russia. Am. J. Clin. Nutr., 75 (2002), pp. 971–977
149. Wetter, A.C., Goldberg, J.P., King, A.C., Sigman-Grant, M., Baer, R., Crayton, E., Devine, C., Drewnowski, A., Dunn, A., et al., 2001. How and why do individuals make food and physical activity choices? Nutr Rev 59:S11-20; discussion S57-65.
150. M.C. Whitt-Glover, S.K. Kumanyika. Systematic review of interventions to increase physical activity and physical fitness in African-Americans. Am. J. Health Promot., 23 (2009), pp. S33–S56
151. WHO Expert Panel Appropriate body-mass index for Asian populations and its implications for policy and intervention strategies. Lancet, 363 (2004), pp. 157–163
152. J.D. Williams, D. Crockett, R.L. Harrison, K.D. Thomas. The role of food culture and marketing activity in health disparities. Prev. Med (2012) http://dx.doi.org/10.1016/j.ypmed.2011.12.021
153. A. Wilson, A.M. Renzaho, M. McCabe, B. Swinburn. Towards understanding the new food environment for refugees from the Horn of Africa in Australia. Health Place, 16 (2010), pp. 969–976

154. World Health Organisation. The SuRF Report 2: Surveillance of Chronic Disease Risk Factors. WHO, Geneva (2005)
155. World Health Organization. Obesity. Preventing and managing the global epidemic. Report of a WHO Expert CommitteeWorld Health Organization, Geneva (2000)
156. World Health Organization. Global Strategy on Diet, Physical Activity and Health. World Health Organization, Geneva (2003)
157. Y. Wu. Overweight and obesity in China. BMJ (2006), p. 333
158. A.K. Yancey, M.G. Ory, S.M. Davis. Dissemination of physical activity promotion interventions in underserved populations. Am. J. Prev. Med., 31 (2006), pp. S82–S91
159. A.K. Yancey, B.L. Cole, R. Brown et al.. A cross-sectional prevalence study of ethnically targeted and general audience outdoor obesity-related advertising. Milbank Q., 87 (2009), pp. 155–184

CHAPTER 3

A GENOME-WIDE ASSOCIATION STUDY ON OBESITY AND OBESITY-RELATED TRAITS

KAI WANG, WEI-DONG LI, CLARENCE K. ZHANG, ZUOHENG WANG, JOSEPH T. GLESSNER, STRUAN F. A. GRANT, HONGYU ZHAO, HAKON HAKONARSON, and R. ARLEN PRICE

3.1 INTRODUCTION

Obesity is the sixth most important risk factor contributing to the overall burden of disease worldwide [1]. Affected subjects have reduced life expectancy, and they suffer from several adverse consequences such as cardiovascular disease, type 2 diabetes and several cancers. Many studies have shown that body weight and obesity are strongly influenced by genetic factors, with heritability estimates in the range of 65–80% [2], [3]. Genetic variants in several genes are known to influence BMI, but these mutations are rare and often cause severe monogenic syndromes with obesity [4]. With the development of high-throughput genotyping techniques and the implementation of genome-wide association studies (GWAS), common variations, such as those in *FTO* [5] and *MC4R* [6], have been associated with obesity and body mass index (BMI). Recent large-scale meta-analysis of multiple GWAS identified additional genes harboring common SNPs that associate with BMI [7]–[10]. GWASs have also found associations with measures of body fat distribution [9], [11], [12]. By far the largest GWAS to date included almost 250 thousand individuals and 2.8 million SNPs [13]. Associations of BMI with 28 loci reached genome wide significance, including 10 that were reported previously and 18 that were newly identified. Four additional loci were associated with body fat distribution, all of which had been identified previously. However, even this major expansion of sample size has not explained much variation, 1.39% for BMI and 0.16% for body fat distribution. On the other hand, confirmation of existing BMI loci, and detailed analysis on their association with obesity as a binary trait and with other obesity-related quantitative traits, are important at the current stage to move GWAS signals forward and understand their functional consequences.

A few studies utilized samples with early-onset or morbid obesity for discovery, and replicated previously reported association signals on BMI [7], [14]–[16], or implicated specific genetic variants such as a recurrent 16p11.2 deletion [17]. Utilizing extreme phenotypes increases the odds ratio of association, with improved power to identify novel association signals under fixed genotyping budgets and fixed sample sizes. We have collected a large cohort of obese cases and families ascertained from tails of BMI distribution together with detailed phenotype measures on multiple obesity-related traits. In addition, we have adult controls who have never been overweight. However, given fixed genotyping budget, instead of genotyping all these samples by whole-genome SNP arrays, we elected to perform a case-control GWAS, and then follow up the top signals by candidate SNP genotyping on the entire set of samples including family members. Therefore, the unique dataset provides an opportunity to examine GWAS associations in a combined sample of cases, family members, and controls.

3.2 RESULTS

We analyzed genotype data for 520 cases and 540 control subjects, and performed a GWAS on obesity as a binary trait. We observed a strong association of obesity to the *FTO* gene, with the most significantly associated marker being rs3751812 ($P = 2.01\times10^{-8}$, odds ratio = 1.64). All association signals with $P<10^{-5}$ are shown in Table 3, and the Manhattan plot is shown in Figure 1. No additional loci with genome-wide significance were identified in the GWAS; nevertheless, the fact that *FTO* readily reached genome-wide significance in a small data set confirmed the high quality of the phenotypes within the sample collection. It also illustrated how a small sample ascertained from extreme phenotypes have high power to detect genuinely associated genes, compared to quantitative trait association analysis conducted on population-based samples.

Considering the possibility that some obesity-associated genes may be enriched among the top ranked genes in GWAS, we next followed up selected association signals (~500 top SNPs) by iSelect genotyping on 2,256 cases, family members and controls. Additionally, we also performed dense genotyping of 49 SNPs in the *FTO* gene itself, including 7 from the original top 500 and 42 spanning the entire gene. We used the MQLS software for the association analysis, to account for the familial relationships. Interestingly, the significance for *FTO* SNPs increased by several orders of magnitude (P-values range from 10−9 to 10−12), suggesting that genotyping additional family members increased power to detect genuine associations (Table 4).

We next completed exploratory analyses of quantitative measures of obesity. In part because of the extreme bimodality of the phenotype distributions based on sample ascertainment, we controlled for case/control status. Moreover, this approach makes it possible to assess the potential effects of genes on the extent of obesity in extremely obese individuals. The complete set of results ($P<1\times10^{-6}$) were given in Table 5. We note that a few markers reached $P<5\times10^{-8}$, notably waist circumference (chromosome 21, rs11088859, $p = 3.75\times10^{-8}$, nearest gene *NCAM2*), and waist to hip ratio (chromosome 14, rs11624704, $p = 2.67\times10^{-9}$, nearest gene *NRXN3*), but the *NCAM2* locus cannot be regarded as genome-wide significant considering the need to adjust for multiple phenotypes being tested. Therefore, these exploratory results were provided as potentially interesting findings worthy of additional replication efforts.

Table S1 summarizes our results with respect to previously reported associations with obesity related traits. As noted, only *FTO* and *NRXN3*

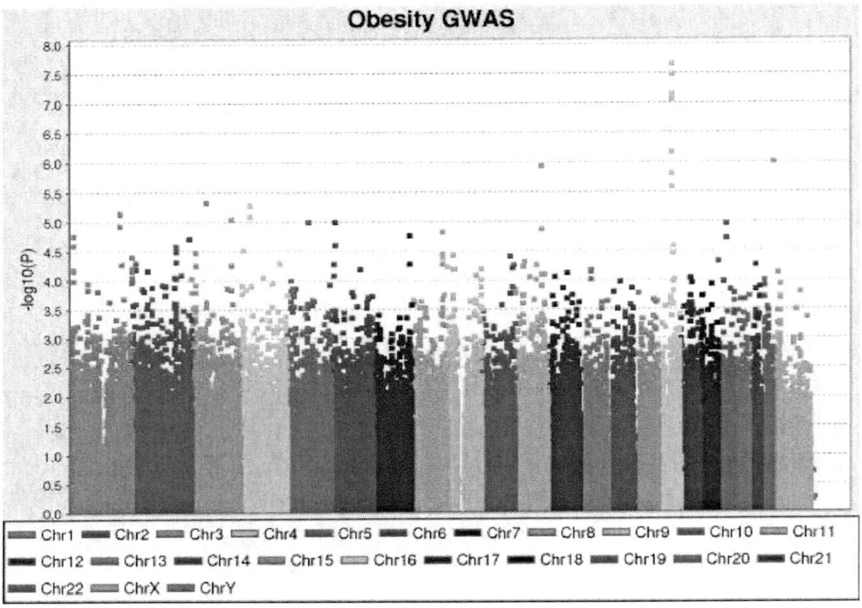

FIGURE 1. Manhattan plot (logarithm of P-values versus chromosome coordinates) for SNP association on obesity. The *FTO* locus on 16q12.2 reached genome-wide significance.

reached genome wide significance. Three genes, including SH2B1, *MC4R* and KCTD15, showed trends towards significance in the case/control association tests (P-value ranges from 0.015 to 0.065), but they did not pass multiple testing thresholds (based on number of genes tested). For quantitative traits, we cannot estimate the power of our study, since previously published studies utilized population samples for quantitative trait association with BMI [18]. Nevertheless, in our data, it is interesting to see that *MC4R* and *FTO* are the two genes with the strongest effect sizes (risk allele odds ratio >1.2), probably explaining why they were the first two genes identified in GWAS for BMI [5], [6].

3.3 DISCUSSION

In the current study, we performed a GWAS on obesity and obesity-related traits. The *FTO* gene reached genome-wide significance in this cohort with an odds ratio of 1.6. The *MC4R* gene is the second gene found by GWAS to be associated with BMI [6], and, while only marginally associated with obesity in our study, its odds ratio was 1.3. Given our modest sample size in GWAS, we estimate that the power to detect association (with perfect SNP tagging) at $P<5\times10^{-8}$ is 78.8% and 0.18% for *FTO* and *MC4R*, respectively. These odds ratio estimates in our data are higher than previous reports, for example, odds ratio for *FTO* is 1.3 in a study for early-onset obesity [5], for *FTO* and *MC4R* are 1.46 and 1.02 in a study for extreme obesity [14], or 1.25 and 1.26 in a study on morbidly obese adults with familial obesity [15], or 1.27 and 1.12 for obesity [10]. We note that the Hinney et al report investigated early onset extreme obesity and reported an odds ratio of 1.67 for *FTO* [16], comparable to our study. Therefore, the increased effect size could be due to the specific sample ascertainment scheme that we have used, that is, we sampled from the extreme tails of a quantitative trait distribution based on BMI. Even with the augmented sample of cases, family members and controls, no other SNPs reached genome wide significance. The results therefore strongly suggest that *FTO* and *MC4R* might be the only two major-effect genes for obesity with common variants in populations of European ancestry. Our study also represents an example where enrichment of extreme cases and controls can lead to increased odds ratio, and subsequently leads to improved power to detect associations.

The association between waist to hip ratio and the *NRXN3* gene is of interest, as this is the third time the gene has been associated with body fat distribution [12], [13]. Neurexins are expressed in nervous tissue and are thought to be involved in cell adhesion during synapse formation [19]. Besides fat distribution, *NRXN3* has been associated with several other traits, including addictions and schizophrenia [20]–[22]. Identifying the specific causal variant may be difficult because *NRXN3* is an extremely large gene (~1.5 Mb) [19]. It is controlled by two promoters and has multiple transcripts. The SNPs associated with weight and fat distribution lie in different parts of the gene and will likely involve different transcripts with potentially different functions. The associated SNP in our study, rs11624704, appears to be about 85 kb upstream of the first exon, while those for the previous two studies, rs10150332 and rs10146997, appear to be about 8 kb apart near exon 11.

In conclusion, we have assayed a sample collection of obese cases, families and never-overweight controls, and performed association analysis on obesity and multiple quantitative phenotype measures. We obtained strong support for *FTO* as well as suggestive confirmation of several previously identified BMI-associated genes in obesity. Another outcome of our study is the identification of new candidate genes for obesity-related traits. Of particular interest is the association of *NRXN3* with body fat distribution among extremely obese individuals.

TABLE 1: Sample characteristics of 1,060 cases and controls in GWAS.

cases	N	Minimum	Maximum	Mean	SD
488 females	32 males				
BMI[1]	520	35.57	96.95	49.39	8.78
%FAT	467	30.70	70.70	49.88	6.03
WEIGHT	512	77.05	273.64	138.13	26.91
HEIGHT	509	135.60	198.30	167.07	7.87
WAIST	509	74.40	224.79	122.11	15.32
HIP	509	67.00	276.00	148.49	18.16
WHR	508	0.61	1.46	0.83	0.09
AGE	520	18.	64	41.06	9.35
AGEONSET[2]	411	0.5	55.0	13.63	9.02
controls					
532 females	8 males				
BMI*	540	15.97	24.93	20.75	1.76
%FAT	530	6.90	40.00	23.70	5.45
WEIGHT	539	37.50	90.00	55.52	6.39
HEIGHT	539	133.90	194.00	163.49	6.53
WAIST	539	40.20	100.00	72.89	5.76
HIP	539	56.90	110.10	86.51	6.51
WHR	538	0.50	1.33	0.84	0.07
AGE	540	16	65	43.10	8.81

[1] *Self reported maximum BMI were used in 11 cases and 1 control.*
[2] *AGEONSET refers to the age of onset for the obesity diagnosis*

TABLE 3: Top association results ($P<5\times10^{-8}$) for GWAS on obesity.

SNP	Chr	Position	Closest Gene	SNP-gene distance	MAF (case)	MAF (control)	P-value	Odds ratio	P-value (case+control+family)
rs3751812	16	52375961	*FTO*	0	0.4836	0.3632	2.01×10^{-8}	1.642	4.2×10^{-12}
rs8050136	16	52373776	*FTO*	0	0.4836	0.3657	3.01×10^{-8}	1.631	4.7×10^{-12}
rs9941349	16	52382989	*FTO*	0	0.499	0.3826	6.53×10^{-8}	1.607	6.1×10^{-11}
rs9930333	16	52357478	*FTO*	0	0.5144	0.3983	7.90×10^{-8}	1.6	2.0×10^{-11}
rs10852521	16	52362466	*FTO*	0	0.4088	0.5166	6.34×10^{-7}	0.647	1.4×10^{-11}
rs10991096	11	109767953	*FDX1*	38 kb	0.0904	0.0383	1.03×10^{-6}	2.494	0.0045
rs7190492	16	52386253	*FTO*	0	0.3064	0.4067	1.46×10^{-6}	0.644	7.8×10^{9}
rs8044769	16	52396636	*FTO*	0	0.4117	0.5139	2.36×10^{-6}	0.662	4.9×10^{-10}
rs9813516	3	60268044	*FHIT*	0	0.3004	0.2127	4.34×10^{-6}	1.59	N/A
rs7697609	4	40651331	*APBB2*	0	0.2587	0.1766	4.71×10^{-6}	1.627	0.11
rs6857327	4	40649029	*APBB2*	0	0.2658	0.1848	7.76×10^{-6}	1.597	0.14
rs3912607	3	163981452	*OTOL1*	1.3 Mb	0.3721	0.4677	8.34×10^{-6}	0.675	N/A
rs6921953	6	16127094	*MYLIP*	110 kb	0.0212	0.0594	9.13×10^{-6}	0.344	0.00054
rs274916	5	87566009	*TMEM161B*	0	0.1965	0.2787	9.15×10^{-6}	0.633	0.0022

TABLE 4: Most significantly associated SNPs in the combined case/control and family cohort.

SNP	Chr	Loc	Closest Gene	P(MQLS)
rs17817449	16	52370868	*FTO*	2.34×10^{12}
rs3751812	16	52375961	*FTO*	4.22×10^{12}
rs9935401	16	52374339	*FTO*	4.36×10^{-12}
rs8050136	16	52373776	*FTO*	4.71×10^{-12}
rs1121980	16	52366748	*FTO*	9.50×10^{-12}
rs10852521	16	52362466	*FTO*	1.38×10^{-11}
rs1861866	16	52361841	*FTO*	1.41×10^{-11}
rs9937053	16	52357008	*FTO*	1.56×10^{-11}
rs9930333	16	52357478	*FTO*	2.02×10^{-11}
rs9931494	16	52384680	*FTO*	4.24×10^{11}
rs9941349	16	52382989	*FTO*	6.08×10^{11}
rs8044769	16	52396636	*FTO*	4.86×10^{10}
rs7206790	16	52355409	*FTO*	6.08×10^{-10}
rs1477196	16	52365759	*FTO*	9.33×10^{-9}
rs7190492	16	52386253	*FTO*	9.79×10^{-9}
rs3751813	16	52376209	*FTO*	1.63×10^{-8}
rs16867321	2	181070624	*UBE2E3*	1.63×10^{-6}
rs2887180	2	181157550	*UBE2E3*	2.44×10^{-6}
rs4784323	16	52355066	*FTO*	3.88×10^{-6}
rs925642	4	187915860	*FAT1/MTNR1A*	7.37×10^{-6}

The associated tests were performed by MQLS.

3.4 MATERIALS AND METHODS

3.4.1 STUDY PARTICIPANTS

The current GWAS study includes 520 cases and 540 control subjects, who were non-Hispanic Caucasians. Cases were obese (BMI≥35 kg/m^2) with a lifetime BMI>40 kg/m^2. Among them, 32 were male while the rest were female subjects. Independent controls were selected who had a current and lifetime BMI$\leq$25 kg/m^2. The individuals in the samples were of approximately the same age but differed in average BMI by 29 kg/m^2 (Table 1). After performing the GWAS, a combined sample of cases, controls and family members (N = 2,256), including all the study participants in the GWAS, were included for genotyping the top ~500 most significant SNPs based on genotyping budget. Subject characteristics of family members were shown in Table 2. Note that this is a study originally designed for investigating obesity genes in female subjects, but over time we have included a small fraction of males during the recruitment. All subjects gave written informed consent, and the protocol was approved by the Committee on Studies Involving Human Beings at the University of Pennsylvania.

3.4.2 PHENOTYPE MEASURES

Anthropomorphic phenotypes were directly measured in field settings. Percent fat was estimated using a bioelectric impedance (BIA) measure. The complete list of measures examined in this study is described in Table 1 and Figure S1. Body mass index was calculated from measured height and weight by the standard formula, Weight (kg) divided by Height (m^2). Measurements were taken of subjects dressed in light clothing. Height was measured from a standing position using a stadiometer. Weight was measured by a scale with a maximum weight of 600 pounds (270 kg) (Tanita TBF310 Pro Body Composition Analyzer, Tanita, Arlington Heights, IL). Body composition was estimated by bioelectric impedance using the same Tanita scale. Waist circumference was measured while standing at the height of the iliac crest. Hip circumference was taken while standing at the maximum extension of the buttocks. Waist to hip ratio (WHR) was calculated by measured waist circumference divided by measured hip circumference. Age of Obesity Onset was the age at which the subject reported having first become overweight.

3.4.3 GENOTYPING

DNA was extracted from whole blood or lymphoblastoid cell lines using a high salt method. All cases and control subjects were genotyped on the Illumina HumanHap550 SNP arrays (Illumina, San Diego, CA) with ~550,000 SNP markers, at the Center for Applied Genomics, Children's Hospital of Philadelphia. Standard data normalization procedures and canonical genotype clustering files were used to process the genotyping signals and generate genotype calls. In addition, the combined sample of cases, controls and family members (N = 2,256, Table 2) were genotyped for the top 500 SNPs from the GWAS using the Illumina ISelect platform. All cases, family members, and controls were non-Hispanic Caucasians, and we further utilized multi-dimensional scaling to confirm the ethnicity status of cases and control subjects. A subset of the whole-genome genotype data were previously described in a CNV study on obesity [23].

3.4.4 ASSOCIATION ANALYSIS

The PLINK software version 1.07 was used to conduct association tests between SNP genotypes and specific phenotypes of interest. For traits that are approximately normally distributed, we utilized standard linear regression for assessing association but including age, sex and disease status as covariates. We attempted to exclude samples with genotyping rate less than 95% but none of the samples met this criterion. SNPs were excluded in analysis if the minor allele frequency was less than 1% (23298 SNPs were excluded), or if the Hardy-Weinberg Equilibrium P-value was less than 1×10^{-6} in control subjects (1366 SNPs were excluded), or if the genotype missing rate is higher than 5% (8190 SNPs were excluded). The study participants are of European ancestry as evaluated in previous studies [24]; given whole-genome data, we also performed multi-dimensional scaling analysis on SNPs not in LD ($r2<0.2$) with each other and confirmed that all cases and control subjects were of genetically inferred European ancestry (Figure S2). The QQ plot for the obesity GWAS is given in Figure S3, and the genomic control inflation factor was 1.05.

The combined dataset of cases, family members and controls was next analyzed using MQLS. MQLS utilizes a quasi-likelihood score test approach developed by Thornton and McPeek [25] that treats the data as a case-control analysis consisting of related and unrelated individuals. This combined approach has substantially more power than separate analyses using either case-control or family based methods. However, we acknowledge that since the candidate SNP genotyping study is not independent of the GWAS, the P-value distributions will be biased and therefore our study cannot be regarded as a standard "2-stage" analysis. The MQLS (b) statistic incorporates parental data in the estimation of case genotypes. We restricted these analyses to obesity status, since the method currently is adapted only for dichotomous phenotypes.

REFERENCES

1. Haslam DW, James WP (2005) Obesity. Lancet 366: 1197–1209. doi: 10.1016/s0140-6736(05)67483-1.
2. Malis C, Rasmussen EL, Poulsen P, Petersen I, Christensen K, et al. (2005) Total and regional fat distribution is strongly influenced by genetic factors in young and elderly twins. Obes Res 13: 2139–2145. doi: 10.1038/oby.2005.265.
3. Stunkard AJ, Foch TT, Hrubec Z (1986) A twin study of human obesity. Jama 256: 51–54. doi: 10.1001/jama.256.1.51.
4. Farooqi IS (2006) Genetic aspects of severe childhood obesity. Pediatr Endocrinol Rev 3: Suppl 4528–536.
5. Frayling TM, Timpson NJ, Weedon MN, Zeggini E, Freathy RM, et al. (2007) A common variant in the *FTO* gene is associated with body mass index and predisposes to childhood and adult obesity. Science 316: 889–894. doi: 10.1126/science.1141634.
6. Loos RJ, Lindgren CM, Li S, Wheeler E, Zhao JH, et al. (2008) Common variants near *MC4R* are associated with fat mass, weight and risk of obesity. Nat Genet 40: 768–775.
7. Scherag A, Dina C, Hinney A, Vatin V, Scherag S, et al. (2010) Two New Loci for Body-Weight Regulation Identified in a Joint Analysis of Genome-Wide Association Studies for Early-Onset Extreme Obesity in French and German Study Groups. PLoS Genet 6: e1000916. doi: 10.1371/journal.pgen.1000916.
8. Willer CJ, Speliotes EK, Loos RJ, Li S, Lindgren CM, et al. (2009) Six new loci associated with body mass index highlight a neuronal influence on body weight regulation. Nat Genet 41: 25–34.
9. Lindgren CM, Heid IM, Randall JC, Lamina C, Steinthorsdottir V, et al. (2009) Genome-wide association scan meta-analysis identifies three Loci influencing adiposity and fat distribution. PLoS Genet 5: e1000508.
10. Thorleifsson G, Walters GB, Gudbjartsson DF, Steinthorsdottir V, Sulem P, et al. (2009) Genome-wide association yields new sequence variants at seven loci that associate with measures of obesity. Nat Genet 41: 18–24. doi: 10.1038/ng.274.
11. Heid IM, Jackson AU, Randall JC, Winkler TW, Qi L, et al. (2010) Meta-analysis identifies 13 new loci associated with waist-hip ratio and reveals sexual dimorphism in the genetic basis of fat distribution. Nat Genet 42: 949–960.

12. Heard-Costa NL, Zillikens MC, Monda KL, Johansson A, Harris TB, et al. (2009) *NRXN3* is a novel locus for waist circumference: a genome-wide association study from the CHARGE Consortium. PLoS Genet 5: e1000539. doi: 10.1371/journal.pgen.1000539.
13. Speliotes EK, Willer CJ, Berndt SI, Monda KL, Thorleifsson G, et al. (2010) Association analyses of 249,796 individuals reveal 18 new loci associated with body mass index. Nat Genet 42: 937–948.
14. Cotsapas C, Speliotes EK, Hatoum IJ, Greenawalt DM, Dobrin R, et al. (2009) Common body mass index-associated variants confer risk of extreme obesity. Hum Mol Genet 18: 3502–3507. doi: 10.1093/hmg/ddp292.
15. Meyre D, Delplanque J, Chevre JC, Lecoeur C, Lobbens S, et al. (2009) Genome-wide association study for early-onset and morbid adult obesity identifies three new risk loci in European populations. Nat Genet 41: 157–159. doi: 10.1038/ng.301.
16. Hinney A, Nguyen TT, Scherag A, Friedel S, Bronner G, et al. (2007) Genome wide association (GWA) study for early onset extreme obesity supports the role of fat mass and obesity associated gene (*FTO*) variants. PLoS ONE 2: e1361. doi: 10.1371/journal.pone.0001361.
17. Walters RG, Jacquemont S, Valsesia A, de Smith AJ, Martinet D, et al. (2010) A new highly penetrant form of obesity due to deletions on chromosome 16p11.2. Nature 463: 671–675.
18. Willer CJ, Sanna S, Jackson AU, Scuteri A, Bonnycastle LL, et al. (2008) Newly identified loci that influence lipid concentrations and risk of coronary artery disease. Nat Genet 40: 161–169. doi: 10.1038/ng.76.
19. Rowen L, Young J, Birditt B, Kaur A, Madan A, et al. (2002) Analysis of the Human Neurexin Genes: Alternative Splicing and the Generation of Protein Diversity. Genomics 79: 587–597. doi: 10.1006/geno.2002.6734.
20. Hishimoto A, Liu QR, Drgon T, Pletnikova O, Walther D, et al. (2007) Neurexin 3 polymorphisms are associated with alcohol dependence and altered expression of specific isoforms. Hum Mol Genet 16: 2880–2891. doi: 10.1093/hmg/ddm247.
21. Lachman HM, Fann CSJ, Bartzis M, Evgrafov OV, Rosenthal RN, et al. (2007) Genomewide suggestive linkage of opioid dependence to chromosome 14q. Human Molecular Genetics 16: 1327–1334. doi: 10.1093/hmg/ddm081.
22. Novak G, Boukhadra J, Shaikh SA, Kennedy JL, Le Foll B (2009) Association of a polymorphism in the *NRXN3* gene with the degree of smoking in schizophrenia: a preliminary study. World J Biol Psychiatry 10: 929–935. doi: 10.1080/15622970903079499.
23. Wang K, Li WD, Glessner JT, Grant SF, Hakonarson H, et al. (2010) Large copy number variations are enriched in cases with moderate to extreme obesity. Diabetes 59: 2690–2694. doi: 10.2337/db10-0192.
24. Price RA, Li WD, Zhao H (2008) *FTO* gene SNPs associated with extreme obesity in cases, controls and extremely discordant sister pairs. BMC Med Genet 9: 4. doi: 10.1186/1471-2350-9-4.
25. Thornton T, McPeek MS (2007) Case-control association testing with related individuals: a more powerful quasi-likelihood score test. Am J Hum Genet 81: 321–337. doi: 10.1086/519497.

There are two tables and some online supporting information that is not included in this version of the article. To see these additional files, please use the citation in the beginning of the chapter to view the original article.

CHAPTER 4

DIFFERENCES BETWEEN ADIPOSITY INDICATORS FOR PREDICTING ALL-CAUSE MORTALITY IN A REPRESENTATIVE SAMPLE OF UNITED STATES NON-ELDERLY ADULTS

HENRY S. KAHN, KAI MCKEEVER BULLARD, LAWRENCE E. BARKER, and GIUSEPPINA IMPERATORE

5.1 INTRODUCTION

The best clinical measures of adiposity for predicting future health risks are not clear. Ascending categories of body mass index (BMI, kg/m^2) generally define increasing degrees of adiposity [1], but this widely employed indicator cannot account for the weight contributions made by different organs, lean and fat tissues, or the physiology of body-fat distribution [2]. A recent Scientific Statement from the American Heart Association acknowledged substantial heterogeneity in adult body fatness at a given BMI, but it also recognized assessment opportunities related to body-fat distribution and ectopic fat deposition [3]. The review's authors endorsed the use both of BMI measurements (at cutpoints 25, 30, 35, and 40) and of waist circumference (WC) as tools for assessing health risk associated

This chapter was originally published under the Creative Commons Attribution License. Kahn HS, Bullard KM, Barker LE, and Imperatore G. Differences between Adiposity Indicators for Predicting All-Cause Mortality in a Representative Sample of United States Non-Elderly Adults. PLoS ONE *7,11 (2012), doi:10.1371/journal.pone.0050428.*

with adiposity. They drew attention, however, to an absence in the literature of established WC cutpoints that would be specific to BMI level, sex, age, or ancestral groups.

We have explored how the BMI, WC, and four other adiposity indicators were associated with the all-cause mortality experienced by a representative sample of US non-elderly adults. In conventional, sex-stratified analyses we evaluated each adiposity indicator linearly as a continuous variable. Since we could not assume the existence of linear mortality relationships, we also evaluated each indicator as a categorical variable defined by comparing subgroups of adults (ordinal quartiles) defined by the boundary of each indicator's 25th percentile (p25) or the boundary of its 75th percentile (p75) in the sex-stratified, overall population. By evaluating all six adiposity indicators in this manner, we hoped to identify differences in mortality prediction by these indicators when applied to non-elderly men, women, and population subgroups defined by various characteristics.

5.2 POPULATION AND METHODS

5.2.1 STUDY POPULATION

Our baseline sample came from participants in the third National Health and Nutrition Examination Survey (NHANES III), a complex multistage, clustered, stratified probability sample of the US civilian, noninstitutionalized population in 1988–1994 [4]. The analytic cohort included adults who were aged 18–64 years, not pregnant, had complete anthropometric data, and had no history of cancer (with the exception of nonmelanoma skin cancer). We included eligible persons whose self-identified race and ethnicity placed them in one of three categories: non-Hispanic black, Mexican-American (both oversampled in NHANES III), or non-Hispanic white. In this paper we hereafter refer to these categories as "ancestries" [5] to acknowledge the complex contributions of historical, sociocultural, and biological factors. We excluded persons who identified themselves by other races or ethnicities due to their small numbers and heterogeneous descriptions. We also excluded persons who were ineligible for mortality ascertainment (0.1% of sample) because of insufficient personal identifying information [6]. Our remaining analytic cohort contained 5,514 men and 5,923 women.

5.2.2 BASELINE VARIABLES

Participants completed a household interview and an examination with standardized measurements of weight, height, standing WC (in the horizontal plane at the level just above the iliac crest, at minimal respiration), standing hip circumference (at the maximum extension of the buttocks), and midthigh circumference (in seated position at the midpoint of the right thigh) [7]. Height and circumferences were reported to the nearest 0.1 cm. From these measurements we calculated each participant's BMI, waist-to-height ratio (WHtR), waist-to-hip ratio (WHR), and waist-to-thigh ratio (WTR).

From a subset of the analytic cohort whose serum had been assayed for fasting triglyceride concentration (n = 6,890, fast durations 8–24 hours) we calculated an additional index, the lipid accumulation product (LAP). LAP is a non-conventional adiposity indicator for adults that incorporates an anthropometric estimate of central adiposity and a laboratory assay of circulating lipid fuels in order to extend the physiological concept of lipid excess [8]. Earlier literature has described several phenotypes of the "hypertriglyceridemic waist," each defined as a dichotomous indicator [9], [10]. The LAP indicator extends this concept in the form of a continuous variable. Increased values of LAP have been associated with prevalent type 2 diabetes [11]–[13], incident type 2 diabetes [12], [14], hepatic steatosis [15], and insulin resistance [16]. For this calculation we used the formulas:

LAP for men = (WC[cm] – 65) x (triglyceride concentration [mmol/L])

LAP for women = (WC[cm] – 58) x (triglyceride concentration [mmol/L])

TABLE 1: Selected baseline characteristics of U.S. adults aged 18–64 years, NHANES 1988–1994.

Characteristic		Total	Alive		Deceased	
			Men	Women	Men	Women
Sample size, n[a]		11,437	4,858	5,498	656	425
Population estimate, n[b]		128.3	59.0	59.9	5.6	3.9
Follow-up interval, mean y (SE)		14.7 (0.2)	15.2 (0.2)	15.1 (0.3)	9.2 (0.4)	9.6 (0.3)
Age, % (SE)	18–29 y	29.2 (0.9)	31.4 (1.1)	30.0 (1.1)	12.6 (2.5)	7.9 (2.5)
	30–44 y	40.2 (1.0)	42.6 (1.2)	41.2 (1.3)	20.9 (2.9)	18.7 (3.2)
	45–64 y	30.6 (1.0)	26.0 (1.2)	28.9 (1.2)	66.5 (3.3)	73.4 (3.7)
Age, mean y (SE)		38.1 (0.3)	36.7 (0.3)	37.6 (0.3)	47.7 (0.8)	51.0 (1.0)
Ancestry, % (SE)	Non-Hispanic white	81.0 (0.9)	81.9 (1.0)	80.7 (1.1)	76.8 (2.3)	78.7 (2.2)
	Non-Hispanic black	12.6 (0.8)	11.1 (0.7)	13.5 (0.9)	17.3 (2.0)	17.0 (2.0)
	Mexican American	6.3 (0.6)	7.0 (0.7)	5.8 (0.5)	5.9 (0.8)	4.3 (0.8)
<HS education, % (SE)		20.2 (1.0)	20.3 (1.0)	17.6 (1.1)	34.9 (3.1)	38.3 (3.2)
<200% poverty ratio, % (SE)		31.4 (1.1)	28.6 (1.1)	32.7 (1.4)	40.4 (2.6)	41.9 (3.5)
Tobacco exposure, % (SE)		36.1 (1.0)	39.5 (1.0)	29.8 (1.1)	56.3 (3.2)	52.4 (2.5)
Prevalent diabetes, % (SE)		4.6 (0.3)	3.7 (0.4)	3.5 (0.4)	16.8 (1.6)	16.7 (1.9)

NHANES = National Health and Nutrition Examination Survey, SE = standard errorm HS = high school
[a]*Unweighted*
[b]*In millions*

In addition to considering age and three ancestral groups, we adjusted for baseline low socioeconomic position and tobacco exposure since these factors contribute substantially to variation in both adiposity and mortality. For dichotomous indicators of socioeconomic position, we considered both the household poverty-income ratio and the self-reported educational attainment [17], [18]. The poverty-income ratio was determined from household interview questions, and missing poverty-income information (8.5% of analytic cohort) was imputed using 5 imputation files prepared by the National Center for Health Statistics [19]. We dichotomized the poverty-income ratio at less than 200% of poverty, a threshold consistent with recent mortality analyses for the US [17], [20], and we dichotomized attained education at less than high school completion [17], [18]. As sole adjustments for low socioeconomic position, our men's models included only the poverty-income ratio marker and our women's models included only the high-school completion marker. As shown in Table 1, these choices reflected the sex-specific, relative strengths of these alternative risk factors for mortality.

Dichotomous active tobacco exposure was inferred for participants whose serum cotinine assay was >10 ng/ml [21], [22]. For participants with missing cotinine assays (5.1% of cohort) we imputed tobacco exposure from variables (including self-reported smoking history) contained in the 5 imputation files.

In our primary, multiply-adjusted models we included no terms for physiologic risk markers at baseline (e.g., diabetes, hypercholesterolemia, hypertension, inflammatory cytokines) because these characteristics can evolve or fluctuate more rapidly than adiposity, their relation to mortality may represent a downstream consequence of increased adiposity, or their inclusion may depend on uncommon laboratory assays. However, we conducted one sub-analysis in which diabetes baseline status was included so that we could determine if results varied by diabetes status. We defined baseline diabetes from self-reports or a concentration of glycated hemoglobin (HbA1c)≥6.5% [23].

5.2.3 ASCERTAINMENT OF DEATHS

The mortality status of the NHANES III participants was ascertained through probabilistic record matching with the National Death Index, a centralized database of all US deaths [6]. Of the original 11,437 eligible cohort members, 1,081 (9.5%) were determined to have died by 31 December 2006. We computed the survival time for each deceased participant from the exact dates of the NHANES III exam and of death from the restricted-use, linked mortality files of the National Center for Health Statistics. Those not deemed to have died by the end of 2006 were treated as alive for these analyses.

5.2.4 STATISTICAL ANALYSIS

Sampling weights from the NHANES III examinations were used with SAS programs (Release 9.2.2, SAS Institute, Cary, NC) and SUDAAN (Release 10.0.1, Research Triangle Institute, Research Triangle, NC) to estimate the size and characteristics of the represented US non-elderly adult population and the sex-specific, statistical distributions of the six adiposity indicators. The sampling weights employed in SUDAAN accounted for the NHANES III unequal selection probabilities (clustered design, planned oversampling, and differential nonresponse) [24]. For each adiposity indicator, we defined a sex-specific midrange to include those persons in quartiles 2 plus 3 (half of the described population) whose adiposity put them between the indicator's p25 and p75.

We used PROC SURVIVAL (SUDAAN) to fit Cox proportional-hazard models that estimated each adiposity indicator's associations with time from baseline examination to death. Sex-specific models evaluated:

1. a linear association with the standardized adiposity indicator (per 1 SD of the continuous variable);
2. a categorical mortality risk associated with being above adiposity boundary p25 (midrange compared with quartile 1 adiposity, ignoring the remote quartile 4); and
3. a categorical mortality risk associated with being above adiposity boundary p75 (quartile 4 adiposity compared with midrange, ignoring the remote quartile 1).

For (1) we used log-transformations of BMI, WC, WHtR, WTR and LAP to bring these variables closer to a normal distribution; log-transformation was not necessary for WHR. In all models we considered results with $p<0.05$ significant.

To estimate p25 and p75 for each adiposity indicator we first assessed the empirical effects of baseline age by fitting sex-specific cubic models (function of age, age^2, and age^3). Cubic models were considered because they are a flexible family of non-linear curves. The value of all the indicators rose with increased age up to about 45 years old, but, at older ages, the men's age relationship was generally more curvilinear (inverted U shape) than that observed for the women. We therefore estimated p25 and p75 for four subpopulations represented by the cross-class of sex and age groups 18–44 or 45–64 years.

These linear and categorical associations are reported as sex-specific hazard ratios (HRs) either unadjusted or multiply adjusted for age, ancestry and specified dichotomous variables. Because some of the adjusted Cox models for men included a significant term for age^2, we, to maintain consistency, included an age^2 term for all men's adjusted models (but not for women's adjusted models). With inclusion of three categories of ancestry in our models we identified interactions of adiposity with non-Hispanic black ancestry (compared to non-Hispanic whites) but not with Mexican Americans; we therefore collapsed non-Hispanic white and Mexican American into one category because there was little difference between them.

5.3 RESULTS

Our analytic sample represented a US population of 128 million non-elderly adults with a baseline mean age of 38.1 years (Table 1). During the follow-up period (up to 18.1 years), deaths occurred among an estimated 8.7% of the men (baseline mean age of 47.7 years) and 6.1% of the women (baseline mean age of 51.0 years). Deaths were more likely among non-Hispanic blacks, those with education less than high school (especially women), those with income below 200% of the poverty threshold (especially men), and those with baseline tobacco exposure.

At baseline, irrespective of sex and the adiposity indicator used, the older participants (ages 45–64) had greater adiposity than the younger participants (Table 2). At p25, p50 and p75 the men had higher adiposity values than women for WC, WHR, WTR and LAP, but this sex difference was not consistently seen for BMI or WHtR.

TABLE 2: Median (p50) and interquartile boundary values (p25, p75) for baseline adiposity indicators by age group and sex among U.S. adults, 1988–1994.

Adiposity indicator	Total			18–44 years						45–64 years					
				Men			Women			Men			Women		
	p25	p50	p75	p25	p50	p75	p25	p50	p75	p25	p50	p75	p25	p50	p75
BMI, kg/m^2	22.4	25.3	29.2	22.8	25.2	28.2	21.0	23.6	28.4	24.3	26.7	29.9	23.4	26.8	31.5
WC, cm	79.2	89.5	100.0	82.1	90.4	99.3	73.0	80.7	91.6	92.0	98.5	106.3	83.0	92.3	103.3
WHtR	0.47	0.52	0.58	0.47	0.51	0.56	0.45	0.49	0.56	0.52	0.56	0.61	0.51	0.57	0.64
WHR	0. 83	0.89	0.95	0.87	0.91	0.96	0.77	0.82	0.87	0.94	0.98	1.03	0.83	0.88	0.94
WTR	1.60	1.72	1.87	1.63	1.73	1.84	1.50	1.61	1.72	1.84	1.93	2.04	1.66	1.79	1.95
LAP[a], cm x mmol/L	15.9	30.3	60.1	15.6	28.8	56.6	11.5	20.8	38.4	30.2	50.2	84.9	25.3	47.6	82.8

[a]*LAP = lipid accumuation product (estimates derived from fasting participants; n = 6,890)*

TABLE 3: Hazard ratios (95% CI) for all-cause mortality associated with 6 adiposity indicators presented as linear continuous models and categorical models at boundaries p25 or p75 for US nonelderly men.

Indicator	Unadjusted models			Multiply adjusted models[a]		
	Linear HRs	Categorical HRs		Linear aHRs	Categorical aHRs	
	Continuous (per SD)	*At p25*[b]	*At p75*[c]	*Continuous (per SD)*	*At p25*[b]	*At p75*[c]
BMI	1.32 (1.15–1.51)	0.78 (0.57–1.06)	1.50 (1.16–1.94)	1.24 (1.06–1.45)	0.78 (0.56–1.09)	1.54 (1.18–2.01)
WC	1.52 (1.32–1.75)	0.83 (0.62–1.10)	1,62 (1.23–2.14)	1.27 (1.08–1.51)	0.85 (0.63–1.15)	1.54 (1.18–2.02)
WHtR	1.62 (1.39–1.88)	0.97 (0.68–1.38)	1.79 (1.35–2.36)	1.33 (1.11–1.59)	0.91 (0.63–1.31)	1.70 (1.31–2.19)
WHR	1.71 (1.51–1.94)	1.17 (0.87–1.58)	1.19 (0.92–1.53)	1.27 (1.09–1.48)	1.03 (0.75–1.42)	1.23 (0.94–1.61)
WTR	2.11 (1.78–2.49)	1.51 (1.09–2.09)	1.38 (1.03–1.87)	1.43 (1.20–1.71)	1.38 (0.98–1.93)	1.13 (0.86–1.49)
LAP	1.49 (1.21–1.83)	1.03 (0.74–1.45)	1.10 (0.64–1.89)	1.22 (0.95–1.55)	1.03 (0.72–1.49)	1.11 (0.66–1.85)
P-value[d]	<0.001	0.042	0.25	0.86	0.22	0.18

HR = hazard ratio, aHR = multiply adjusted hazard ratio

[a]*Models for men were adjusted for age, age^2, black ancestry, tobacco exposure, and income <200% of poverty threshold.*

[b]*Risk comparing midrange vs. quartile 1*

[c]*Risk comparing quartile 4 vs. midrange*

[d]*P-values determined from chi-squared test evaluating 6 adiposity indicators (5 degrees of freedom)*

Table 4. Hazard ratios (95% CI) for all-cause mortality associated with 6 adiposity indicators presented as linear continuous models and categorical models at boundaries p25 or p75 for US nonelderly women.

Indicator	Unadjusted models			Multiply adjusted models[a]		
	Linear HRs	Categorical HRs		Linear aHRs	Categorical aHRs	
	Continuous (per SD)	*At p25[b]*	*At p75[c]*	*Continuous (per SD)*	*At p25[b]*	*At p75[c]*
BMI	1.50 (1.39–1.62)	1.30 (0.91–1.85)	1.42 (1.08–1.86)	1.32 (1.19–1.47)	1.24 (0.87–1.77)	1.54 (1.18–2.00)
WC	1.86 (1.71–2.03)	1.85 (1.37–2.49)	1.65 (1.31–2.08)	1.47 (1.29–1.67)	1.50 (1.06–2.13)	1.64 (1.30–2.07)
WHtR	1.88 (1.73–2.05)	1.83 (1.26–2.66)	1.63 (1.24–2.14)	1.45 (1.29–1.64)	1.39 (0.98–1.99)	1.65 (1.26–2.17)
WHR	1.43 (1.25–1.63)	1.90 (1.08–3.34)	2.33 (1.81–3.00)	1.30 (1.17–1.46)	1.23 (0.71–2.14)	1.80 (1.42–2.27)
WTR	2.41 (2.09–2.77)	1.73 (1.10–2.72)	2.23 (1.69–2.93)	1.53 (1.31–1.78)	1.20 (0.79–1.82)	1.72 (1.28–2.31)
LAP	1.80 (1.55–2.08)	1.89 (1.11–3.20)	1.53 (0.95–2.46)	1.27 (1.02–1.57)	1.26 (0.75–2.15)	1.48 (0.90–2.43)
P-value[d]	<0.001	0.70	0.053	0.35	0.96	0.95

HR = hazard ratio, aHR = multiply adjusted hazard ratio

[a]*Models for women were adjusted for age, black ancestry, tobacco exposure, and education <high school graduation.*

[b]*Risk comparing midrange vs. quartile 1*

[c]*Risk comparing quartile 4 vs. midrange*

[d]*P-values determined from chi-squared test evaluating 6 adiposity indicators (5 degrees of freedom)*

Population-based cross-tabulations demonstrated that, when comparing any two adiposity indicators, substantial portions of US non-elderly adults had discordant assignments to quartile 1, midrange, or quartile 4 (see supplementary appendix).

5.3.1 UNADJUSTED MORTALITY PREDICTION

In our unadjusted models each linear adiposity indicator was positively associated with mortality. The hazard ratios (HRs, per 1 SD adiposity increment) ranged from 1.3 [95%CI 1.2–1.5] (men's BMI) to HR 2.4 [2.1–2.8] (women's WTR). WTR was a stronger linear predictor than other adiposity indicators among both men (Table 3) and women (Table 4).

Evaluated categorically, WTR was the only indicator that significantly predicted mortality for both sexes at the p25 boundary (midrange vs quartile 1, HRs 1.5–1.7) and the p75 boundary (quartile 4 vs midrange, HRs 1.4–2.2).

5.3.2 MULTIPLY ADJUSTED MORTALITY PREDICTION

The linear associations with mortality were attenuated in models adjusted for age, black ancestry, tobacco exposure and socioeconomic position (Tables 3 and 4). In these adjusted models we found little variation in linear risk among indicators (adjusted hazard ratios [aHRs] 1.2–1.4 for men, 1.3–1.5 for women). For both sexes WTR was marginally stronger than the other continuous indicators.

At the p25 boundary five of the men's adiposity indicators had no significant categorical association with increased mortality (aHRs 0.8–1.0), but WTR showed a modest increased risk (aHR 1.4 [1.0–1.9]) (Table 3 and Figure 1). For women overall at the p25 boundary the mortality risks were similar for each indicator (aHRs 1.2–1.5) (Table 4). However, when black women were assessed by BMI, WC, or WHtR they were not at significantly increased risk (aHRs 0.7–0.8 vs 1.4–1.6 for non-Black women) (Figure 1).

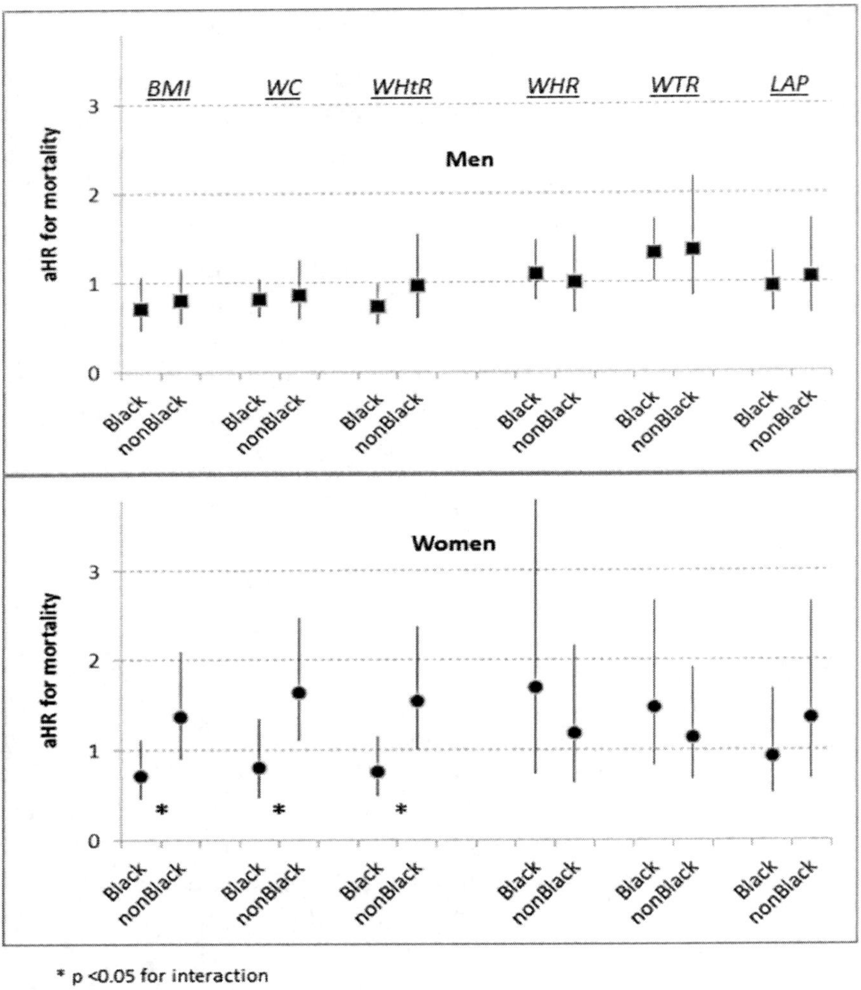

FIGURE 1: Interactions with ancestral group for mortality risk at p25, by 6 adiposity indicators. (aHR = multiply adjusted hazard ratio).

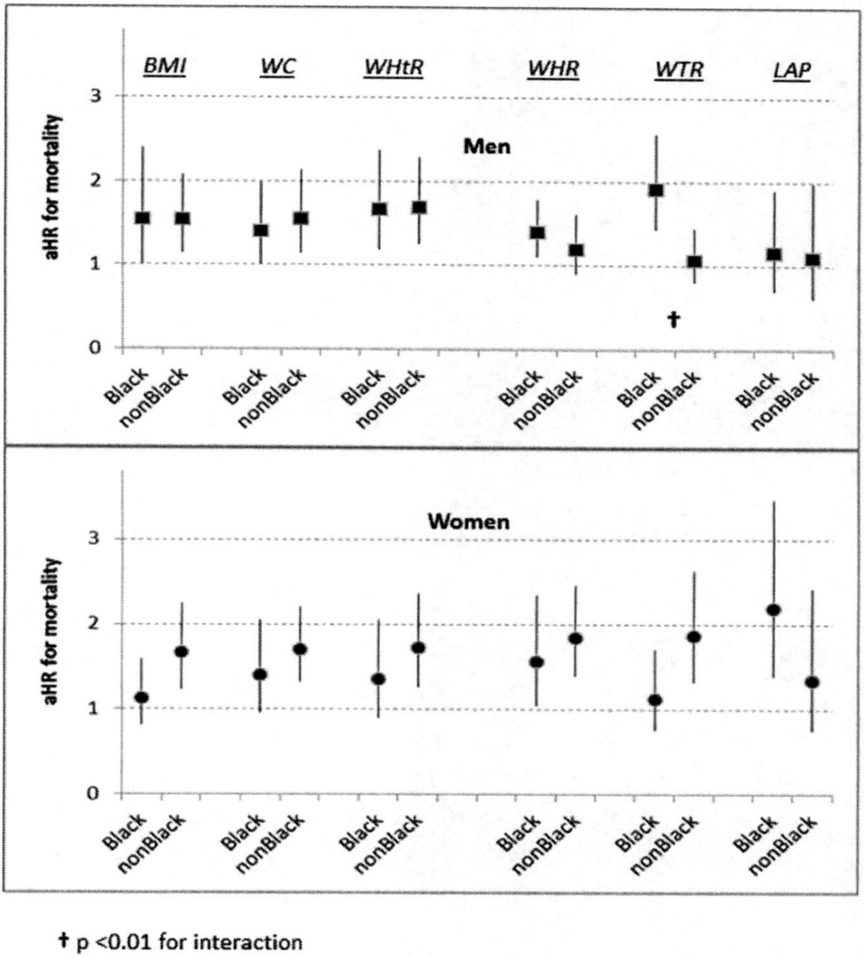

FIGURE 2: Interactions with ancestral group for mortality risk at p75, by 6 adiposity indicators. (aHR = multiply adjusted hazard ratio).

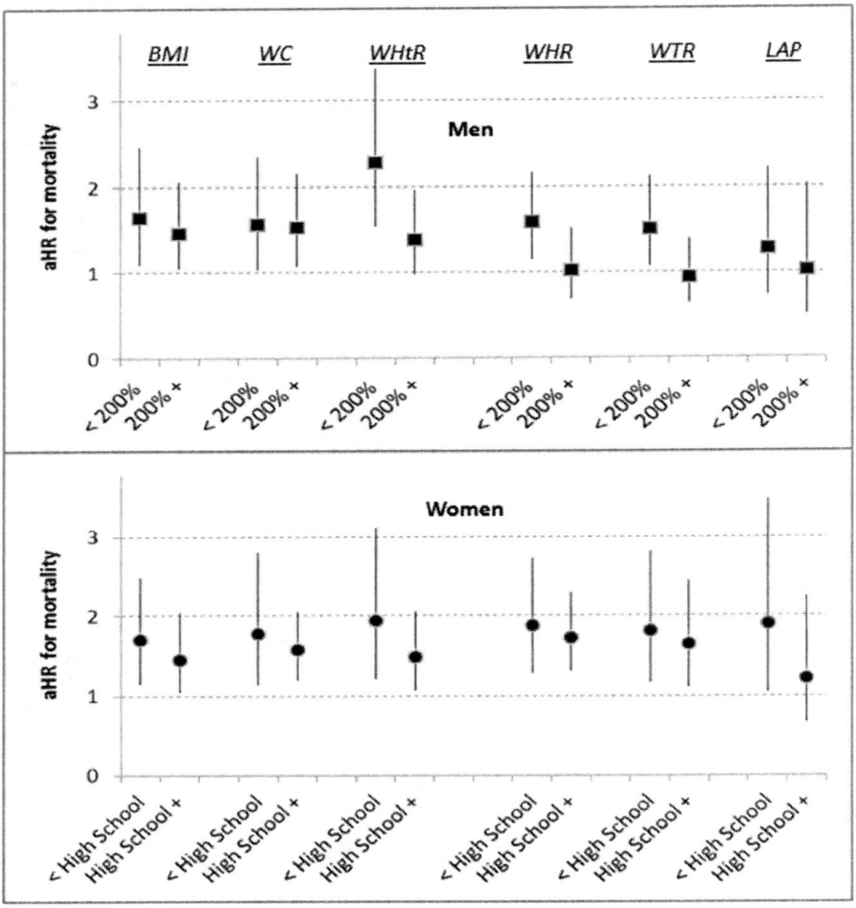

FIGURE 3: Interactions with socioeconomic position (poverty-income ratio or high-school completion) for mortality risk at p75, by 6 adiposity indicators. (aHR = multiply adjusted hazard ratio).

At the p75 boundary the significant associations of BMI, WC, and WHtR with mortality were similar for men and women (aHRs 1.5–1.7) (Tables 3 and 4), and we found no interactions between these indicators and ancestral group (Figure 2). However, for low-income men, compared to men with higher income, quartile 4 of WHtR appeared to have a greater increased risk (aHR 2.3 [1.5–3.4]) (Figure 3; p = 0.07 for interaction).

With assessment by WHR at adiposity p75 the increased mortality risk for men overall was weak (aHR 1.2 [0.9–1.6]) (Table 3), but for low-income men the risk by WHR was possibly increased (aHR 1.6 [1.2–2.2]) (Figure 3; p = 0.085 for interaction). For women overall at p75 WHR was strongly associated with risk (Table 4) irrespective of ancestry (Figure 2) or socioeconomic position (Figure 3).

Assessment by WTR at p75 for men overall was not significantly associated with mortality risk (Table 3). For black men, however, WTR at p75 was strongly associated with mortality (aHR 1.9 [1.4–2.6]) (Figure 2), and low-income men also had an increased risk (aHR 1.5 [1.1–2.1]) (Figure 3; p = 0.08 for interaction) For women overall, WTR at p75 was associated with substantial mortality risk (aHR 1.7 [1.3–2.3]) (Table 4), but this risk estimated by WTR was much less for black women (aHR 1.1 [0.8–1.7]) (Figure 2; p = 0.07 for interaction). By contrast, black women assessed by LAP at p75 had a high mortality risk (aHR 2.2 [1.4–3.5]) (Figure 2).

At p75, for both sexes and all indicators, higher adiposity was associated with greater mortality risks among persons with tobacco exposure than without (Figure 4). The interactions with tobacco exposure were only significant for adiposity assessed by LAP.

In all categorical models with multiple adjustments there were substantial mortality risks associated with tobacco exposure (aHRs 1.9–3.3), men's poverty status (aHRs 1.7–1.8) and women's low educational attainment (aHRs 1.5–1.7). The aHRs for these binary risk factors were generally larger than those associated with terms for categorical adiposity at either p25 or p75 (data not shown).

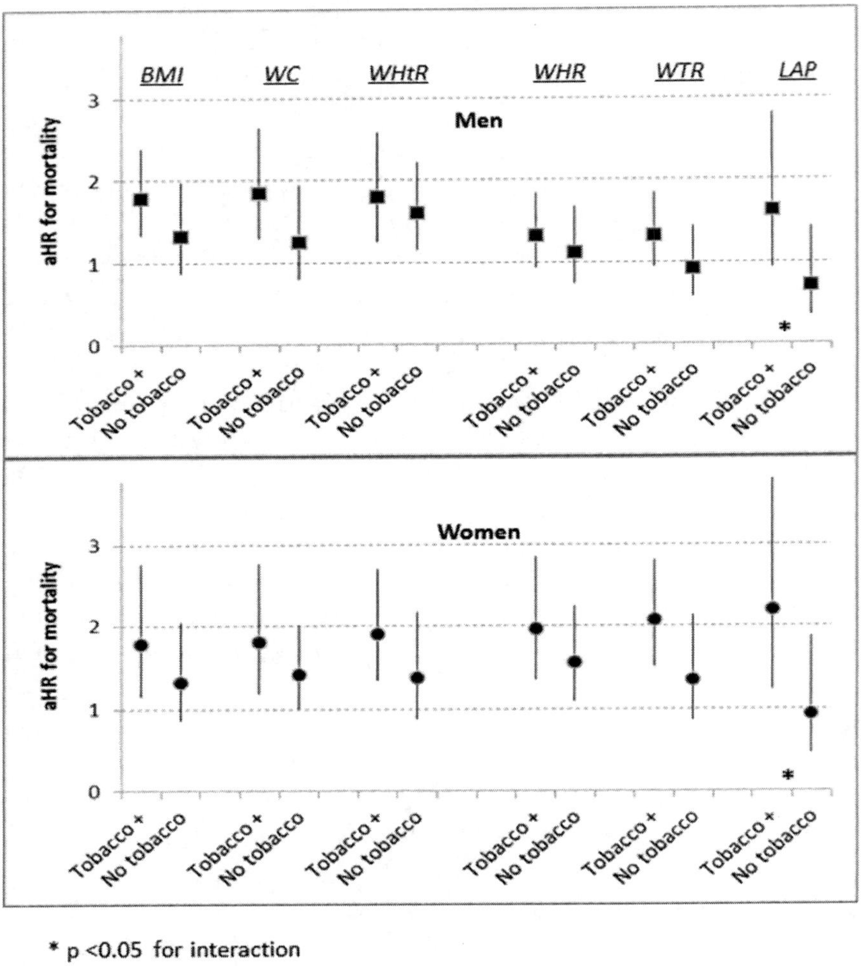

FIGURE 4: Interactions with tobacco exposure for mortality risk at p75, by 6 adiposity indicators. (aHR multiply adjusted hazard ratio).

5.3.3 DIFFERENCES RELATED TO BASELINE DIABETES STATUS OR AGE GROUP

In expanded categorical models that included a term for baseline diabetes status, we found that WC and WHtR at the p75 boundary were significantly associated with increased mortality for non-diabetic men and women (aHRs 1.6–1.7), but not for those who had diabetes (aHRs 0.7–1.1) (Figure 5). At p25 we identified no differences in mortality risk by baseline diabetes and any of the adiposity indicators.

In expanded models with a term for baseline age groups 18–44 vs 45–64 years (but retaining also continuous terms for age) we found no age-group interaction for either sex at p25 or for women at p75. However, WTR for men at p75 was unrelated to mortality for the younger age group (aHR 1.0 [0.8–1.4]), but it carried a high risk for men ages 45–64 (aHR 2.4 [1.5–3.8]) (not shown in a figure; $p = 0.002$ for interaction).

5.4 DISCUSSION

Previous prospective studies of community-based, non-elderly adults have described how all-cause mortality was associated with measured BMI [25]–[35], WC [26]–[30], [33], [34], [36], [37], WHtR [26], [33], [34], WHR [26]–[28], [30], [33], [34], [36], [38] or WTR [29], [30]. Most of the cohorts occurred in Europe, Asia or Australia. One report was a large meta-regression in which 27% of the participants came from the US, but BMI was the only indicator analyzed in that study [31]. The other cited articles with US participants were earlier analyses of participants in the NHANES III examination [25], [30]; our report from the same baseline population benefits from six additional years of mortality experience.

We believe ours is the first analysis of nationally representative data to include all-cause mortality estimates associated with these five conventional adiposity indicators, and we have also included mortality estimates associated with LAP. Some of these six indicators had distinctly non-linear associations with all-cause mortality. Therefore, in order to simplify

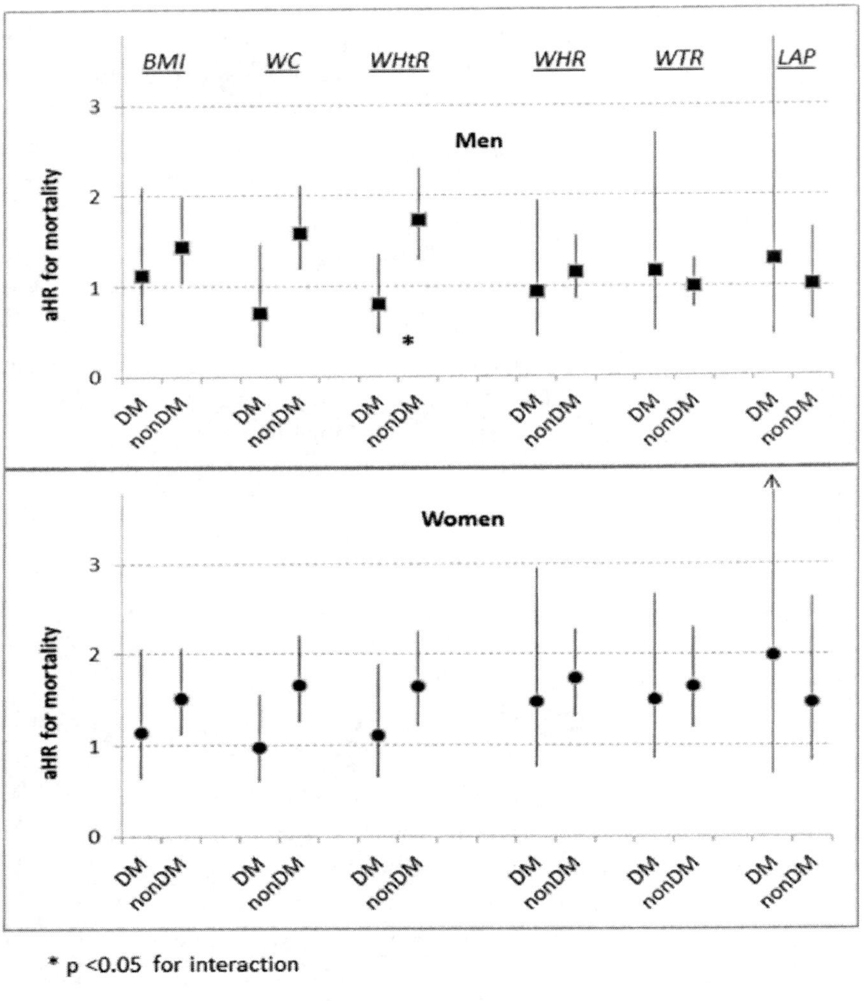

FIGURE 5: Interactions with baseline diabetes for mortality risk at p75, by 6 adiposity indicators. (aHR = multiply adjusted hazard ratio).

the comparison of all six indicators, we have reported categorical hazard ratios that predicted mortality for persons in each indicator's midrange (compared to those below p25) and for persons above the indicator's p75 (compared to those in the midrange).

Among the continuous, unadjusted adiposity indicators WTR had the strongest association with mortality, and this ranking was preserved in the multiply adjusted models. These results mirror an earlier prospective analysis of WTR and mortality in the Canadian Fitness Survey [29]. Despite different anthropometric protocols, both the Canadian Fitness Survey and our NHANES analysis demonstrated that information on thigh size relative to waist size can enhance mortality prediction. These enhancements in risk estimation depended, however, on sex and whether our categorical analysis was made at adiposity boundary p25 or p75. Among men at p25, an increase in waist size alone was not significantly associated with increased mortality, but the incorporation of information about thigh size (in the denominator of WTR) substantially increased their estimated risk (Table 3 and Figure 1). We infer that the men's increased mortality risk in the WTR midrange is not related primarily to an expanded WC but to a relatively diminished thigh circumference. As a corollary inference, men in quartile 1 of WTR are protected against mortality by their large thighs relative to their waists.

Thigh expansion among men is less common than among women, but for both sexes an increase in thigh size has been associated with reduced all-cause mortality [29], [39]. In contrast to upper-body adipose tissue, the volume of fat in the lower body tends to be less responsive to short-term variations in nutrient intake [40]. The existence of metabolic benefits associated with large thighs is supported by cross-sectional studies of non-elderly adults that demonstrated larger leg-fat mass was associated with lower levels of circulating triglycerides and total cholesterol/HDL cholesterol, and higher levels of HDL-cholesterol and insulin sensitivity [41], [42]. Other benefits of an enlarged subcutaneous depot of gluteofemoral adipose tissue may include decreased circulating inflammatory cytokines, increased adiponectin, and an enhanced capacity of lower-body adipocytes to buffer or sequester fatty acids that would otherwise contribute to harmful deposition of lipid metabolites in ectopic (non-adipose) tissues [43]–[45].

Adults above the p75 boundary of WTR might include many persons with limited expandability of the adipose tissue in their thighs. We note with interest that black men in quartile 4 of WTR have markedly increased mortality risk, but this adverse association was not found for black women in quartile 4 (Figure 2).

The reduced mortality observed among men with BMI, WC, or WHtR in the midrange relative to quartile 1 (Table 3) is consistent with the previous international literature showing a J-shaped risk curve for both sexes at the lower values of these three adiposity indicators [27], [28], [30], [31], [34]–[37]. Contrary to expectation, the women in our cohort tended to have increased mortality risk in adiposity midrange assessed by BMI, WC, or WHtR (Table 4), but these increased risk estimates above p25 applied specifically to non-Black women (Figure 1). It is possible that some US women examined in NHANES III—primarily those non-Black—were different from women with baseline body measurements described in earlier cohorts or from other countries. The US Cancer Prevention Study II that began a decade before NHANES III reported little difference in all-cause mortality experience between white women with baseline BMI <22 kg/m2 (comparable to our BMI quartile 1) and those with BMI 22.0 to 29.9 (comparable to our BMI midrange) [46]. This large, often cited cohort, however, depended on self-reported weight and height, had no objective indicator of tobacco use, excluded participants <30 years old, and under-represented persons with low educational level. Non-elderly women in BMI quartile 1 from other environments possibly shared unfavorable nutritional or social circumstances that were associated with an increased mortality risk. By contrast, non-Black women in BMI quartile 1 from our US cohort may have included many who benefited from substantial social privilege despite having low levels of adiposity. A recent cohort reported from Mauritius has also found that women in WC quartile 1 had reduced risk of mortality if they were of South Asian ancestry (absent J-shape) but increased mortality risk if they were of African ancestry [37]. Mauritian men in WC quartile 1 of either ancestry had comparably increased mortality risk.

Conventional assessments of increased adult adiposity depend on a BMI threshold value ≥30 kg/m^2 ("obesity") irrespective of age, sex or clinical circumstances [1], [3]. This threshold is close to the BMI value for p75 in our NHANES III sample of non-elderly US adults (Table 2). At this upper boundary of adiposity midrange the BMI associations with all-cause mortality (aHR 1.5 for men or women) suggest that adiposity's impact on long-term health could have been assessed at least as well by the WC or WHtR (Tables 3 and 4). However, despite categorical risk estimates that were similar for BMI, WC, and WHtR at p75, the individuals located in the midrange or quartile 4 were frequently different depending on the indicator used (see the estimated prevalences of discordance in the supplementary appendix). More recent surveys of non-elderly adults in Finland suggest that discordances between these 3 adiposity indicators may have increased since about 1997 [47].

Given that "obese" individuals located in quartile 4 of BMI might be located in the midrange of an abdominal adiposity indicator (or vice versa), our mortality predictions at p75 for BMI could be interpreted in conjunction with mortality predictions at the p75 values for an alternative adiposity indicator. The availability of population-based p75 values of WC or WHtR, for example, begins to respond to the American Heart Association's request for abdominal adiposity cutoff values specific to BMI, age, and sex [3].

Among adults aged 18–44 years with a BMI of ~30 kg/m^2 a supplementary health-risk estimate might depend on a men's WC p75 threshold value of ~99 cm and women's WC p75 threshold value of ~92 cm (Table 2). For adults 45–64 years old, a supplementary health-risk estimate might depend on a men's WC p75 threshold of ~106 cm and women's WC p75 threshold of ~103 cm. For black women, a BMI value above 30 is associated with only a weakly increased risk (aHR 1.1 [0.8–1.6]; Figure 2). Indeed, contemporary estimates from other sources suggest that the cardiometabolic risk [48] and mortality risk [49] for US black women begin to rise significantly only above ~33 kg/m^2. Assessing black women's risk by the p75 WC threshold instead of the BMI threshold might better clarify their true risk. An alternative assessment for black women using the p75 threshold value for LAP instead of BMI could provide a substantially higher risk estimate (Figure 2). For persons of ancestries other than non-Hispanic white, non-Hispanic black, or Mexican Americans we cannot be certain whether different adiposity thresholds would be better markers of health risk.

Similar to supplementary assessments using WC, the WHtR could likewise provide refined risk estimates for persons with BMI ~30 kg/m^2. Since the p75 for WHtR ranges from ~0.56 to ~0.64 for all non-elderly adults (Table 2), a practical, simplified estimate of health risk among persons with BMI ~30 kg/m^2 could depend on rounding the WHtR p75 threshold value to 0.60 irrespective of sex and age. The same "pragmatic" WHtR threshold value has recently been proposed to identify a "Take Action" adiposity level associated with increased health risk [50].

Among men and women with diabetes at baseline we found that neither WC nor WHtR above p75 was associated with increased mortality risk (Figure 5). Recent, large, observational studies including older participants have described a similar "obesity paradox" in which the diabetic adults with BMI ≥30, compared to the diabetic persons in lower BMI categories, had mortality risks that were reduced [51], [52] or similar [53]. Compared to the risk for non-diabetic adults, the attenuation of relative risk in quartile 4 may occur because diabetes itself already carries an increased risk of mortality, and thus adiposity contributes very little further detriment to health. However, risk estimation for diabetic patients using thresholds of LAP at p75 would provide higher relative-risk estimates than those provided by WC or WHtR. Use of WTR thresholds would also yield a similarly increased relative-risk estimate, possibly because reduced thigh size is associated with an increase in circulating triglycerides [41]. These advantages of LAP and WTR raise interesting issues about the pathophysiological consequences for diabetic patients of having an increased concentration of circulating triglycerides. An older cohort of high-risk patients from the US found that LAP predicted mortality better among persons without diabetes [54], whereas one from Germany found that LAP predicted mortality better among patients with diabetes [13]. Our community-based US cohort cannot resolve this conflict regarding baseline diabetes status in clinic-derived cohorts.

The weak association between LAP and all-cause mortality in our cohort overall is compatible with recent reports from smaller cohorts of older adults [13], [55]. However, at the p75 boundary increased LAP predicted mortality relatively well among persons with tobacco exposure (Figure 4). Among heavy smokers the concentration of circulating triglycerides is increased [56], [57], and, since the definition of LAP extends the concept of lipid overload by including a laboratory assay of circulating triglycerides, the value of the LAP expression is closely tied to hypertriglyceridemia. Quartile 4 of LAP, therefore, likely includes an excess of heavy smokers. The increased mortality for tobacco-exposed persons above LAP p75 probably reflects their risk linked to smoking levels beyond what was captured by our binary adjustment for tobacco exposure.

The limited ability of LAP to predict mortality might be explained to some degree by LAP's association with hepatic steatosis [15]. A recent analysis of over 11,000 adult NHANES III participants reported that fatty liver (as assessed from ultrasound images of the gallbladder) had no association with increased mortality [58]. This unexpected finding tends to support the recent concept that some persons with fatty livers may indeed be "good fat storers" [59] who can sequester excessive lipid fuel as relatively benign triglycerides. Consistent with LAP's relation to type 2 diabetes and similar clinical states [11]–[16], it has been proposed that triglyceride storage in liver tissue might be a marker of hepatic insulin resistance and diabetes risk, but these adverse effects of neutral triglyceride storage could be balanced by the protection it provides against lipotoxic damage to hepatocytes caused by some non-triglyceride fatty acids and their derivatives [59], [60]. In other non-adipose (ectopic) tissues there could be distinct roles for lipid storage. The functional consequences of increased intramyocellular lipid in skeletal muscle may differ depending on factors related to body fat distribution, ancestral origin, or habitual physical activity [61], [62].

Our study has limitations. We measured adiposity at only one point in time, so our estimates could not account for changes in adiposity. Our models also lacked information about changes in diet, physical activity or co-morbidities that might well have modified the likelihood of mortality. In addition, our use of circumferences at the waist, hip, and thigh was limited to the NHANES' specific anthropometric protocols. Other studies or clinical settings may employ different protocols for measuring the waist, hip, or thigh. Our analytic sample provided no genetic markers of ancestral admixture, and we included only persons who described themselves as non-Hispanic whites, non-Hispanic blacks, and Mexican-Americans. It is possible that persons of other ancestries might experience different mortality outcomes in relation to their baseline adiposity indicators. Our

NHANES sample of persons with LAP values (restricted to fasting participants) underrepresented high-risk diabetic patients because insulin users were not asked to fast before their NHANES exam.

Despite these limitations, our identification of some differences in health risk associated with adiposity indicators may help to focus research questions for the future. Indeed, the concept of LAP emerged initially from an intention to estimate inexpensively how lipid metabolites were accumulated ectopically with increasing age [8]. Basic research may increasingly focus on variations in the qualitative aspects and limits of lipid storage and how these characteristics may vary between tissues, regional depots, and organs. There will be complementary interests in the metabolic alterations and functional losses ("lipotoxicity") that occur when the benign accumulation limits are exceeded [63]. As new technologies describe the quantities and actions of specific fatty-acid derivatives in various anatomic locations, future epidemiologic studies may then clarify how specific regional depots of adipose tissue are related positively or negatively to lipotoxic consequences in the liver, skeletal muscle, pancreas, and other non-adipose tissues. These emerging insights should improve our ability to recognize and address health risks in population subgroups defined by sex, age, or other characteristics.

REFERENCES

1. World Health Organization Expert Committee on Physical Status (1995) Physical Status: The Use and Interpretation of Anthropometry - Report of a WHO Expert Committee. Geneva: WHO technical report series; 854. Available: http://helid.digicollection.org/en/d/Jh0211e/#Jh0211e. Accessed 30 March 2012.
2. Dulloo AG, Jacquet J, Solinas G, Montani JP, Schutz Y (2010) Body composition phenotypes in pathways to obesity and the metabolic syndrome. Int J Obes 34: S4–S17. doi: 10.1038/ijo.2010.234.
3. Cornier MA, Despres JP, Davis N, Grossniklaus DA, Klein S, et al. (2011) Assessing adiposity: A scientific statement from the American Heart Association. Circulation 124: 1996–2019. doi: 10.1161/CIR.0b013e318233bc6a.
4. National Center for Health Statistics - Office of Analysis and Epidemiology (1994) Plan and Operation of the Third National Health and Nutrition Examination Survey, 1988–1994. Hyattsville, MD. Available: http://www.cdc.gov/nchs/data/series/sr_01/sr01_032.pdf. Accessed 30 March 2012.

5. Hahn RA, Truman BI, Barker ND (1996) Identifying ancestry: The reliability of ancestral identification in the United States by self, proxy, interviewer, and funeral director. Epidemiology 7: 75–80. doi: 10.1097/00001648-199601000-00013.
6. National Center for Health Statistics - Office of Analysis and Epidemiology (2009) The Third National Health and Nutrition Examination Survey (NHANES III) Linked Mortality File, Mortality follow-up through 2006: Matching Methodology. Hyattsville, MD. Available: http://www.cdc.gov/nchs/data/datalinkage/matching_methodology_nhanes3_final.pdf. Accessed 30 Mar 2012.
7. National Center for Health Statistics (1988) National Health and Nutrition Examination III: Body Measurements (Anthropometry). Rockville, MD. Available: http://www.cdc.gov/nchs/data/nhanes/nhanes3/cdrom/NCHS/MANUALS/anthro.pdf. Accessed 30 Mar 2012.
8. Kahn HS (2005) The "lipid accumulation product" performs better than the body mass index for recognizing cardiovascular risk: a population-based comparison. BMC Cardiovasc Disord 5: 26. Available: http://www.biomedcentral.com/1471-2261/5/26. Accessed 31 Jul 2012.
9. Arsenault BJ, Lemieux I, Despres JP, Wareham NJ, Kastelein JJ, et al. (2010) The hypertriglyceridemic-waist phenotype and the risk of coronary artery disease: results from the EPIC-Norfolk prospective population study. CMAJ 182: 1427–1432. doi: 10.1503/cmaj.091276.
10. Kahn HS, Valdez R (2003) Metabolic risks identified by the combination of enlarged waist and elevated triacylglycerol concentration. Am J Clin Nutr 78 928–934.
11. Kahn HS (2006) The lipid accumulation product is better than BMI for identifying diabetes: a population-based comparison. Diabetes Care 29: 151–153. doi: 10.2337/diacare.29.01.06.dc05-1805.
12. Bozorgmanesh M, Hadaegh F, Azizi F (2010) Diabetes prediction, lipid accumulation product, and adiposity measures; 6-year follow-up: Tehran lipid and glucose study. Lipids Health Dis 9: 45. Available: http://dx.doi.org/10.1186/1476-511X-9-45. Accessed 30 Mar2012.
13. Wehr E, Pilz S, Boehm BO, Marz W, Obermayer-Pietsch B (2011) The lipid accumulation product is associated with increased mortality in normal weight postmenopausal women. Obesity (Silver Spring) 19: 1873–1880. doi: 10.1038/oby.2011.42.
14. Yang C, Guo ZR, Hu XS, Zhou ZY, Wu M (2010) [A prospective study on the association between lipid accumulation product or body mass index and diabetes.]. Zhonghua Liu Xing Bing Xue Za Zhi 31: 5–8.
15. Bedogni G, Kahn HS, Bellentani S, Tiribelli C (2010) A simple index of lipid overaccumulation is a good marker of liver steatosis. BMC Gastroenterol 10: 98. Available: http://www.biomedcentral.com/1471-230X/10/98. Accessed 30 Mar 2012.
16. Xia C, Li R, Zhang S, Gong L, Ren W, et al.. (2012) Lipid accumulation product is a powerful index for recognizing insulin resistance in non-diabetic individuals. Eur J Clin Nutr 66: : 1035–1038.
17. Muennig P, Fiscella K, Tancredi D, Franks P (2010) The relative health burden of selected social and behavioral risk factors in the United States: implications for policy. Am J Public Health 100: 1758–1764. doi: 10.2105/AJPH.2009.165019.

18. Galea S, Tracy M, Hoggatt KJ, Dimaggio C, Karpati A (2011) Estimated deaths attributable to social factors in the United States. Am J Public Health 101: 1456–1465. doi: 10.2105/AJPH.2010.300086.
19. National Center for Health Statistics (2001) Third National Health and Nutrition Examination Survey (NHANES III, 1988–1994): Multiply Imputed Data Set. Series 11. Available: ftp://ftp.cdc.gov/pub/Health_Statistics/NCHS/nhanes/nhanes3/7a/miuserguide.pdf. Accessed 30 Mar 2012.
20. Dowd JB, Albright J, Raghunathan TE, Schoeni RF, Leclere F, et al. (2011) Deeper and wider: income and mortality in the USA over three decades. Int J Epidemiol 40: 183–188. doi: 10.1093/ije/dyq189.
21. Pirkle JL (1996) Exposure of the US population to environmental tobacco smoke: the Third National Health and Nutrition Examination Survey, 1988 to 1991. JAMA 275: 1233–1240. doi: 10.1001/jama.275.16.1233.
22. Centers for Disease Control and Prevention (2011) Million hearts: strategies to reduce the prevalence of leading cardiovascular disease risk factors–United States, 2011. MMWR Morb Mortal Wkly Rep 60: 1248–1251. Available: http://www.cdc.gov/mmwr/preview/mmwrhtml/mm6036a4.htm. Accessed 30 Mar 2012.
23. American Diabetes Association (2011) Diagnosis and Classification of Diabetes Mellitus. Diabetes Care 34: S62–S69. doi: 10.2337/dc11-S062.
24. Mohadjer L, Montaquila J, Waksberg J, Bell B, James P, et al.. (1996) National Health and Nutrition Examination Survey III, Weighting and Estimation Methodology. Available: http://www.cdc.gov/nchs/data/nhanes/nhanes3/cdrom/NCHS/MANUALS/WGT_EXEC.PDF. Accessed 30 Mar 2012.
25. Flegal KM, Graubard BI, Williamson DF, Gail MH (2005) Excess deaths associated with underweight, overweight, and obesity. JAMA 293: 1861–1867. doi: 10.1001/jama.293.15.1861.
26. Welborn TA, Dhaliwal SS (2007) Preferred clinical measures of central obesity for predicting mortality. Eur J Clin Nutr 61: 1373–1379. doi: 10.1038/sj.ejcn.1602656.
27. Simpson JA, MacInnis RJ, Peeters A, Hopper JL, Giles GG, et al. (2007) A comparison of adiposity measures as predictors of all-cause mortality: the Melbourne Collaborative Cohort Study. Obesity (Silver Spring) 15: 994–1003. doi: 10.1038/oby.2007.622.
28. Pischon T, Boeing H, Hoffmann K, Bergmann M, Schulze MB, et al. (2008) General and abdominal adiposity and risk of death in Europe. N Engl J Med 359: 2105–2120. doi: 10.1056/nejmoa0801891.
29. Mason C, Craig CL, Katzmarzyk PT (2008) Influence of central and extremity circumferences on all-cause mortality in men and women. Obesity 16: 2690–2695. doi: 10.1038/oby.2008.438.
30. Reis JP, Araneta MR, Wingard DL, Macera CA, Lindsay SP, et al. (2009) Overall obesity and abdominal adiposity as predictors of mortality in U.S. white and black adults. Ann Epidemiol 19: 134–142. doi: 10.1016/j.annepidem.2008.10.008.
31. Prospective Studies Collaboration (2009) Body-mass index and cause-specific mortality in 900 000 adults: collaborative analyses of 57 prospective studies. Lancet 373: 1083–1096. doi: 10.1016/S0140-6736(09)60318-4.
32. Taylor AE, Ebrahim S, Ben-Shlomo Y, Martin RM, Whincup PH, et al. (2010) Comparison of the associations of body mass index and measures of central adiposity and

fat mass with coronary heart disease, diabetes, and all-cause mortality: a study using data from 4 UK cohorts. Am J Clin Nutr 91: 547–556. doi: 10.3945/ajcn.2009.28757.
33. Schneider HJ, Friedrich N, Klotsche J, Pieper L, Nauck M, et al. (2010) The predictive value of different measures of obesity for incident cardiovascular events and mortality. J Clin Endocrinol Metab 95: 1777–1785. doi: 10.1210/jc.2009-1584.
34. Petursson H, Sigurdsson JA, Bengtsson C, Nilsen TI, Getz L (2011) Body configuration as a predictor of mortality: comparison of five anthropometric measures in a 12 year follow-up of the Norwegian HUNT 2 Study. PLoS ONE 6: e26621. Available: http://dx.doi.org/10.1371/journal.pone.0026621. Accessed 30 Mar 2012.
35. Chen Z, Yang G, Offer A, Zhou M, Smith M, et al. (2012) Body mass index and mortality in China: a 15-year prospective study of 220 000 men. Int J Epidemiol 41: 472–481. doi: 10.1093/ije/dyr208.
36. Bigaard J, Frederiksen K, Tjonneland A, Thomsen BL, Overvad K, et al. (2004) Waist and hip circumferences and all-cause mortality: usefulness of the waist-to-hip ratio? Int J Obes Relat Metab Disord 28: 741–747. doi: 10.1038/sj.ijo.0802635.
37. Cameron AJ, Magliano DJ, Shaw JE, Zimmet PZ, Carstensen B, et al. (2012) The influence of hip circumference on the relationship between abdominal obesity and mortality. Int J Epidemiol 41: 484–494. doi: 10.1093/ije/dyr198.
38. Zhang X, Shu XO, Yang G, Li H, Cai H, et al. (2007) Abdominal adiposity and mortality in Chinese women. Arch Intern Med 167: 886–892. doi: 10.1001/archinte.167.9.886.
39. Heitmann BL, Frederiksen P (2009) Thigh circumference and risk of heart disease and premature death: prospective cohort study. BMJ 339: b3292. doi: 10.1136/bmj.b3292.
40. Singh P, Somers VK, Romero-Corral A, Sert-Kuniyoshi FH, Pusalavidyasagar S, et al. (2012) Effects of weight gain and weight loss on regional fat distribution. Am J Clin Nutr 96: 229–233. doi: 10.3945/ajcn.111.033829.
41. Boorsma W, Snijder MB, Nijpels G, Guidone C, Favuzzi AMR, et al. (2008) Body composition, insulin sensitivity, and cardiovascular disease profile in healthy Europeans. Obesity 16: 2696–2701. doi: 10.1038/oby.2008.433.
42. Hunter GR, Chandler-Laney PC, Brock DW, Lara-Castro C, Fernandez JR, et al. (2010) Fat distribution, aerobic fitness, blood lipids, and insulin sensitivity in African-American and European-American women. Obesity (Silver Spring) 18: 274–281. doi: 10.1038/oby.2009.229.
43. Manolopoulos KN, Karpe F, Frayn KN (2010) Gluteofemoral body fat as a determinant of metabolic health. Int J Obes (Lond) 34: 949–959. doi: 10.1038/ijo.2009.286.
44. Virtue S, Vidal-Puig A (2010) Adipose tissue expandability, lipotoxicity and the metabolic syndrome - An allostatic perspective. Biochim Biophys Acta 1801: 338–349. doi: 10.1016/j.bbalip.2009.12.006.
45. Karastergiou K, Smith SR, Greenberg AS, Fried SK (2012) Sex differences in human adipose tissues - the biology of pear shape. Biology of Sex Differences 3: 13. Available: http://www.bsd-journal.com/content/3/1/13. Accessed 30 Jun 2012.
46. Calle EE, Thun MJ, Petrelli JM, Rodriguez C, Heath CW Jr (1999) Body-mass index and mortality in a prospective cohort of U.S. adults. N Engl J Med 341: 1097–1105. doi: 10.1056/NEJM199910073411501.
47. Lahti-Koski M, Harald K, Saarni SE, Peltonen M, Männistö S (2012) Changes in body mass index and measures of abdominal obesity in Finnish adults between 1992

and 2007, the National FINRISK Study. Clinical Obesity 2: 57–63. Available: http://dx.doi.org/10.1111/j.1758-8111.2012.00035.x. Accessed 30 Mar 2012.
48. Katzmarzyk PT, Bray GA, Greenway FL, Johnson WD, Newton RL Jr, et al. (2011) Ethnic-specific BMI and waist circumference thresholds. Obesity (Silver Spring) 19: 1272–1278. doi: 10.1038/oby.2010.319.
49. Lakoski SG, Le AH, Muntner P, Judd SE, Safford MM, et al. (2011) Adiposity, inflammation, and risk for death in black and white men and women in the United States: the Reasons for Geographic and Racial Differences in Stroke (REGARDS) Study. J Clin Endocrinol Metab 96: 1805–1814. doi: 10.1210/jc.2010-3055.
50. Ashwell M (2011) Charts based on body mass index and waist-to-height ratio to assess the health risks of obesity: A review. Open Obes J 3: 78–84. Available: http://dx.doi.org/10.2174/1876823701103010078. Accessed 30 March 2012.
51. Kokkinos P, Myers J, Faselis C, Doumas M, Kheirbek R, et al. (2012) BMI–mortality paradox and fitness in African American and Caucasian men with type 2 diabetes. Diabetes Care 35: 1021–1027. doi: 10.2337/dc11-2407.
52. Jerant A, Franks P (2012) Body mass Index, diabetes, hypertension, and short-term mortality: a population-based observational study, 2000–2006. The Journal of the American Board of Family Medicine 25: 422–431. doi: 10.3122/jabfm.2012.04.110289.
53. McEwen LN, Karter AJ, Waitzfelder BE, Crosson JC, Marrero DG, et al. (2012) Predictors of mortality over 8 years in type 2 diabetic patients: Translating Research Into Action for Diabetes (TRIAD). Diabetes Care 35: 1301–1309. doi: 10.2337/dc11-2281.
54. Ioachimescu AG, Brennan DM, Hoar BM, Hoogwerf BJ (2010) The lipid accumulation product and all-cause mortality in patients at high cardiovascular risk: A PreCIS database study. Obesity (Silver Spring) 18: 1836–1844. doi: 10.1038/oby.2009.453.
55. Bozorgmanesh M, Hadaegh F, Azizi F (2010) Predictive performances of lipid accumulation product vs. adiposity measures for cardiovascular diseases and all-cause mortality, 8.6-year follow-up: Tehran lipid and glucose study. Lipids Health Dis 9: 100. Available: http://dx.doi.org/10.1186/1476-511X-9-100. Accessed 30 Mar 2012.
56. Craig WY, Palomaki GE, Haddow JE (1989) Cigarette smoking and serum lipid and lipoprotein concentrations: an analysis of published data. BMJ 298: 784–788. doi: 10.1136/bmj.298.6676.784.
57. Zaratin AC, Quintao EC, Sposito AC, Nunes VS, Lottenberg AM, et al. (2004) Smoking prevents the intravascular remodeling of high-density lipoprotein particles: implications for reverse cholesterol transport. Metabolism 53: 858–862. doi: 10.1016/j.metabol.2004.02.005.
58. Lazo M, Hernaez R, Bonekamp S, Kamel IR, Brancati FL, et al.. (2011) Non-alcoholic fatty liver disease and mortality among US adults: prospective cohort study. BMJ 343. Available: http://www.bmj.com/content/343/bmj.d6891. Accessed 30 March 2012.
59. Trauner M, Arrese M, Wagner M (2010) Fatty liver and lipotoxicity. Biochim Biophys Acta 1801: 299–310. doi: 10.1016/j.bbalip.2009.10.007.
60. Chavez JA, Summers SA (2010) Lipid oversupply, selective insulin resistance, and lipotoxicity: Molecular mechanisms. Biochim Biophys Acta 1801: 252–265. doi: 10.1016/j.bbalip.2009.09.015.

61. Ingram KH, Lara-Castro C, Gower BA, Makowsky R, Allison DB, et al. (2011) Intramyocellular lipid and insulin resistance: differential relationships in European and African Americans. Obesity (Silver Spring) 19: 1469–1475. doi: 10.1038/oby.2011.45.
62. Muoio DM (2010) Intramuscular triacylglycerol and insulin resistance: guilty as charged or wrongly accused? Biochim Biophys Acta 1801: 281–288. doi: 10.1016/j.bbalip.2009.11.007.
63. Sørensen TI (2011) Obesity defined as excess storage of inert triglycerides–do we need a paradigm shift? Obes Facts 4: 91–94. Available: http://dx.doi.org/10.1159/000328198. Accessed 30 Mar 2012.

There is various online supporting information that is not included in this version of the article. To see these additional files, please use the citation in the beginning of the chapter to view the original article.

CHAPTER 5

A NEW BODY SHAPE INDEX PREDICTS MORTALITY HAZARD INDEPENDENTLY OF BODY MASS INDEX

NIR Y. KRAKAUER and JESSE C. KRAKAUER

5.1 INTRODUCTION

According to the World Health Organization (WHO), overweight and obesity are increasing in prevalence and rank fifth as worldwide causes of death among risk factors, behind high blood pressure, tobacco use, high blood glucose, and physical inactivity. In high and middle income countries, where the prevalence of overweight and obesity among the adult population already exceeds 50%, overweight and obesity occupy third place as risk factors causing death, behind high blood pressure and tobacco use. WHO defined overweight as body mass index (BMI; weight divided by height^2) at or above 25 kg m^{-2}, with obesity defined as BMI $\geq$ 30 kg m^{-2} [1]. Guidelines published by the USA National

This chapter was originally published under the Creative Commons Attribution License. Krakauer NY and Krakauer JC. A New Body Shape Index Predicts Mortality Hazard Independently of Body Mass Index. PLoS ONE *7,7 (2012), doi:10.1371/journal.pone.0039504.*

Institutes of Health, using the same definition, considered that overweight and obesity are the second leading cause of preventable death in the USA, behind smoking [2].

These BMI-based obesity guidelines have been accompanied by doubt as to the validity of BMI as an indicator of dangerous obesity. BMI does not distinguish between muscle and fat accumulation [3]–[6], and there is evidence that whereas higher fat mass is associated with greater risk of premature death, higher muscle mass reduces risk [7]. As well, BMI does not distinguish between fat locations, when central or abdominal fat deposition is thought to be particularly perilous [8]–[11]. Waist circumference (WC) has emerged as a leading complement to BMI for indicating obesity risk. A number of studies have found that WC predicted mortality risk better than BMI [12]–[17]. A recent WHO report summarized evidence for WC as an indicator of disease risk, and suggests that WC could be used as a alternative to BMI [18].

A key limitation, mentioned in the WHO report, of using WC as a proxy for abdominal fat distribution is that it is sensitive to body size (height and weight) as well as to fat percentage and distribution. In fact, WC is highly correlated with BMI, to the extent that differentiating the two as epidemiological risk factors can be difficult [19]. According to a consensus statement on the clinical usefulness of WC [20], "Further studies are needed to establish WC cut points that can assess cardiometabolic risk, not adequately captured by BMI and routine clinical assessments." Scaling WC via allometric analysis to produce a quantity that is independent of BMI offers one means of separating the impact on health of body shape (degree of central bulge, presumably correlating with abdominal fat deposits) from that of body size (as measured by height, weight, and BMI). In this paper, our objectives are (1) develop A Body Shape Index (ABSI) based on WC that is approximately independent of height, weight, and BMI; and (2) evaluate ABSI as a predictor of mortality across age, sex, ethnicity, and BMI categories in a population sample, compared to the conventional predictors BMI and WC.

5.2 METHODS

5.2.1 DESCRIPTION OF DATA

We employed public-use releases of baseline interview and medical examination and mortality outcome data from the National Health and Nutrition Examination Survey (NHANES) 1999–2004. NHANES 1999–2004 was designed to sample the civilian noninstitutionalized USA population using a cluster approach. Mexicans and blacks, people 12–19 years of age and 60 years or older, low-income whites, and pregnant women were oversampled to better understand the health status of these groups. The survey included a home interview followed by a physical examination at a mobile examination center. Mortality outcomes based on the National Death Index were available through the end of 2006, representing 2–8 years of follow-up. NHANES 1999–2004 was approved by the National Center for Health Statistics (NCHS) Research Ethics Review Board under Protocol #98–12, and written informed consent was obtained from participants [21].

Basic demographic variables included baseline age (because of privacy concerns, this was given as 85 for all those 85 or older), sex, and ethnicity (given as Mexican, other Hispanic, white, black, or other). Body measurements including height, weight, and waist circumference were obtained by trained health technicians following standardized procedures. Standing height was measured using a digital stadiometer with a fixed vertical backboard and an adjustable head piece. Weight in an examination gown was measured on a digital scale. Waist circumference at the end of a normal exhalation was measured to the nearest 0.1 cm with a steel tape positioned just above the uppermost lateral border of the ilium. All instruments were calibrated following uniform protocols. These body measurements were generally not taken for people confined to wheelchairs [22].

We considered adults (age $\geq$ 18) with height, weight, and waist circumference measurements, excluding women determined to be pregnant by self-report or urine pregnancy test. Of the 14,123 individuals meeting these criteria, 14,105 had valid mortality follow-up data. The follow-up period for those remaining alive averaged 4.8 yr, and there were 828 deaths.

Additional variables we considered were smoking status (coded as yes if reported smoking cigarettes in last 5 days or smoking 'every day' or 'some days'), diabetes status (coded yes if reported a diabetes diagnosis or taking insulin or diabetes pills), and systolic and diastolic blood pressure and serum total and HDL cholesterol from the medical examination. A total of 12,044 individuals in our sample had all these variables available, with 647 deaths during follow-up.

We used the NHANES mobile examination center sample weights, which adjust for targeted oversampling and nonresponse, as well as information on which cluster each sampled individual belonged to, following the analytic guidance provided by NCHS [23]. Thus, the average ABSI values and risk estimates we compute can be taken to hold for the wider nonpregnant adult USA population insofar as NHANES was successful in sampling it. Looking at the consistency of responses across subgroups within the sample can also provide some guidance on the wider applicability of our results.

5.2.2 CONSTRUCTION OF THE BODY SHAPE INDEX

We performed linear least-squares regression on log(WC) as a function of log(height) and log(weight) for the entire nonpregnant adult sample. (Pregnant woman averaged bigger WC for a given height and weight.) Expressing WC and height in m and weight in kg, the results were.

$$\log(WC) = (-2.589 \pm 0.020) + (0.6807 \pm 0.0052)\log(\text{weight}) - (0.814 \pm 0.020)\log(\text{height}) \quad (1)$$

($R^2 = 0.829$), where the given uncertainties are standard errors. Approximating the obtained regression coefficients with ratios of small integers, we have,

$$\text{WC} \propto \text{weight}^{2/3}\text{height}^{-5/6} \quad (2)$$

We defined A Body Shape Index (ABSI) to be proportional to the ratio of actual WC to the WC expected from the regression allometry:

$$\text{ABSI} \equiv \text{WC weight}^{-2/3}\text{height}^{5/6} = (\text{WC}) / (\text{BMI}^{2/3}\text{height}^{1/2}) \quad (3)$$

The sample mean and standard deviation of ABSI thus defined is $(0.0808 \pm 0.0053)\text{m}^{11/6}\ \text{kg}^{-2/3}$.

Correlation coefficients of ABSI with height, weight, BMI and WC in the NHANES sample are shown in Table 1. It can be seen that most variability in WC reflects variability in BMI ($r \approx 0.9$) and that unlike BMI, WC also has some correlation with height ($r \approx 0.2$), consistent with earlier findings [24]–[26]. On the other hand, ABSI shows little correlation with height, weight, or BMI ($|r| < 0.1$). Its correlation with WC is modest ($r \approx 0.4$), since most variability in WC is correlated with BMI and therefore excluded from ABSI.

5.2.3 CONVERSION TO Z SCORES

To control for age and sex differences in mean ABSI, we entered it into proportional hazards regression for mortality as a z score:

$$\text{ABSI z score} = (\text{ABSI} - \text{ABSI}_{mean}) / \text{ABSI}_{SD} \quad (4)$$

where the population ABSI mean and standard deviation depend on age and sex. To estimate $ABSI_{mean}$ and $ABSI_{SD}$, we first computed the sample mean and standard deviation for each age, separately for males and females and using the NHANES sample weights (markers in Figure 1a-b). Then we smoothed the $ABSI_{mean}$(age) and $ABSI_{SD}^2$(age) curves for each sex using Tikhonov regularization with a regularization matrix that approximates a second derivative operator and a regularization parameter chosen so that the mean square residual between the curve and the sample values, scaled by the estimated standard error of the sample values, is equal to 1 [27]. These smoothed values (curves in Figure 1) were used for converting ABSI to z scores following Eq. 4. Individuals age 85 and over (for whom the exact age was not available) were not included in the smoothing, and their ABSI values were converted to z scores using the sample mean and standard deviation (asterisks near right edges of panels in Figure 1). The age and sex specific $ABSI_{mean}$ and $ABSI_{SD}$ used for computing ABSI z scores are tabulated as (Table S1).

TABLE 1: Correlations between body size and shape.

	Height	Weight	BMI	WC	ABSI
Height	1	0.452	–0.040	0.174	0.040
Weight	0.380	1	0.867	0.874	0.049
BMI	0.007	0.922	1	0.881	0.019
WC	0.163	0.908	0.918	1	0.439
ABSI	0.041	0.020	0.007	0.361	1

Mean ABSI increased steadily from midlife into old age (Figure 1a). Mean ABSI was consistently higher in males than females after young adulthood (Figure 1a), while the scatter in ABSI at a given age was greater in females than in males (Figure 1b). The age- and sex-specific BMI and WC means (Figure 1c,e), calculated using the same approach, showed different behavior than ABSI, falling after about age 60. Mean WC was higher in males while mean BMI was higher in females, consistent with the higher mean ABSI in males compared to females. As with ABSI, variability in BMI and WC was higher in females than in males (Figure 1d,f).

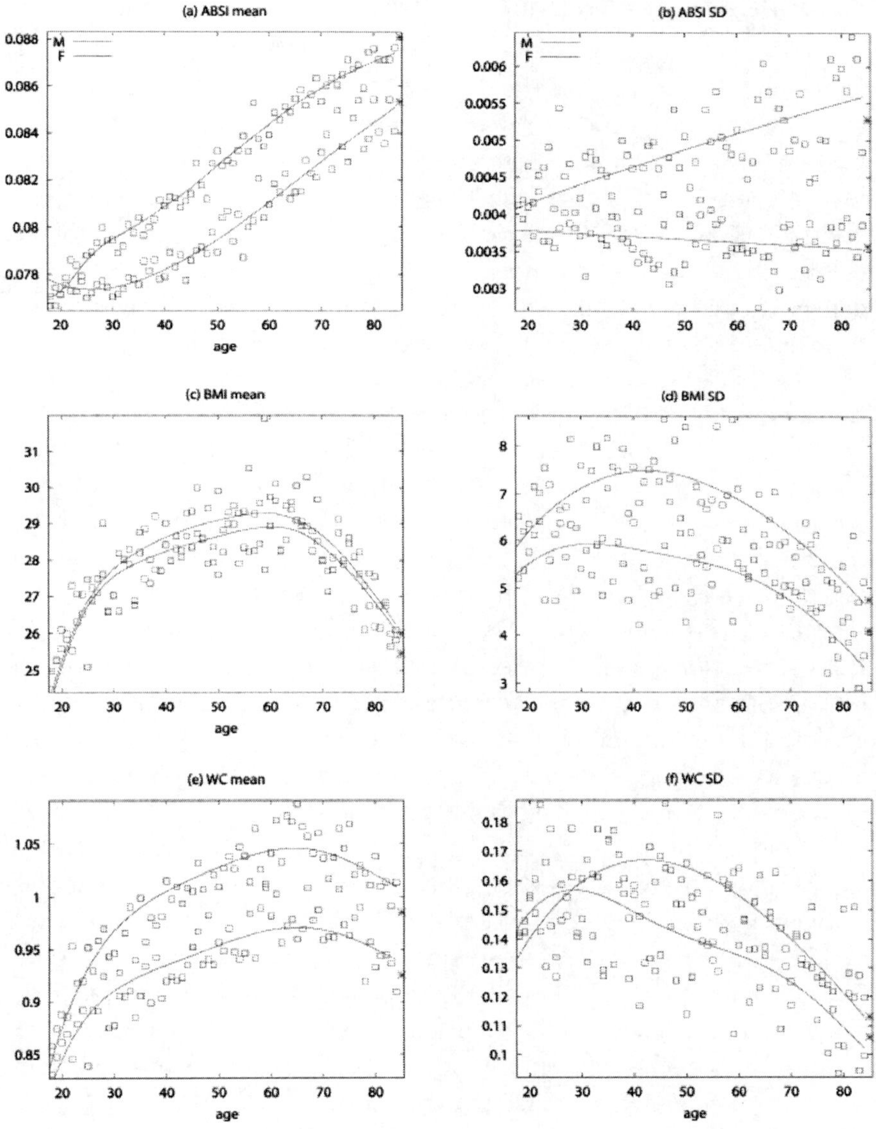

FIGURE 1: Mean and standard deviation of ABSI, BMI, and WC by age and sex. Markers show the sample quantities for each age; the smooth curves shown were used to convert values to z scores. Units are $m^{11/6}$ $kg^{-2/3}$ for ABSI, kg m^{-2} for BMI, and m for WC.

5.2.4 MORTALITY HAZARD MODELING

To quantify the association of baseline ABSI with death rate, we employed Cox proportional hazard modeling for mortality with age as the time scale [28]. In this approach, log death rate is modeled as a nonparametric function of age plus fitted coefficients that multiply the values of predictors, such as baseline ABSI. Predictors may be entered as continuous variables or discretized into two or more categories (such as quantiles of ABSI), depending on their nature and the desired model. ABSI and the other anthropometric variables (BMI, WC) were entered as z scores relative to age- and sex-specific normals, obtained as described above, to avoid confounding by age and sex differences in body size and shape.

Two types of models were employed. In one ('unadjusted'), the anthropometric variable of interest (ABSI, BMI, or WC) was the only predictor entered. In the second ('adjusted'), additional predictors corresponding to other known major risk factors were entered. Comparing the unadjusted and adjusted model coefficients showed to what extent the mortality risk associated with higher ABSI, BMI, or WC changed when these other risk factors are controlled for. The additional factors considered were sex, ethnicity, smoking status, presence of diabetes, blood pressure, and serum cholesterol. Sex, ethnicity, smoking status, and presence of diabetes were all entered as binary variables. Ethnicity was entered as 1 for blacks and 0 for all others, since we found that blacks had significantly elevated death rates compared to the other four ethnicities, whose death rates were not significantly different from each other. Systolic and diastolic blood pressure and total and HDL cholesterol levels were each entered as z scores relative to age- and sex-specific normals, obtained as described for ABSI. Because not all individuals with anthropometric measurements also had the other data needed for the adjusted analysis, the unadjusted analyses were run twice—once for the full sample with available anthropometry (n = 14105) and once restricted to the sample used for the adjusted analysis (n = 12044).

We also determined the mortality risk associated with ABSI, BMI, and WC for subgroups of the NHANES sample, in order to test the robustness and range of applicability of coefficients determined for the entire sample. Subgroups included males and females; people younger and older than 65 yr at baseline; the three largest ethnic groupings (whites, blacks, and Mexicans); and people with BMI above and below the age- and sex-specific mean. As another check of whether these attributes impact the association with mortality, we checked the significance in the proportional hazard model of interaction terms of ABSI (BMI, WC) with sex, age, ethnicity variables (white, black, or Mexican), and BMI. To address the question of whether ABSI predicts medium-term as compared to short-term mortality, we conducted an additional analysis where the modeled follow-up period started 3 yr after the baseline, thus excluding from consideration all deaths within 3 yr of examination.

In Cox proportional hazard modeling, the relationship between hazard (here, death rate) and continuous variables, such as ABSI here, is most commonly estimated on the assumption that the logarithm of the hazard is a linear function of the variable; this yields a single regression coefficient that summarizes the strength of the relationship between the variable and log hazard. A recommended test of this linearity assumption is to fit an alternative model where the dependence of log hazard on the variable is described by a smoothing spline, with the degree of smoothing determined to optimize the Akaike Information Criterion [29], [30]. Linearity is rejected if the nonlinear terms in the fitted smoothing spline are different from zero with low p value. Our testing showed that the linearity assumption did not hold for ABSI, BMI or WC. In showing results from the models described above, we retained the linearity assumption for all three variables to facilitate comparing mortality hazards across populations and population subgroups. In separate analyses, we also fit smoothing splines to the association with mortality risk of ABSI, BMI, and WC in order to visualize it as accurately as possible. To quantify in a simpler form the nonlinear relationship between ABSI (BMI, WC) and log mortality, we also carried out analyses where risk was computed separately for each quintile of the ABSI (BMI, WC) z score, relative to the middle quintile.

A measure of the fraction of the total population mortality hazard predicted by high values of ABSI (BMI, WC) was calculated as.

$$\text{Fraction population mortality hazard from high values} = \frac{\sum_{i,high} f_i(R_i - 1)}{\sum_{i,all} f_1 R_i} \quad (5)$$

where f_i is the fraction of the population in each quantile and R_i is the relative risk in each quantile. The quantiles we used for this calculation were the top 40%, middle 20%, and bottom 40%, with the top 40% regarded as the 'high' range included in the numerator, and risks were relative to the middle quintile. Uncertainty in this expression was approximated as being due only to uncertainty in the numerator R_i.

While converting variables to z scores before entering them into a hazard regression model may be methodologically preferable given the nonlinear effects of age and sex on mean ABSI, BMI, and WC (Figure 1), we also conducted the same proportional hazard modeling using the original variables, rather than z scores, as predictors. For these analyses, sex was included as a predictor even for the unadjusted models, in order to control for the sex differences in ABSI, BMI, and WC distributions.

Proportional hazard modeling, including differential sample weighting and adjustment for the cluster survey design, was carried out using the survey package in the computer language R [31]. For all analyses, $P < 0.05$ (two-tailed) was taken as the threshold for statistical significance. This corresponds to the 95% confidence interval of the exponent of a linear regression log hazard coefficient not including 1 (as would be the case under the null hypothesis that the variable has no effect on the death rate).

5.3 RESULTS

5.3.1 HIGHER MORTALITY HAZARD FOR INCREASING ABSI

Table 2 shows the impact of ABSI z score, as a continuous variable, on death rate, along with results for BMI and WC z scores. ABSI clearly has distinct impacts on mortality compared to BMI and WC: if we model the relationship between the z scores and log mortality risk as linear, the regression coefficients imply that uniformly increasing the population ABSI by one standard deviation would result in a significant increase of 33% (95% confidence interval: +20% – +48%), while the corresponding linear regression coefficients for BMI and WC are not significantly different from zero. Because the proportional hazard regression coefficients for

ABSI, BMI, and WC showed little impact – generally shifting by less than their standard error – from either restricting the sample to those with data for the other risk factors (sex, ethnicity, smoking, diabetes, blood pressure, and serum cholesterol; middle column of Table 2) or from adjusting for the other risk factors (right column of Table 2), we carried out the analyses described below with unadjusted models.

TABLE 2: Body size and shape z scores and mortality hazard.

	Hazard ratio per SD increase		
	Unadjusted	Restricted	Adjusted
ABSI	1.33 (1.20–1.48)	1.37 (1.23–1.53)	1.30 (1.16–1.44)
BMI	0.98 (0.89–1.08)	0.98 (0.88–1.09)	0.96 (0.86–1.08)
WC	1.07 (0.98–1.16)	1.08 (0.98–1.20)	1.05 (0.94–1.17)

Results of Cox proportional hazard modeling for mortality risk with ABSI, BMI, or WC z scores taken as linear predictors. Ranges in parantheses are 95% confidence intervals. The restricted models are unadjusted but included only those people who had all the measurements required for the adjusted model. The adjusted models included as additional predictors sex, ethnicity, smoking, presence of diabetes, blood pressure, and serum cholesterol.
SD = standard deviation

5.3.2 MORTALITY HAZARD FROM INCREASING ABSI BY SUBGROUP

Restricting our analysis to males or females within the sample does not significantly change the impact of increasing ABSI on mortality (Table 3); the change in mortality hazard per standard deviation increase in ABSI is + 32% (95% confidence interval: +15% – +50%) for males and +35% (95% confidence interval:+18% – +54%) for females. Further, high ABSI predicts similar elevation of relative mortality hazard for younger (age <65 yr at baseline) and older (age ≥65 yr) individuals, with narrower confidence intervals for the older group because of their much higher absolute death rate over the follow-up period (Table 3). ABSI predicted mortality among individuals with above-mean BMI about as well as it did for individuals with below-mean BMI (Table 3). Among the three main ethnic groups in the sample, ABSI predicted mortality in both whites and blacks, while ABSI was not a significant predictor of mortality in Mexicans (Table 3).

TABLE 3. Mortality hazard by subgroup.

	Hazard ratio			
	Deaths/N	ABSI	BMI	WC
All	828/14105	1.33 (1.20–1.48)	0.98 (0.89–1.08)	1.07 (0.98–1.16)
Male	502/7133	1.32 (1.15–1.50)	0.92 (0.81–1.06)	1.00 (0.88–1.14)
Female	326/6972	1.35 (1.18–1.54)	1.04 (0.91–1.19)	1.14 (1.01–1.30)
<65 yr	213/10728	1.37 (1.12–1.69)	1.05 (0.84–1.31)	1.12 (0.91–1.39)
≥ 65 yr	615/3377	1.31 (1.18–1.45)	0.94 (0.87–1.02)	1.04 (0.96–1.12)
White	483/6709	1.43 (1.26–1.62)	1.02 (0.92–1.13)	1.12 (1.02–1.24)
Black	165/2882	1.21 (1.02–1.43)	0.68 (0.54–0.85)	0.76 (0.63–0.91)
Mexican	134/3392	1.11 (0.95–1.29)	0.78 (0.61–0.99)	0.84 (0.63–1.12)
High BMI	356/6011	1.37 (1.19–1.59)	1.20 (1.01–1.42)	1.39 (1.21–1.62)
Low BMI	472/8094	1.31 (1.12–1.51)	0.50 (0.40–0.62)	0.80 (0.64–1.00)
≥ 3 yr follow up	408/11346	1.32 (1.15–1.52)	1.01 (0.90–1.14)	1.10 (1.00–1.22)
Interaction term p-values				
*female		0.81	0.24	0.17
*age		0.93	0.28	0.58
*white		+, 0.005	0.11	0.052
*black		0.21	–, <0.001	–, <0.001
*mexican		0.07	0.16	0.16
*bmi		0.36	+, <0.001	+, <0.001

Cox proportional hazard modeling for mortality hazard ratio per unit of ABSI, BMI, or WC z score (standard deviation). Ranges in parentheses are 95% confidence intervals. The sign of significant interaction terms is given. High BMI is defined as exceeding the age- and sex-specific population mean.

These conclusions from subgroup analysis were largely borne out by checking the significance of interaction terms added to the Cox proportional hazard model. $ABSI_{age}$, $ABSI_{sex}$, and $ABSI_{BMI}$ interactions were not significant, confirming that high ABSI predicts mortality across these categories. By contrast, the impact of increasing BMI and WC depended strongly on BMI (Table 3), consistent with U-shaped relationships where lower weight would increase mortality at low BMI and decrease it at high BMI. Interaction with ABSI of an indicator variable for white ethnicity were significantly positive, implying that whites with high ABSI show greater relative risk elevation than other USA ethnicities.

High ABSI continued to be a significant predictor of death even when the first 3 yr of the follow-up period were excluded (Table 3), suggesting that the correlation of higher ABSI with death rate is not merely due to a propensity of acutely ill people to have high ABSI.

5.3.3 MORTALITY HAZARD BY ABSI QUANTILE

To examine the correlation of different levels of ABSI with death rate, we stratified the population into quintiles by ABSI z score, where the middle (third) quintile included those near the population mean ABSI, and conducted proportional hazard modeling with ABSI quintiles, rather than ABSI z score, as the predictor variables, with hazard ratios expressed relative to the middle quintile. We found that people with low ABSI (first and second quintiles) had nonsignificantly decreased mortality risk relative to the middle quintile, while ABSI in the fourth and fifth quintiles was associated with progressively and significantly increased mortality risk (Table 4).

TABLE 4. Mortality by quintile.

	Hazard ratio		
Quintile	ABSI	BMI	WC
1 (lowest)	0.97 (0.69–1.37)	1.88 (1.44–2.45)	1.51 (1.12–2.03)
2	0.93 (0.64–1.35)	1.23 (0.89–1.69)	1.31 (0.92–1.87)
3 (reference)	1	1	1
4	1.46 (1.08–1.99)	1.37 (0.95–1.97)	1.30 (0.95–1.77)
5 (highest)	1.93 (1.39–2.68)	1.71 (1.22–2.39)	1.72 (1.28–2.32)

Cox proportional hazard modeling for mortality risk with ABSI, BMI, or WC z score quintiles taken as the predictors. Hazard ratios are relative to the middle quintile in each case. Ranges in parentheses are 95% confidence intervals. The between-quintile cut points are –0.868, –0.272, +0.229, +0.798 for ABSI; –.759, –0.337, +0.113, +0.746 for BMI; and –0.826, –0.346, +0.120, +0.775 for WC

Similar analyses were conducted with BMI and WC quintiles. BMI and WC in the first quintile were both associated with significantly greater

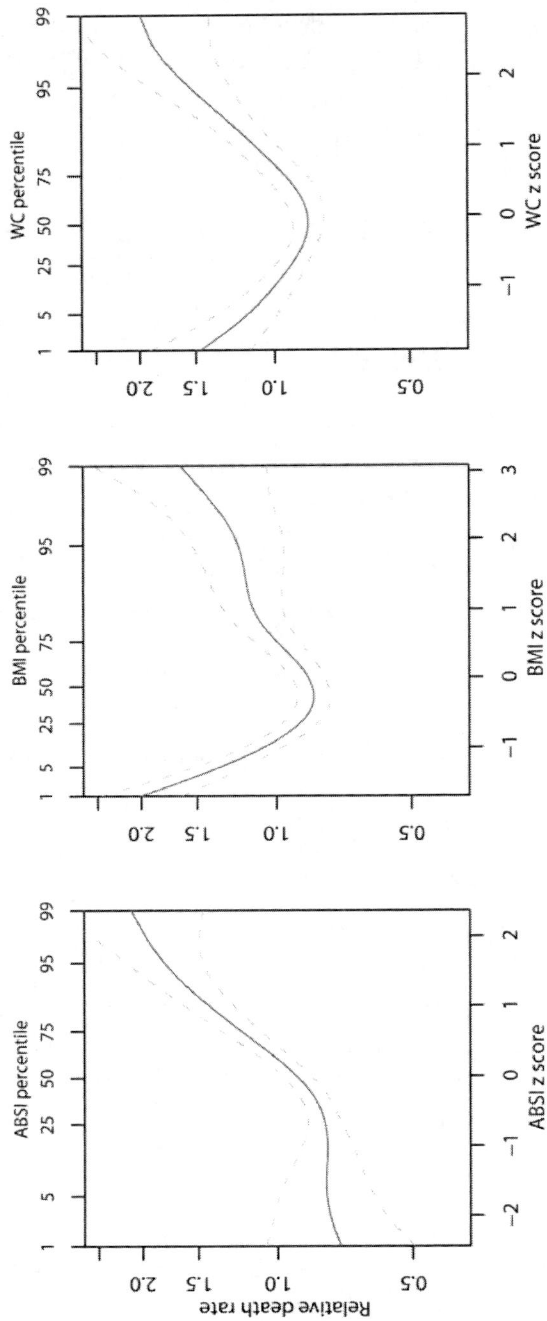

FIGURE 2: Mortality hazard by ABSI, BMI, and WC z score relative to age and sex specific normals. Estimates are from proportional hazard modeling where log mortality hazard is a smoothing-spline function in ABSI, BMI, or WC. Dashed curves show 95% confidence intervals. Corresponding population percentiles are given in the top axis; the range shown is the 1st through 99th percentiles. The vertical axis is logarithmic.

mortality hazard than for the middle quintile. Significantly increased death rate compared to the middle quintile was also seen for WC and BMI in the fifth quintile (Table 4). Comparing the excess mortality hazard from high ABSI (top two quintiles) with that posed by high BMI and WC as a fraction of the total population death rate, we found that 22% (8%–41%) of the population mortality hazard was attributable to high ABSI, compared to 15% (3% – 30%) for BMI and 15% (4% – 29%) for WC. Plotting estimated mortality risk by percentile from models with ABSI, BMI, or WC as continuous predictor variables (Figure 2), with smoothing splines used to represent their nonlinear associations with mortality, gives results consistent with the quantile analyses. While risk increases progressively with increasing ABSI, BMI and WC risk is lowest near the population median and increases for both high and low values.

Figure 3 shows the estimated relative mortality risk taking both body size (BMI) and shape (ABSI) z score into account. These estimates are based on the lack of interaction we found between BMI and ABSI as predictors of mortality, so that the estimated mortality risk given both values is the product of that due to each separately (Figure 2a, b). Lowest risk is found at below-average ABSI and near average BMI (lower middle of plot), while risk elevations of above 100% are found at high ABSI and BMI either below or above average (upper left and upper right corners of plot).

We found that our main results continued to hold when the original variables, rather than their z scores, were used as mortality predictors. Log mortality risk increased steadily with ABSI, while decreasing for increasing BMI and WC up to values around the population median (Figure 4). The association of ABSI with mortality hazard remained after adjusting for other known risk factors (Table 5).

5.4 DISCUSSION

The newly developed and applied ABSI is based on WC, weight and height, where high ABSI indicates that WC is higher than expected for a given height and weight and corresponds to a more central concentration of body volume. Applying ABSI along with BMI as a predictor variable

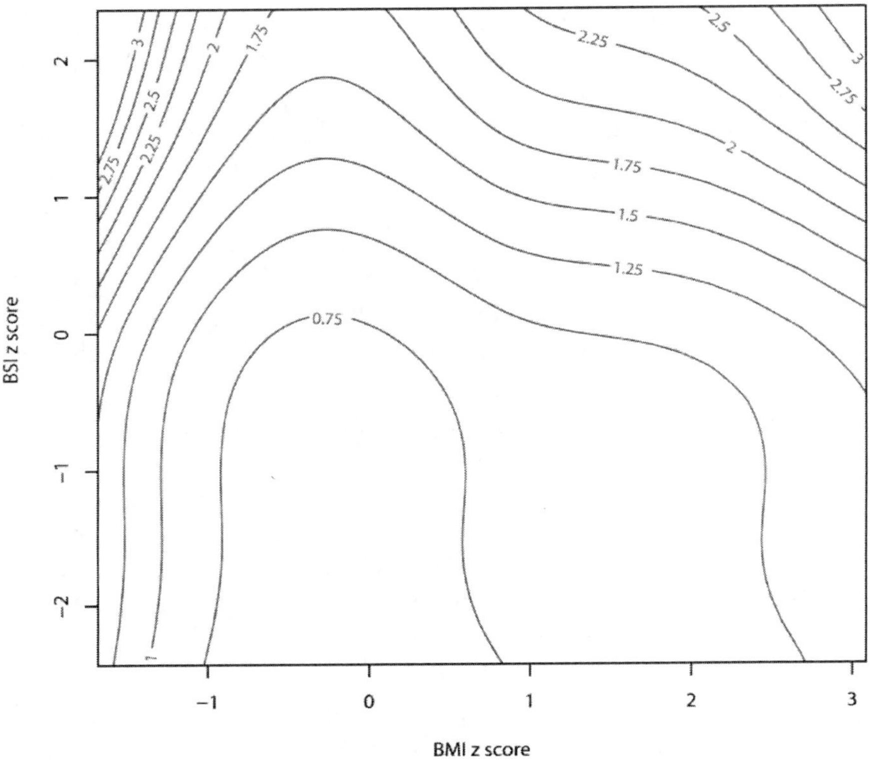

FIGURE 3: Estimated mortality hazard (relative to the population mean) by combination of BMI and ABSI z score. The ranges of BMI and ABSI shown correspond to the 1st through 99th percentiles. The contour interval is 0.25.

separates the influence of the component of body shape measured by WC from that of body size. Our finding that higher ABSI predicts mortality hazard is thus quite analogous to the outcome of analyses which have adjusted WC for BMI without invoking ABSI. Thus, an analysis of mortality outcomes in an elderly (≥ 65 yr) USA cohort found that including both BMI and WC as continuous variables in a Cox proportional hazard model for mortality results in a direct correlation between WC and mortality and an inverse correlation between BMI and mortality [12]. In a large multination European cohort, stratifying by BMI category transformed the curve of mortality risk as a function of WC from U-shaped to more linear,

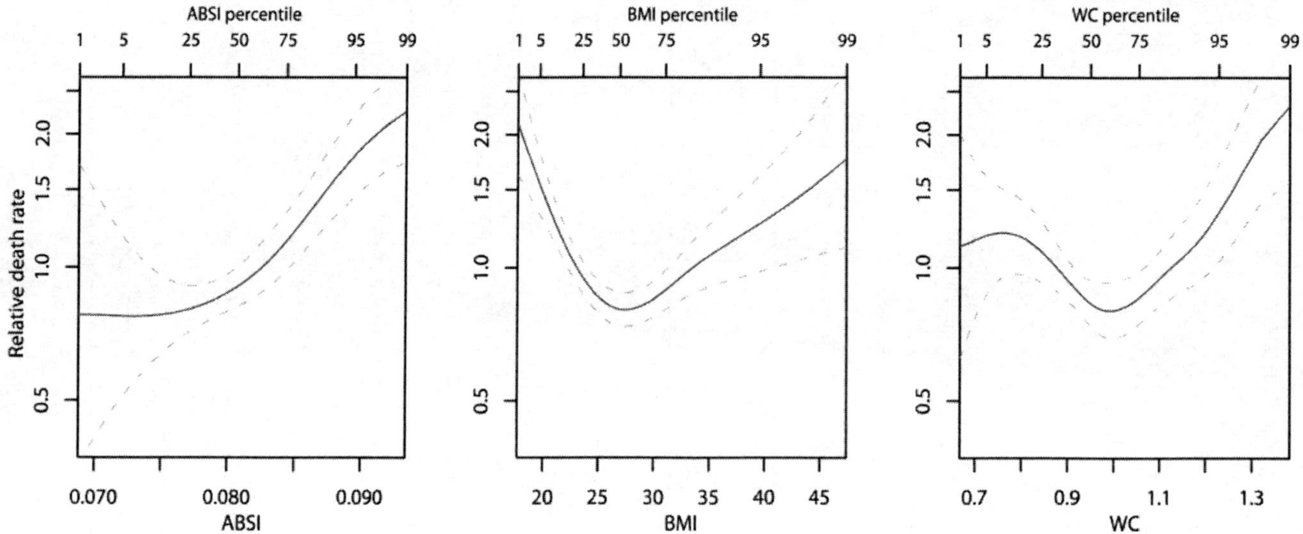

FIGURE 4: Mortality hazard by ABSI, BMI, and WC. Estimates are from proportional hazard modeling where log mortality hazard is a smoothing-spline function in ABSI, BMI, or WC. Dashed curves show 95% confidence intervals. Corresponding population percentiles are given in the top axis; the range shown is the 1st through 99th percentiles. The vertical axis is logarithmic. This is the same as Figure 2, but with ABSI, BMI, or WC, rather than their z scores, used as predictors. Units are $m^{11/6}$ $kg^{-2/3}$ for ABSI, kg m+-2 for BMI, and for WC.

similar to our curve of mortality risk as a function of ABSI quantile [14]. Our work also follows on findings that dividing WC by height increases its ability to predict cardiometabolic risk factors [32]–[35]. Some conceptual advantages of introducing ABSI are that it accounts for the sublinear increase of WC with BMI (i.e. WC $\propto$ BMI$^{2/3}$) along with the nonlinear association of WC with height, and that using it instead of WC avoids inflation of regression uncertainty associated with the near collinearity of WC and BMI.

In the USA population as sampled in NHANES, ABSI predicted mortality risk across age, sex, and weight, although the ethnic difference found suggests that analysis of more cohorts is needed to delineate the limits of ABSI's utility. A logical next step would be to investigate the association of ABSI with longer-term mortality risk, as well as its ability to predict morbidity and impaired quality of life.

TABLE 5: Body size and shape and mortality hazard.

	Hazard ratio per SD increase		
	Unadjusted	Restricted	Adjusted
ABSI	1.39 (1.23–1.57)	1.44 (1.26–1.63)	1.34 (1.18–1.51)
BMI	1.00 (0.88–1.13)	0.99 (0.87–1.13)	0.97 (0.84–1.12)
WC	1.08 (0.97–1.21)	1.10 (0.97–1.25)	1.06 (0.93–1.22)

Results of Cox proportional hazard modeling for mortality risk with ABSI, BMI, or WC, as well as sex, taken as linear predictors. Ranges in parentheses are 95% confidence intervals. The restricted models are unadjusted but included only those people who had all the measurements required for the adjusted model.The adjusted models included as additional predictors ethnicity, smoking, presence of diabetes, blood pressure, and serum cholesterol. This is the same as Table 2, but ABSI, BMI, WC, rather than their z scores, used as predictors.

SD = standard deviation. The population standard deviation used here are 0.00535 $m^{11/6}$ $k^{-2/3}$ for ABSI, 6.20 kg m^{-2} for BMI, and 0.155 for WC.

What aspect of human physiology measured by ABSI accounts for its association with death rate? At a given height and weight, high ABSI may correspond to a greater fraction of visceral (abdominal) fat compared to peripheral tissue. As mentioned in the Introduction, excess visceral fat has been associated with a variety of potentially adverse metabolic changes. Equally important may be that individuals with high ABSI have a smaller fraction of mass as limb muscle; lean tissue mass and limb circumference have been shown to have strong negative correlations with mortality risk [7], [36]. Dual energy X-ray absorptimetry body composition data for most of the NHANES 1999–2004 sample is available [37], [38] and could be used to investigate ABSI's associations with muscle, fat and bone fraction by site. For example, we found that ABSI is positively correlated to trunk fat mass as estimated from X-ray scans (r = +0.45 between z score of trunk fat mass adjusted for height and weight and ABSI z score) but negatively correlated with limb lean mass (r = -0.26), consistent with the above hypotheses; by contrast, WC has only weak associations with both trunk fat and limb lean mass after these are adjusted for height and weight (r = -0.04 for both), suggesting that it is a less consistent indicator of changes in body shape and composition not reflected in height and weight.

We found that both low and high BMI increased the mortality hazard compared to near-median BMI (U-shaped curve for mortality hazard vs. BMI and WC in Figure 2). In the studied population, the hazard sustained by low BMI quantiles appears to be at least as great than that sustained by corresponding high BMI quantiles, consistent with the nonsignificantly negative linear regression coefficient for mortality hazard on BMI z score (Table 2). This substantial mortality hazard for low BMI held even though few (292/14105 or 2.1%) of the study population were in the WHO 'underweight' category of BMI < 18.5 kg m^{-2}. The lowest mortality hazard was for the middle quintile of both BMI and WC, although the population median was well in the WHO 'overweight' or 'pre-obese' category [39]: the 40th-60th percentile range for the sample was 25.6 – 28.4 kg m^{-2}, with the exact cutoffs for the middle quintile of BMI z score varying by age and sex (Figure 1c; cf. Figure 4b). Similarly, the 40th-60th percentile range of population WC was 94–101 cm for men and 88–97 cm for women, above most suggested cut-off points for higher mortality hazard [18]. These results add to many previous studies that show high population mortality hazard even in developed countries from underweight compared to overweight, particularly among the elderly and chronically ill [15], [40]–[45], supporting a rethinking of BMI-based obesity thresholds [46]. However, since high ABSI appears to identify increased mortality risk independent of BMI, it could complement either low or high BMI in risk assessment, as illustrated in Figure 3.

In addition to WC, inverse hip circumference, or waist to hip ratio, have been suggested as alternative measures of body shape that predict mortality better than BMI [18], [47]. It is theorized that gluteofemoral fat may benefit health by removing free fatty acids from the bloodstream [48]. Different studies have reached a range of conclusions about whether WC [14], [16] or waist to hip ratio [13], [17] is a better predictor of mortality; a meta-analysis of British studies found them to be equally good predictors [49]. A recent prospective analysis from Mauritius found that higher WC and lower hip circumference both correlated with greater mortality risk, while BMI did not correlate with mortality risk [50]. An analysis of an earlier NHANES cohort (NHANES III, examined 1988–1994) found that neither low nor high waist to hip ratio significantly affected mortality hazard compared to an intermediate reference level, where levels were defined by analogy with WHO obesity categories [41]. That study also found that waist to hip ratio, despite its nondimensional form, was significantly correlated to BMI ($r \approx 0.4 - 0.5$), and we may hypothesize that adjusting hip circumferences or waist to hip ratios for height and weight, as done here for WC, would make them more useful as predictors of mortality hazard. The significance of hip circumference or waist to hip ratio cannot be evaluated with NHANES 1999–2004 data because hip circumference was not measured, though it is possible that adjusting WC for height and weight may indirectly provide similar information to waist to hip ratio – i.e. a wider waist for given height and weight may imply narrower hips, and vice versa. It would be of interest to compare the waist to hip ratio's performance with that of ABSI in suitable data sets, and it may well be that ABSI can be improved as an indicator of hazardous body shape by including hip circumference in addition to height, weight and WC (which is why ABSI for now bears the indefinite article).

This prospective study does not directly address whether interventions aimed at reducing ABSI would reduce mortality risk, independent of weight change, for which large randomized controlled trials would be necessary. If ABSI does reflect malleable body shape and composition attributes, however, we may speculate that the effectiveness of weight loss interventions in improving health outcomes would be affected by how they impact WC relative to weight, since ABSI varies with the ratio WC/BMI$^{2/3}$. Lifestyle change that reduces ABSI, such as an exercise program that builds skeletal muscle, may yield health benefits independent of the amount of weight loss; indeed, exercise has been shown to have beneficial health impacts for obese individuals, including reductions in WC (and hence ABSI), even when weight loss does not occur [51]. Weight loss programs including either low-calorie diets or exercise can also reduce WC, along with BMI, enough to reduce ABSI [52], [53]. As other possible applications, the strong association of ABSI with mortality may be of interest to actuaries [54], and may be used as a selection criterion for enrollment in clinical trials desired to have higher power to detect mortality outcome differences with given sample size. Note that since ABSI varies over a small range (population standard deviation is of order 5%, Figure 1b), it is sensitive to the accuracy of the biometric measurements on which it is based. In particular, WC should be measured according to the NHANES protocol [22] in order to meaningfully compare ABSI with the population normals given here, even though in general the association of WC with health outcomes seems independent of the specified measurement protocol [55].

In summary, body shape, as measured by ABSI, appears to be a substantial risk factor for premature mortality in the general population derivable from basic clinical measurements. ABSI expresses the excess risk from high WC in a convenient form that is complementary to BMI and to other known risk factors.

REFERENCES

1. WHO (2009) Global health risks: Mortality and burden of disease attributable to selected major risks. Technical report, World Health Organization. URL. http://www.who.int/entity/healthinfo/global_burden_disease/GlobalHealthRisks_report_full.pdf.
2. NHLBI (1998) Clinical guidelines on the identification, evaluation, and treatment of overweight and obesity in adults: The evidence report. Technical Report 98–4083, National Heart Lung and Blood Institute, National Institutes of Health. URL. http://www.nhlbi.nih.gov/guidelines/obesity/ob_gdlns.pdf.
3. Nevill AM, Stewart AD, Olds T, Holder R (2006) Relationship between adiposity and body size reveals limitations of BMI. American Journal of Physical Anthropology 129: 151–156. doi: 10.1002/ajpa.20262.

4. Heymsfield SB, Scherzer R, Pietrobelli A, Lewis CE, Grunfeld C (2009) Body mass index as a phenotypic expression of adiposity: quantitative contribution of muscularity in a population-based sample. International Journal of Obesity 33: 1363–1373. doi: 10.1038/ijo.2009.184.
5. Gómez-Ambrosi J, Silva C, Galofré JC, Escalada J, Santos S, et al. (2012) Body mass index classification misses subjects with increased cardiometabolic risk factors related to elevated adiposity. International Journal of Obesity 36: 286–294. doi: 10.1038/ijo.2011.100.
6. Bray GA, Smith SR, de Jonge L, Xie H, Rood J, et al. (2012) Effect of dietary protein content on weight gain, energy expenditure, and body composition during overeating. Journal of the American Medical Association 307: 47–55. doi: 10.1001/jama.2011.1918.
7. Bigaard J, Frederiksen K, Tjonneland A, Thomsen BL, Overvad K, et al. (2004) Body fat and fat-free mass and all-cause mortality. Obesity 12: 1042–1049. doi: 10.1038/oby.2004.131.
8. Ruhl CE, Everhart JE (2010) Trunk fat is associated with increased serum levels of alanine aminotransferase in the United States. Gastroenterology 138: 1346–1356. doi: 10.1053/j.gastro.2009.12.053.
9. Kang SM, Yoon JW, Ahn HY, Kim SY, Lee KH, et al. (2011) Android fat depot is more closely associated with metabolic syndrome than abdominal visceral fat in elderly people. PLoS ONE 6: e27694. doi: 10.1371/journal.pone.0027694.
10. Katzmarzyk PT, Barreira TV, Harrington DM, Staiano AE, Heymsfield SB, et al. (2012) Relationship between abdominal fat and bone mineral density in white and African American adults. Bone 50: 576–579. doi: 10.1016/j.bone.2011.04.012.
11. Lumeng CN, Saltiel AR (2011) Inflammatory links between obesity and metabolic disease. Journal of Clinical Investigation 121: 2111–2117. doi: 10.1172/JCI57132.
12. Janssen I, Katzmarzyk PT, Ross R (2005) Body mass index is inversely related to mortality in older people after adjustment for waist circumference. Journal of the American Geriatrics Society 53: 2112–2118. doi: 10.1111/j.1532-5415.2005.00505.x.
13. Simpson JA, MacInnis RJ, Peeters A, Hopper JL, Giles GG, et al. (2007) A comparison of adiposity measures as predictors of all-cause mortality: the Melbourne Collaborative Cohort Study. Obesity 15: 994–1003. doi: 10.1038/oby.2007.622.
14. Pischon T, Boeing H, Hoffmann K, Bergmann M, Schulze M, et al. (2008) General and abdominal adiposity and risk of death in Europe. New England Journal of Medicine 359: 2105–2120. doi: 10.1056/nejmoa0801891.
15. Kuk JL, Ardern CI (2009) Influence of age on the association between various measures of obesity and all-cause mortality. Journal of the American Geriatrics Society 57: 2077–2084. doi: 10.1111/j.1532-5415.2009.02486.x.
16. Seidell JC (2010) Waist circumference and waist/hip ratio in relation to all-cause mortality, cancer and sleep apnea. European Journal of Clinical Nutrition 64: 35–41. doi: 10.1038/ejcn.2009.71.
17. Petursson H, Sigurdsson JA, Bengtsson C, Nilsen TIL, Getz L (2011) Body configuration as a predictor of mortality: comparison of five anthropometric measures in a 12 year follow-up of the Norwegian HUNT 2 study. PLoS ONE 6: e26621. doi: 10.1371/journal.pone.0026621.

18. WHO (2011) Waist Circumference and Waist-Hip Ratio: Report of a WHO Expert Consultation, Geneva, 8–11 December 2008. Technical report, World Health Organization.
19. Moore SC (2009) Waist versus weight – which matters more for mortality? American Journal of Clinical Nutrition 89: 1003–1004. doi: 10.3945/ajcn.2009.27598.
20. Klein S, Allison DB, Heymsfield SB, Kelley DE, Leibel RL, et al. (2007) Waist circumference and cardiometabolic risk: a consensus statement from Shaping America's Health. Diabetes Care 30: 1647–1652. doi: 10.2337/dc07-9921.
21. NCHS (2011) National Health and Nutrition Examination Survey data. URL. http://www.cdc.gov/nchs/nhanes/nhanes_questionnaires.htm.
22. NHANES (2002) National Health and Nutrition Examination Survey anthropometry procedures manual. Technical report, National Center for Health Statistics. URL. http://www.cdc.gov/nchs/data/nhanes/nhanes_01_02/body_measures_year_3.pdf.
23. NCHS (2006) Analytic and Reporting Guidelines: The National Health and Nutrition Examination Survey (NHANES). Technical report, National Center for Health Statistics, Centers for Disease Control and Prevention, Hyattsville, Maryland. URL. http://www.cdc.gov/nchs/data/nhanes/nhanes_03_04/nhanes_analytic_guidelines_dec_2005.pdf.
24. Burton R (2010) Waist circumference as an indicator of adiposity and the relevance of body height. Medical Hypotheses 75: 115–119. doi: 10.1016/j.mehy.2010.02.003.
25. MacKay N (2010) Scaling of human body mass with height: The body mass index revisited. Journal of Biomechanics 43: 764–766. doi: 10.1016/j.jbiomech.2009.10.038.
26. Heymsfield SB, Heo M, Pietrobelli A (2011) Are adult body circumferences associated with height? Relevance to normative ranges and circumferential indexes. American Journal of Clinical Nutrition 93: 302–307. doi: 10.3945/ajcn.110.005132.
27. Hansen PC (1998) Rank-deficient and Discrete Ill-posed Problems: Numerical Apects of Linear Inversion. SIAM.
28. Kom EL, Graubard BI, Midthune D (1997) Time-to-event analysis of longitudinal follow-up of a survey: choice of the time-scale. American Journal of Epidemiology 145: 72–80. doi: 10.1093/oxfordjournals.aje.a009034.
29. Therneau TM, Grambsch PM (2000) Modeling survival data: extending the Cox model. New York: Springer-Verlag.
30. 30. Keele L (2010) Proportionally difficult: testing for nonproportional hazards in Cox models. Political Analysis 18: 189–205. doi: 10.1093/pan/mpp044.
31. Lumley T (2004) Analysis of complex survey samples. Journal of Statistical Software 9: 8.
32. Hsieh SD, Yoshinaga H, Muto T (2003) Waist-to-height ratio, a simple and practical index for assessing central fat distribution and metabolic risk in Japanese men and women. International Journal of Obesity 27: 610–616. doi: 10.1038/sj.ijo.0802259.
33. Browning LM, Hsieh SD, Ashwell M (2010) A systematic review of waist-to-height ratio as a screening tool for the prediction of cardiovascular disease and diabetes: 0.5 could be a suitable global boundary value. Nutrition Research Reviews 23: 247–269. doi: 10.1017/S0954422410000144.
34. Ashwell M, Gunn P, Gibson S (2012) Waist-to-height ratio is a better screening tool than waist circumference and BMI for adult cardiometabolic risk factors: system-

atic review and meta-analysis. Obesity Reviews 13: 275–286. doi: 10.1111/j.1467-789X.2011.00952.x.

35. Li WC, Chen IC, Chang YC, Loke SS, Wang SH, et al. (2011) Waist-to-height ratio, waist circumference, and body mass index as indices of cardiometabolic risk among 36,642 Taiwanese adults. European Journal of Nutrition.
36. Heitmann BL, Frederiksen P (2009) Thigh circumference and risk of heart disease and premature death: prospective cohort study. British Medical Journal 339: b3292. doi: 10.1136/bmj.b3292.
37. Kelly TL, Wilson KE, Heymsfield SB (2009) Dual energy x-ray absorptiometry body composition reference values from NHANES. PLoS ONE 4: e7038. doi: 10.1371/journal.pone.0007038.
38. Sun Q, van Dam RM, Spiegelman D, Heymsfield SB, Willett WC, et al. (2010) Comparison of dualenergy x-ray absorptiometric and anthropometric measures of adiposity in relation to adiposityrelated biologic factors. American Journal of Epidemiology 172: 1442–1454. doi: 10.1093/aje/kwq306.
39. WHO (2000) Obesity: preventing and managing the global epidemic. Technical Report WHO Obesity Technical Report Series No. 894, World Health Organization.
40. Allison DB, Gallagher D, Heo M, Pi-Sunyer FX, Heymsfield SB (1997) Body mass index and allcause mortality among people age 70 and over: the Longitudinal Study of Aging. International Journal of Obesity 21: 424–431. doi: 10.1038/sj.ijo.0800423.
41. Flegal KM, Graubard BI (2009) Estimates of excess deaths associated with body mass index and other anthropometric variables. American Journal of Clinical Nutrition 89: 1213–1219. doi: 10.3945/ajcn.2008.26698.
42. Gulsvik AK, Thelle DS, Mowé M, Wyller TB (2009) Increased mortality in the slim elderly: a 42 years follow-up study in a general population. European Journal of Epidemiology 24: 683–690. doi: 10.1007/s10654-009-9390-3.
43. Atlantis E, Browning C, Kendig H (2010) Body mass index and unintentional weight change associated with all-cause mortality in older Australians: the Melbourne Longitudinal Studies on Healthy Ageing (MELSHA). Age and Ageing 39: 559–565. doi: 10.1093/ageing/afq073.
44. Cepeda-Valery B, Pressman GS, Figueredo VM, Romero-Corral A (2011) Impact of obesity on total and cardiovascular mortality – fat or fiction? Nature Reviews Cardiology 8: 233–237. doi: 10.1038/nrcardio.2010.209.
45. Nilsson G, Hedberg P, Öhrvik J (2011) Survival of the fattest: unexpected findings about hyperglycaemia and obesity in a population based study of 75-year-olds. BMJ Open 1: e000012. doi: 10.1136/bmjopen-2010-000012.
46. Campos P, Saguy A, Ernsberger P, Oliver E, Gaesse G (2006) The epidemiology of overweight and obesity: public health crisis or moral panic? International Journal of Epidemiology 35: 55–60. doi: 10.1093/ije/dyi254.
47. Heitmann BL, Lissner L (2011) Hip Hip Hurrah! Hip size inversely related to heart disease and total mortality. Obesity Reviews 12: 478–481. doi: 10.1111/j.1467-789X.2010.00794.x.
48. Manolopoulos KN, Karpe F, Frayn KN (2010) Gluteofemoral body fat as a determinant of metabolic health. International Journal of Obesity 34: 949–959. doi: 10.1038/ijo.2009.286.

49. Czernichow S, Kengne AP, Stamatakis E, Hamer M, Batty GD (2011) Body mass index, waist circumference and waist-hip ratio: which is the better discriminator of cardiovascular disease mortality risk? Evidence rom an individual-participant meta-analysis of 82 864 participants from nine cohort studies. Obesity Reviews 12: 680–687. doi: 10.1111/j.1467-789X.2011.00879.x.
50. Cameron AJ, Magliano DJ, Shaw JE, Zimmet PZ, Carstensen B, et al. (2012) The influence of hip circumference on the relationship between abdominal obesity and mortality. International Journal of Epidemiology.
51. King NA, Hopkins M, Caudwell P, Stubbs RJ, Blundell JE (2009) Beneficial effects of exercise: shifting the focus from body weight to other markers of health. British Journal of Sports Medicine 43: 924–927. doi: 10.1136/bjsm.2009.065557.
52. Han TS, Richmond P, Avenell A, Lean MEJ (1997) Waist circumference reduction and cardiovascular benefits during weight loss in women. International Journal of Obesity 21: 127–134. doi: 10.1038/sj.ijo.0800377.
53. Ross R, Dagnone D, Jones PJ, Smith H, Paddags A, et al. (2000) Reduction in obesity and related comorbid conditions after diet-induced weight loss or exercise-induced weight loss in men. Annals of Internal Medicine 133: 92–103. doi: 10.7326/0003-4819-133-2-200007180-00008.
54. Kuh D, Hardy R, Hotopf M, Lawlor DA, Maughan B, et al. (2009) A review of life time risk factors for mortality. British Actuarial Journal 15: 17–64. doi: 10.1017/S135732170000550X.
55. Ross R, Berentzen T, Bradshaw AJ, Janssen I, Kahn HS, et al. (2008) Does the relationship between waist circumference, morbidity and mortality depend on measurement protocol for waist circumference? Obesity Reviews 9: 312–325. doi: 10.1111/j.1467-789X.2007.00411.x.

There is online supporting information that is not included in this version of the article. To see these additional files, please use the citation in the beginning of the chapter to view the original article.

CHAPTER 6

METABOLICALLY HEALTHY AND UNHEALTHY OBESITY PHENOTYPES IN THE GENERAL POPULATION: THE FIN-D2D SURVEY

PIA PAJUNEN, ANNA KOTRONEN, EEVA KORPI-HYLIVΔLTI, SIRKKA KEINΔNEN-KIUKAANNIEMI, HEIKKI OKSA, LEO NISKANEN, TIMO SAARISTO, JUHA T. SALTEVO, JOUKO SUNDVALL, MAUNO VANHALA, MATTI UUSITUPA, and MARKKU PELTONEN

6.1 BACKGROUND

Obesity is a major contributor to the global epidemic of type 2 diabetes [1] to fatty liver disease [2] and to cardiovascular diseases (CVD) [3]. Worldwide, at least 300 million individuals are clinically obese [4] and in Finland, out of those aged 25-74 years, 25% are obese and over half are overweight [5].

Metabolic abnormalities which are usually associated with obesity, do not, however, affect all obese people. Approximately 10-25% of obese people [6] and a fraction of morbidly obese individuals [7] are not affected by metabolic disturbances [8-11]. These "metabolically healthy but obese" subjects are insulin sensitive, have normal blood pressure, a favorable lip-

This chapter was originally published under the Creative Commons Attribution License. Pajunen P, Kotronen A, Hyövälti EK, Kiukaanniemi SK, Oksa H, Niskanen L, Saaristo T, Saltevo JT, Sundvall J, Vanhala M, Uusitupa M, and Peltonen M. Metabolically Healthy and Unhealthy Obesity Phenotypes in the General Population: The FIN-D2D Survey. BMC Public Health ***11**,754 (2011), doi:10.1186/1471-2458-11-754.*

id profile, a lower proportion of visceral fat, less liver fat and a normal glucose metabolism despite having an excessive amount of body fat [9-17].

On the other hand, a subset of normal weight individuals suffer from metabolic disturbances that are characteristic of obesity [18]. These individuals are called "metabolically obese, normal weight individuals" [19,20]. Thus, obesity consists of different subtypes with different metabolic profiles. Although these phenotypes have been recognized by the scientific community, not much data exists on the subject. It has been suggested that metabolically healthy obesity may have a less adverse metabolic profile and outcome than normal weight individuals with metabolic syndrome (MetS). However, there are only a few studies comparing these phenotypes and giving the true estimation of characteristics of these phenotypes in the general population [8,19].

In this study, we examine the prevalence of different metabolic phenotypes of obesity, especially the "metabolically healthy but obese" phenotype, and analyze, by using different risk scores, how the MetS definition discriminates between unhealthy and healthy metabolic phenotypes in different obesity classes in a large population-based cohort of 2,849 individuals.

6.2 METHODS

6.2.1 FIN-D2D SURVEY

As part of evaluation of the implementation project of the national type 2 diabetes prevention programme (FIN-D2D), a survey was carried out in three hospital districts in Finland between October and December 2007 [21]. A random sample of 4,500 subjects aged 45-74 years, stratified according to gender, 10-year age groups (45-54, 55-64, and 65-74 years), and the three geographical areas, was selected from the National Population Register. The overall participation rate was 64%. In addition, 26 subjects were excluded from the present analyses due to missing data on variables needed for defining the MetS (n = 17) or BMI (n = 19). The total number of individuals included was thus 2,849 (63% of the original sample). The study protocol was approved by the Ethical Committee of the Hospital District of Helsinki and Uusimaa and all participants gave their written and informed consent.

6.2.2 CLINICAL EXAMINATION

Subjects were invited by mail to a clinical examination. Together with the invitation, they also received a self-administered questionnaire on medical history and health behaviour. They were asked to complete the questionnaire at home, and bring it with them to the health examination, which was carried out according to the WHO MONICA project protocol [22]. At the study site, trained nurses measured height, weight and waist circumference, as well as BP using a standardized protocol. Height was measured to the nearest 0.1 cm. Body weight of the participants wearing usual light indoor clothing without shoes was measured with a 0.1 kg precision. Blood pressure was measured twice in a sitting position after a minimum of five minutes of acclimatization and before blood sampling using a mercury sphygmomanometer. The mean of the two blood pressure measurements was used in the analyses.

6.2.3 CLASSIFICATION OF OBESITY AND THE METS

BMI was calculated as weight (kg) divided by height × height (m^2). Overweight and obesity were defined as BMI 25-29 kg/m^2 and $\geq$ 30 kg/m^2, respectively. The MetS was defined according to the Harmonization definition [23], which requires three or more of the following five components: large waist circumference ($\geq$ 94 cm in men and $\geq$ 80 cm in women), hypertriglyceridemia ($\geq$ 1.7 mmol/l), HDL cholesterol level < 1.0 mmol/l in men or < 1.3 mmol/l in women, elevated blood pressure (systolic $\geq$ 130 mmHg and/or diastolic $\geq$ 85 mmHg) or antihypertensive drug treatment or history of hypertension, elevated fasting plasma glucose $\geq$ 5.6 mmol/l or drug treatment.

6.2.4 GLUCOSE TOLERANCE STATUS

The glucose tolerance status was classified according to the WHO 1999 criteria [24]. Individuals who already had diagnosed type 2 diabetes were not included in the OGTT and were classified as known diabetic participants. Individuals who had not been diagnosed as diabetic, but who had a fasting plasma glucose level of ≥ 7.0 mmol/l or 2 h plasma glucose ≥ 11.1 were classified as having screen-detected type 2 diabetes. The known diabetic individuals and the screen-detected diabetic individuals were combined to create a group defined as total type 2 diabetics.

6.2.5 BIOCHEMICAL MEASUREMENTS

All assays were performed at the Disease Risk Unit of the National Institute for Health and Welfare, Helsinki, using Architect ci8200 analyzer (Abbott Laboratories, Abbott Park, IL, US). Plasma glucose was determined with a hexokinase method (Abbott Laboratories, Abbott Park, IL) and serum insulin with a chemiluminescent microparticle immunoassay (Abbott Laboratories, Abbott Park, IL, US). Serum total and HDL cholesterol, and triglyceride concentrations were measured with enzymatic kits from Abbott Laboratories (Abbott Park, IL, US). The lipoproteins apoA1 and apoB were determined with an immunoturbidimetric method (Abbott Park, IL, US). The concentrations of LDL cholesterol were calculated using the Friedewald formula [25]. Serum ALT, AST, and γGT concentrations were determined using photometric IFCC (International Federation of Clinical Chemistry) methods (Abbott Laboratories, Abbott Park, IL, US). High-sensitivity C-reactive protein (hsCRP) was measured with an immunoturbidimetric method (Sentinel Diagnostics, Milano, Italy).

6.2.6 RISK SCORES

Cardiovascular risk was estimated with the Framingham [26] and SCORE risk scores [27]. Diabetes risk was assessed with the FINDRISK score

[28]. Non-alcoholic fatty liver disease (NAFLD) was estimated with the NAFLD score [29].

6.2.7 LIFESTYLE DEFINITIONS

The average daily alcohol consumption (g/d) was calculated from the self-reported number of drinks taken during the past week. The estimation of fruit and vegetable consumption was derived from the question: "How often do you eat fruit, vegetables and brown bread (rye- or whole-grain bread)?" The possible answers were: 1) every day, and 2) not every day. Fruit and vegetable consumption was considered scarce if it did not occur daily.

Leisure time physical activity was estimated with the question: "How much do you exercise or exert yourself physically in your leisure time?" Endurance training such as jogging or swimming at least 3 hours per week was classified as "active". Endurance training less than 3 hours per week was considered "inactive".

Weight change during the past year was ascertained from the question:" How much does your weight differ from the weight you had one year ago?" The average amount of sleep was calculated from the question:" How many hours do you sleep on average each night?"

6.2.8 STATISTICAL METHODS

Mean values with standard deviations and proportions were used to describe the characteristics of different obesity subgroups. For continuous variables, analysis of covariance (ANCOVA) was used to test the linear trend between BMI and various characteristics in individuals with and without MetS, respectively. Similarly, logistic regression models were used for analyses of dichotomous variables. ANCOVA and logistic regression models were further used to test the interaction between BMI and MetS when considering the associations. All p-values are two-sided and $p < 0.05$ was considered as statistically significant. Statistical analyses were carried out using the Stata statistical package 10.1 (Stata-Corp. 2007. Stata Statistical Software: Release 10.1. College Station, TX; StataCorp LP).

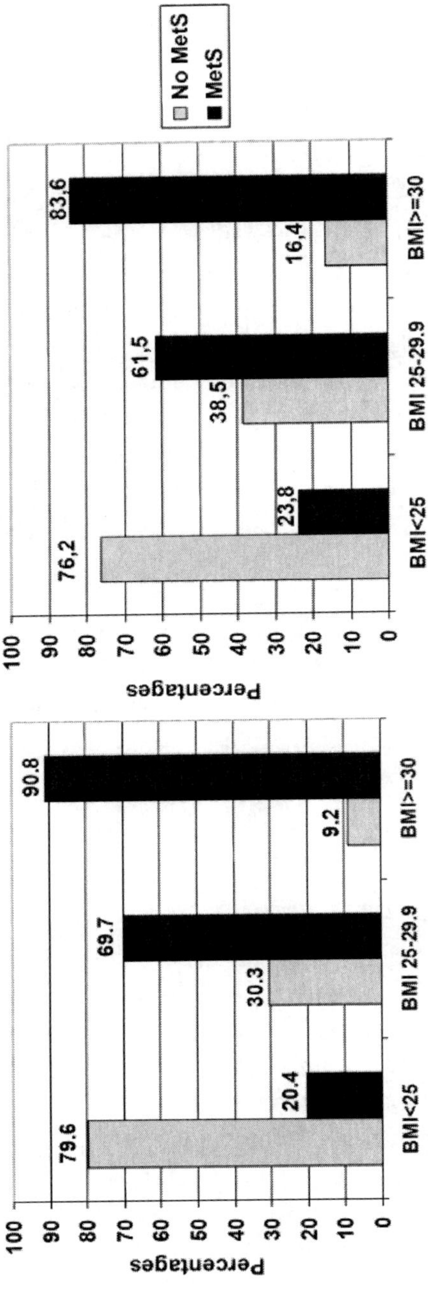

FIGURE 1: Prevalence of persons with and without MetS within each BMI category among men (left panel) and among women (right panel) (total 100% within the BMI class).

TABLE 1: Basic characteristics and components of the metabolic syndrome in individuals with and without metabolic syndrome in different BMI classes

	No MetS				MetS				
	BMI < 25 No MetS (n = 712)	BMI 25-29.9 No MetS (n = 418)	BMI ≥ 30 No MetS (n = 94)	P trend	BMI < 25 MetS (n = 205)	BMI 25-29.9 MetS (n = 811)	BMI ≥ 30 MetS (n = 609)	P trend	P MetS/ BMI Interaction
Population prevalence, %	25.0	14.7	3.3		7.2	28.5	21.3		
Proportion of men, %	43.8	48.6	28.7		39.0	57.6	44.2		
Age (yr)	57.8 ± 8.5	57.6 ± 8.3	58.5 ± 8.2	0.801	60.3 ± 8.1	61.4 ± 7.8	61.3 ± 8.3	0.356	0.593
Height (cm)	168.7 ± 8.7	168.7 ± 8.6	165.8 ± 9.6	0.053	169.1 ± 9.3	170.3 ± 9.2	167.7 ± 9.0	< 0.001	< 0.001
Weight (kg)	64.4 ± 8.7	76.6 ± 8.4	91.4 ± 12.6	< 0.001	68.1 ± 8.5	80.1 ± 9.6	96.2 ± 15.0	< 0.001	0.003
MetS components									
Waist (cm)	81.2 ± 7.5	91.8 ± 7.0	105.1 ± 9.7	< 0.001	88.4 ± 6.7	97.4 ± 7.5	111.1 ± 11.2	< 0.001	0.205
BMI (kg/m2)	22.5 ± 1.7	26.9 ± 1.3	33.2 ± 3.1	< 0.001	23.7 ± 1.1	27.5 ± 1.3	34.1 ± 4.2	< 0.001	< 0.001
SBP (mmHg)	128.8 ± 18.1	127.2 ± 15.5	130.1 ± 16.7	0.589	139.2 ± 16.7	143.3 ± 17.5	144.7 ± 17.3	< 0.001	0.006
DBP (mmHg)	78.1 ± 9.3	78.8 ± 8.4	79.2 ± 7.7	0.077	82.8 ± 8.8	83.7 ± 9.2	84.8 ± 9.5	0.003	0.424
FPG (mmol/l)	5.8 ± 0.88	5.8 ± 0.94	5.8 ± 1.4	0.585	6.2 ± 0.85	6.5 ± 1.2	6.7 ± 1.4	< 0.001	< 0.001
Triglycerides (mmol/l)	0.96 ± 0.34	1.1 ± 0.34	1.2 ± 0.35	< 0.001	1.4 ± 0.68	1.6 ± 0.97	1.8 ± 1.0	< 0.001	< 0.001
HDL cholesterol (mmol/l)	1.6 ± 0.34	1.5 ± 0.31	1.5 ± 0.21	< 0.001	1.4 ± 0.38	1.4 ± 0.33	1.3 ± 0.27	< 0.001	0.029

BMI, body mass index; FPG, fasting plasma glucose; HDL cholesterol, high-density lipoprotein cholesterol; DBP, diastolic blood pressure; SBP, systolic blood pressure. P values adjusted for age and sex (except p for age which is adjusted for sex only).

6.3 RESULTS

A metabolically healthy but obese phenotype was observed in 9.2% of obese men and in 16.4% of obese women (Figure 1). Among all participants, the prevalence of healthy obesity was 2.0% among men and 4.5% among women. Of the normal weight individuals, 20.4% of men and 23.8% of women had the MetS (Figure 1). MetS increased with age in both sexes (data not shown).

Table 1 presents the distribution of the MetS definition components by obesity class in persons with and without MetS. Table 2 shows CVD risk factors, parameters related to glucose metabolism and liver function as well as lifestyle factors by obesity class in persons with and without MetS. Overall, in all weight categories (normal weight BMI < 25, overweight BMI 25-29.9, obese BMI ≥ 30) individuals with MetS had a more adverse metabolic profile and greater cardiovascular and diabetes risk scores compared with the individuals without MetS (Tables 1 and 2).

Fasting plasma glucose levels were not modified by increasing BMI among individuals without MetS ($p = 0.589$ for trend, Table 1), but 2-hour plasma glucose was ($p = 0.013$ for trend, Table 2). Among participants with MetS, there was a significant trend for both higher fasting and 2-hour plasma glucose levels with increasing BMI ($p < 0.001$ for both, Tables 1 and 2). MetS-BMI interaction was significant for 2-hour plasma glucose, fasting plasma insulin and HOMA-IR (< 0.001 for all) (Table 2). The OGTT revealed a significantly higher proportion of previously undetected type 2 diabetes among those with MetS than among those without MetS irrespective of the BMI class (7.9% vs. 3.4%, $p = 0.006$ in BMI < 25 class, 14.4% vs. 3.1%, $p < 0.001$ in BMI 25-29.9 class and 21.5% vs. 4.3% in BMI ≥ 30 class). The prevalence of total diabetes (detected prior to or during survey) was 37.0% in obese individuals with MetS and 4.3% in obese individuals without MetS ($p < 0.001$). MetS-BMI interaction for the FINDRISK score was not significant whereas the Framingham 10 year CVD risk score was significantly higher in those with the MetS irrespective of the BMI class (Table 2).

TABLE 2: Characteristics and laboratory results in individuals with and without metabolic syndrome in different BMI classes

	No MetS				MetS				
	BMI < 25 (n = 712)	BMI 25-29.9 (n = 418)	BMI ≥ 30 (n = 94)	P trend	BMI < 25 (n = 205)	BMI 25-29.9 (n = 811)	BMI ≥ 30 (n = 609)	P trend	P for MetS/BMI Interaction
Glucose metabolism									
2-hour plasma glucose (mmol/l)	6.0 ± 2.1	6.3 ± 1.8	6.5 ± 2.1	0.013	7.1 ± 2.5	7.6 ± 2.7	8.6 ± 3.4	< 0.001	< 0.001
fP-insulin (mU/l)	5.1 ± 4.4	6.0 ± 2.5	8.5 ± 4.2	< 0.001	6.7 ± 4.1	9.8 ± 22.0	14.7 ± 22.6	< 0.001	< 0.001
HOMA-IR	1.4 ± 2.5	1.6 ± 0.76	2.3 ± 2.4	0.001	1.8 ± 1.1	3.3 ± 15	4.7 ± 8.7	< 0.001	< 0.001
FINDRISK diabetes risk score (points)	6.6 ± 3.4	9.8 ± 3.4	13 ± 3.1	< 0.001	10.2 ± 4.0	12.5 ± 3.9	16 ± 4.1	< 0.001	0.518
Total T2DM, %	5.1	3.8	4.3	0.490	14.4	21.3	37.0	< 0.001	< 0.001
Previously diagnosed T2DM, %	1.7	0.7	0	0.064	6.4	6.9	15.5	< 0.001	0.002
T2DM, undetected prior survey, %	3.4	3.1	4.3	0.800	7.9	14.4	21.5	< 0.001	0.075
CVD risk									
Cholesterol (mmol/l)	5.4 ± 0.86	5.5 ± 0.90	5.6 ± 0.98	0.001	5.6 ± 1.1	5.4 ± 1.0	5.4 ± 1.1	0.019	< 0.001
LDL cholesterol (mmol/l)	3.3 ± 0.76	3.5 ± 0.80	3.6 ± 0.87	< 0.001	3.5 ± 0.89	3.3 ± 0.89	3.3 ± 0.96	0.001	< 0.001
Apolipoprotein A1 (g/l)	1.7 ± 0.26	1.6 ± 0.24	1.6 ± 0.19	< 0.001	1.6 ± 0.30	1.5 ± 0.26	1.5 ± 0.23	< 0.001	0.985
Apolipoprotein B (g/l)	0.90 ± 0.19	0.97 ± 0.19	0.98 ± 0.19	< 0.001	1.0 ± 0.23	1.0 ± 0.23	1.0 ± 0.24	< 0.001	< 0.001
hsCRP (mg/l)	1.3 ± 3.8	2.5 ± 8.0	3.1 ± 4.6	< 0.001	3.8 ± 16	2.5 ± 5.0	4.4 ± 8.5	0.118	0.713
Framingham 10 yr CVD (%)	11.9 ± 11.1	11.3 ± 8.4	10.4 ± 8.6	0.067	18.7 ± 13.9	22.8 ± 15	25.1 ± 17.2	< 0.001	< 0.001
SCORE 10 yr fatal CVD (%)	4.5 ± 6.1	3.9 ± 4.3	3.6 ± 4.8	0.002	5.8 ± 5.9	7.2 ± 6.5	6.4 ± 5.8	0.560	0.074
Liver									

TABLE 2: *Cont.*

	No MetS				MetS				
	BMI < 25 (n = 712)	BMI 25-29.9 (n = 418)	BMI ≥ 30 (n = 94)	P trend	BMI < 25 (n = 205)	BMI 25-29.9 (n = 811)	BMI ≥ 30 (n = 609)	P trend	P for MetS/BMI Interaction
Serum ALT (U/l)	21.1 ± 12.8	24.4 ± 10.6	24.6 ± 12.5	< 0.001	24.7 ± 15.4	28.1 ± 15.6	32.9 ± 24.9	< 0.001	0.033
Serum AST(U/l)	24.3 ± 12.4	24.4 ± 7.4	25.6 ± 9.4	0.145	26.1 ± 13.0	26.8 ± 10.7	39.6 ± 17.7	< 0.001	0.045
Serum γGT (U/l)	26.9 ± 27.8	32.0 ± 28.1	33.0 ± 31.8	0.001	40.9 ± 117.5	40.5 ± 45.7	49.5 ± 66.6	0.065	0.636
Alcohol (g/d)	8.2 ± 13	7.6 ± 12	5.8 ± 11	0.168	8.6 ± 24	8.6 ± 14	8.0 ± 13	0.860	0.522
NAFLD score	-2.0 ± 0.96	-1.9 ± 0.57	-1.5 ± 0.84	< 0.001	-0.45 ± 1.0	0.021 ± 3.5	0.97 ± 3.6	< 0.001	< 0.001
Estimated liver fat (%)	2.1 ± 1.1	2.2 ± 0.69	2.7 ± 1.0	< 0.001	4.9 ± 2.2	5.6 ± 3.4	7.8 ± 5.1	< 0.001	< 0.001
Lifestyle									
Not eating fruits/vegetables daily, %	18.3	20.0	18.1	0.535	20.2	23.9	19.8	0.548	0.404
Active leisure time physical activity, %	30.9	27.6	14.1	0.002	20.6	19.3	12.1	< 0.001	0.836
Weight change during past year (kg)	-0.31 ± 0.46	0.43 ± 3.8	0.56 ± 6.9	0.015	0.2 ± 0.40	-0.03	-0.16 ± 5.7	0.588	0.108
Hours slept per night (hours)	7.2 ± 0.99	7.3 ± 1.0	7.4 ± 1.1	0.453	7.4 ± 1.1	7.3 ± 1.1	7.3 ± 1.2	0.795	0.449
Currently smoking, %	18.5	12.8	8.6	0.002	16.3	16.7	10.1	0.002	0.470

ALT: alanine aminotransferase; AST: aspartate aminotransferase; Framingham 10 yr CVD, Framingham 10-year risk score for fatal coronary events; HDL cholesterol, high-density lipoprotein cholesterol; HOMA-IR, homeostasis model assessment of insulin resistance; hsCRP, high-sensitivity C-reactive protein; NAFLD: non-alcoholic fatty liver disease; SCORE 10 yr fatal CVD, SCORE risk score 10-year risk score for fatal coronary events T2DM, type 2 diabetes mellitus; γGT: gamma glutamyltransferase. P values adjusted for age and sex.

Increasing BMI had a greater effect on ALT (MetS-BMI interaction $p = 0.033$), AST (MetS-BMI interaction $p = 0.045$), NAFLD score (MetS-BMI interaction $p < 0.001$) and estimated liver fat % (MetS-BMI interaction $p < 0.001$) in those with MetS compared with those without MetS (Table 2).

Leisure time physical activity diminished with increasing BMI class irrespective of MetS classification (Table 2). Leisure time physical activity did not differ between metabolically healthy and metabolically abnormal obese individuals (14.1% vs. 12.1%, $p = 0.591$). There were no differences in lifestyle variables, i.e. the daily consumption of fruits and vegetables, daily length of sleep, cigarette smoking, or reported alcohol consumption between the individuals with and without MetS.

The survey included 205 individuals (80 men and 125 women) of normal weight who had MetS and 94 (27 men and 67 women) obese individuals without MetS. The metabolically healthy but obese individuals had lower systolic and diastolic blood pressure levels than normal weight individuals with MetS (139.2 ± 16.9 vs. 130.1 ± 16.7, $p < 0.001$ and 82.8 ± 8.8 vs. 79.2 ± 7.7, $p = 0.0007$). The metabolically healthy but obese individuals had lower 2-hour postload glucose levels (6.5 ± 2.1 vs. 7.1 ± 2.5 mmol/l, $p = 0.0030$) than normal weight individuals with MetS. There was no difference in cholesterol or LDL-cholesterol levels but the metabolically healthy but obese individuals had lower triglyceride (1.2 ± 0.35 vs. 1.4 ± 0.68 mmol/l, $p = 0.005$) and higher HDL cholesterol levels (1.5 ± 0.21 vs. 1.4 ± 0.38 mmol/l, $p = 0.007$) than the normal weight subjects with the MetS. No difference was observed in the high-sensitivity CRP or liver enzyme values (data not shown). The metabolically healthy but obese individuals had higher scores in the FINDRISK diabetes risk test (13.3 ± 3.1 vs. 10.2 ± 4.0 points, $p < 0.001$), but lower prevalence of current type 2 diabetes than the normal weight subjects with MetS. The estimated 10-year fatal CVD risk (Framingham 18.7% vs. 10.4%, $p < 0.001$ and SCORE 5.8 vs. 3.6%, $p = 0.002$) was higher in the normal weight individuals with MetS than in metabolically healthy but obese individuals. The NAFLD score and estimated liver fat percentage (2.7 ± 1.0 vs. 4.9 ± 2.2, $p < 0.001$) were lower in the metabolically healthy but obese individuals than in normal weight individuals with MetS.

6.4 DISCUSSION

In this study we used the most recent criteria of the MetS [23] to identify metabolically healthy obese individuals and normal weight individuals with MetS. Among the Finnish population aged 45-74 years, the prevalence of the metabolically healthy but obese phenotype was 2.0% among men and 4.5% among women. Of the obese, about one tenth had the metabolically healthy phenotype. As there are currently no international unified criteria for defining healthy obesity, it is difficult to compare these results with the studies from other countries. Indeed, the prevalence estimates of the healthy obese phenotype vary considerably from 3.3% to 43% depending on the criteria used [6,8,14,30-34].

The clinical value, biological basis and usefulness of the MetS has been severely debated [35]. In the present study, the MetS definition discriminated well between unhealthy and healthy metabolic phenotypes in different obesity classes beyond those included in the MetS criteria. Among those with the Mets, the OGTT which was performed as part of the survey revealed a significantly higher proportion of previously undetected type 2 diabetes irrespective of BMI class. The MetS-BMI interaction was significant for fasting glucose, 2-hour plasma glucose, fasting plasma insulin and HOMA-IR, indicating that the metabolic consequences of obesity seem to be more adverse among individuals with MetS. Furthermore, increasing BMI had a significantly greater effect on estimates of liver fat among those with the MetS compared with participants without MetS. The average NAFLD liver fat score was lower in those without MetS irrespective of BMI class. Not surprisingly, NAFLD has previously been shown to predict type 2 diabetes independent of obesity [2].

In accordance with earlier data from the US [8], the metabolically healthy but obese phenotype was associated with an overall better metabolic profile than observed in normal weight individuals with MetS. Obese individuals without MetS had lower fasting plasma glucose and 2-hour postload glucose levels than normal weight individuals with MetS. In addition, they had a better lipid profile and lower CVD risk scores, less estimated liver fat and less often previously undetected diabetes compared with normal weight individuals with the MetS. In clinical work, it is thus important not only to estimate the degree of obesity but also the presence of metabolical abnormalities which are present in a significant proportion of the normal weight individuals.

Some studies from other countries have suggested that a metabolically healthy but obese phenotype would be associated with decreased risk of nonfatal and fatal cardiovascular events [31,36]. This may lie behind the finding that while CVD incidence has been declining in Finland during the past decades [37], the mean BMI has increased significantly [38,39]. MetS irrespective of BMI class may confer increased CVD risk. Even though we do not have the data to study future CVD risk in the present cross-sectional analysis, we have recently shown [40] that the 2009 Harmonization definition of MetS is a significant predictor of future incident CVD and diabetes both in men and in women. In the present study, the Framingham 10-year fatal CVD risk score was significantly lower in individuals without MetS than in those with MetS irrespective of BMI class. As shown by other researchers [8,10,12] and observed in the present study, the metabolically healthy but obese individuals had a slightly less atherogenic lipid profile than normal weight individuals with MetS. However, we did not have data on lipid subclasses or other more detailed biomarkers. No difference was observed in inflammation estimated with the highly sensitive CRP. Longitudinal studies with long enough follow-up periods are needed to reveal the long-term CVD risk related to different obesity phenotypes. However, unlike some earlier data (31, 36), a recent Swedish study with a 30-year follow-up, suggested that increased risk of CVD related to healthy obesity may be detected after only 10 years of follow-up [33].

Different mechanisms behind the different obesity phenotypes include genetic, socioeconomic and behavioral factors, some of which may be modifiable [12,19,20]. In our study, obese individuals without MetS reported similar amount of leisure time physical activity as did the obese individuals with MetS. Contrary to our findings, a US study found leisure time physical activity to be associated with a metabolically healthy obese phenotype [8]. More advanced measures of physical activity may have captured the possible differences in physical activity between the groups in the present study. There were no differences in sleeping patterns between any of the groups. Neither could we detect any differences in consumption of fruit and vegetables. However, more sophisticated methods may be needed to estimate true differences in dietary habits.

To improve comparability of data on healthy obesity, unified criteria for definition of metabolically healthy obesity are urgently needed [30]. These criteria should be suitable for use in population surveys. In the present study we used BMI and the most recent definition of MetS to characterize metabolically healthy obesity. However, BMI does not take into account body composition and amount of body fat. In addition to the need for a definition of healthy obesity, there is a need to develop valid and reliable methods of measuring body composition in population surveys.

The strengths of the present study include a population-based approach and a large and representative sample of middle-aged individuals studied in three districts of Finland. The survey methods have been carefully standardised and comply with international recommendations [22]. However, as previously mentioned, our results are based on cross-sectional data and we cannot determine the future diabetes and CVD risk related to different obesity phenotypes. More sophisticated measures may have captured differences in behavioural factors, but they are labour-intensive to carry out in a population-based survey.

6.5 CONCLUSIONS

This cross-sectional population-based study, demonstrated a prevalence of 9-16% of a metabolically healthy phenotype among obese individuals. Metabolic consequences of obesity seem to be more adverse among individuals with MetS. Undetected type 2 diabetes was more prevalent among those with MetS irrespective of BMI class. Increasing BMI had a significantly greater effect on estimates of liver fat and future CVD risk among those with MetS compared with participants without MetS. The healthy obese phenotype was associated with a better overall metabolic profile than that observed in normal weight individuals with MetS.

REFERENCES

1. Zimmet P, Alberti KG, Shaw J: Global and societal implications of the diabetes epidemic. Nature 2001, 414:782-787.
2. Kotronen A, Yki-Järvinen H: Fatty liver: a novel component of the metabolic syndrome. Arterioscler Thromb Vasc Biol 2008, 28:27-38.
3. van Dis I, Kromhout D, Geleijnse JM, Boer JM, Verschuren WM: Body mass index and waist circumference predict both 10-year nonfatal and fatal cardiovascular disease risk: study conducted in 20 000 Dutch men and women aged 20-65 years. Eur J Cardiovasc Prev Rehabil 2009, 16:729-734.
4. WHO: Report of a WHO Consultation. Geneva: World Health Organization; 2000.
5. Saaristo TE, Barengo NC, Korpi-Hyövälti E, Oksa H, Puolijoki H, Saltevo JT, Vanhala M, Sundvall J, Saarikoski L, Peltonen M, Tuomilehto J: High prevalence of obesity, central obesity and abnormal glucose tolerance in the middle-aged Finnish population. BMC Public Health 2008, 8:423.
6. Bluher M: The distinction of metabolically 'healthy' from 'unhealthy' obese individuals. Curr Opin Lipidol 2010, 21:38-43.
7. Soverini V, Moscatiello S, Villanova N, Ragni E, Di Domizio S, Marchesini G: Metabolic Syndrome and Insulin Resistance in Subjects with Morbid Obesity. Obes Surg 2010, 20:295-301.
8. Wildman RP, Muntner P, Reynolds K, McGinn AP, Rajpathak S, Wylie-Rosett J, Sowers MR: The obese without cardiometabolic risk factor clustering and the normal weight with cardiometabolic risk factor clustering: prevalence and correlates of 2 phenotypes among the US population (NHANES 1999-2004). Arch Intern Med 2008, 168:1617-1624.
9. Karelis AD, Faraj M, Bastard JP, St-Pierre DH, Brochu M, Prud'homme D, Rabasa-Lhoret R: The metabolically healthy but obese individual presents a favorable inflammation profile. J Clin Endocrinol Metab 2005, 90:4145-4150.
10. Brochu M, Tchernof A, Dionne IJ, Sites CK, Eltabbakh GH, Sims EA, Poehlman ET: What are the physical characteristics associated with a normal metabolic profile despite a high level of obesity in postmenopausal women? J Clin Endocrinol Metab 2001, 86:1020-1025.
11. Stefan N, Kantartzis K, Machann J, Schick F, Thamer C, Rittig K, Balletshofer B, Machicao F, Fritsche A, Häring HU: Identification and characterization of metabolically benign obesity in humans. Arch Intern Med 2008, 168:1609-1616.
12. Karelis AD, Brochu M, Rabasa-Lhoret R, Garrel D, Poehlman ET: Clinical markers for the identification of metabolically healthy but obese individuals. Diabetes Obes Metab 2004, 6:456-457.
13. Karelis AD, St-Pierre DH, Conus F, Rabasa-Lhoret R, Poehlman ET: Metabolic and body composition factors in subgroups of obesity: what do we know? J Clin Endocrinol Metab 2004, 89:2569-2575.
14. Aguilar-Salinas CA, Garcia EG, Robles L, Riano D, Ruiz-Gomez DG, Garcia-Ulloa AC, Melgarejo MA, Zamora M, Guillen-Pineda LE, Mehta R, Canizales-Quinteros

S, Tusie Luna MT, Gomez-Perez FJ: High adiponectin concentrations are associated with the metabolically healthy obese phenotype. J Clin Endocrinol Metab 2008, 93:4075-4079.
15. Lynch LA, O'Connell JM, Kwasnik AK, Cawood TJ, O'Farrelly C, O'Shea DB: Are natural killer cells protecting the metabolically healthy obese patient? Obesity (Silver Spring) 2009, 17:601-605.
16. Sims EA: Are there persons who are obese, but metabolically healthy? Metabolism 2001, 50:1499-1504.
17. Messier V, Karelis AD, Robillard ME, Bellefeuille P, Brochu M, Lavoie JM, Rhabasa-Lhoret R: Metabolically healthy but obese individuals: relationship with hepatic enzymes. Metabolism 2010, 59:20-24.
18. Reaven GM, Lithell H, Landsberg L: Hypertension and associated metabolic abnormalities--the role of insulin resistance and the sympathoadrenal system. N Engl J Med 1996, 334:374-381.
19. Ruderman N, Chisholm D, Pi-Sunyer X, Schneider S: The metabolically obese, normal-weight individual revisited. Diabetes 1998, 47:699-713.
20. Conus F, Rabasa-Lhoret R, Peronnet F: Characteristics of metabolically obese normal-weight (MONW) subjects. Appl Physiol Nutr Metab 2007, 32:4-12.
21. Saaristo T, Peltonen M, Keinänen-Kiukaanniemi S, Vanhala M, Saltevo J, Niskanen L, Oksa H, Korpi-Hyövälti E, Tuomilehto J: National type 2 diabetes prevention programme in Finland: FIN-D2D. Int J Circumpolar Health 2007, 66:101-112.
22. WHO MONICA Project Principal Investigators: The World Health Organization MONICA Project (monitoring trends and determinants in cardiovascular disease): a major international collaboration. J Clin Epidemiol 1988, 41:105-114.
23. Alberti KG, Eckel RH, Grundy SM, Zimmet PZ, Cleeman JI, Donato KA, Fruchart JC, James WP, Loria CM, Smith SC Jr: Harmonizing the metabolic syndrome: a joint interim statement of the International Diabetes Federation Task Force on Epidemiology and Prevention; National Heart, Lung, and Blood Institute; American Heart Association; World Heart Federation; International Atherosclerosis Society; and International Association for the Study of Obesity. Circulation 2009, 120:1640-1645.
24. WHO: Definition, Diagnosis and Classification of Diabetes Mellitus and its Complications: Report of a WHO Consultation. Part 1. Diagnosis and Classification of Diabetes Mellitus 1999.
25. Friedewald WT, Levy RI, Fredrickson D: Estimation of the concentration of low-density lipoprotein cholesterol in plasma, without use of the preparative ultracentrifuge. Clin Chem 1972, 18:499-502.
26. D'Agostino RB Sr, Vasan RS, Pencina MJ, Wolf PA, Cobain M, Massaro JM, Kannel WB: General cardiovascular risk profile for use in primary care: the Framingham Heart Study. Circulation 2008, 117:743-753.
27. Conroy RM, Pyörälä K, Fitzgerald AP, Sans S, Menotti A, De Backer G, De Bacquer D, Ducimetière P, Jousilahti P, Keil U, Njølstad I, Oganov RG, Thomsen T, Tunstall-Pedoe H, Tverdal A, Wedel H, Whincup P, Wilhelmsen L, Graham IM, SCORE project group: Estimation of ten-year risk of fatal cardiovascular disease in Europe: the SCORE project. Eur Heart J 2003, 24:987-1003.

28. Lindström J, Tuomilehto J: The diabetes risk score: a practical tool to predict type 2 diabetes risk. Diabetes Care 2003, 26:725-731.
29. Kotronen A, Peltonen M, Hakkarainen A, Sevastianova K, Bergholm R, Johansson LM, Lundbom N, Rissanen A, Ridderstråle M, Groop L, Orho-Melander M, Yki-Järvinen H: Prediction of non-alcoholic fatty liver disease and liver fat using metabolic and genetic factors. Gastroenterology 2009, 137:865-872.
30. Velho S, Paccaud F, Waeber G, Vollenweider P, Marques-Vidal P: Metabolically healthy obesity: different prevalences using different criteria. Eur J Clin Nutr 2010, 64:1043-51.
31. Meigs JB, Wilson PW, Fox CS, Vasan RS, Nathan DM, Sullivan LM, D'Agostino RB: Body mass index, metabolic syndrome, and risk of type 2 diabetes or cardiovascular disease. J Clin Endocrinol Metab 2006, 91:2906-2912.
32. Karelis AD, Messier V, Brochu M, Rabasa-Lhoret R: Metabolically healthy but obese women: effect of an energy-restricted diet. Diabetologia 2008, 51:1752-1754.
33. Ärnlöv J, Ingelsson E, Sundström J, Lind L: Impact of Body Mass Index and the Metabolic Syndrome on the Risk of Cardiovascular Disease and Death in Middle-Aged Men. Circulation 2010, 121:230-236.
34. Calori G, Lattuada G, Piemonti L, Garancini MP, Ragogna F, Villa M, Mannino S, Crosignani P, Bosi E, Luzi L, Ruotolo G, Perseghin G: Prevalence, metabolic features and prognosis of metabolically healthy obese Italian individuals: the Cremona Study. Diabetes Care 2011, 34:210-215.
35. Kahn R, Buse J, Ferrannini E, Stern M: The metabolic syndrome: time for a critical appraisal: joint statement from the American Diabetes Association and the European Association for the Study of Diabetes. Diabetes Care 2005, 28:2289-2304.
36. St-Pierre AC, Cantin B, Mauriege P, Bergeron J, Dagenais GR, Despres JP, Lamarche B: Insulin resistance syndrome, body mass index and the risk of ischemic heart disease. CMAJ 2005, 172:1301-1305.
37. Pajunen P, Pääkkönen R, Juolevi A, Hämäläinen H, Keskimäki I, Laatikainen T, Moltchanov V, Niemi M, Rintanen H, Salomaa V: Trends in fatal and non-fatal coronary heart disease events in Finland during 1991-2001. Scand Cardiovasc J 2004, 38:340-344.
38. Lahti-Koski M, Seppänen-Nuijten E, Männistö S, Härkänen T, Rissanen H, Knekt P, Rissanen A, Heliövaara M: Twenty-year changes in the prevalence of obesity among Finnish adults. Obes Rev 2010, 11:171-176.
39. Vartiainen E, Laatikainen T, Peltonen M, Juolevi A, Männistö S, Sundvall J: Thirty five year trends in cardiovascular risk factors in Finland: results from the National FINRISK Study. Int J Epidemiol 2010, 39:504-518.
40. Pajunen P, Rissanen H, Härkänen T, Jula A, Reunanen A, Salomaa V: The metabolic syndrome as a predictor of incident diabetes and cardiovascular events in the Health 2000 Study.

CHAPTER 7

LIVER AND MUSCLE IN MORBID OBESITY: THE INTERPLAY OF FATTY LIVER AND INSULIN RESISTANCE

MARIANA VERDELHO MACHADO, DUARTE M.S. FERREIRA, RUI E. CASTRO, ANA RITA SILVESTRE, TERESINHA EVANGELISTA, JOГO COUTINHO, FБTIMA CAREPA, ADHLIA COSTA, CECHLIA M. P. RODRIGUES, and HELENA CORTEZ-PINTO

7.1 INTRODUCTION

Nonalcoholic fatty liver disease (NAFLD) is a condition characterized by fat accumulation in the liver, not related with alcohol consumption. It represents a wide spectrum of pathological subgroups, from benign simple steatosis to nonalcoholic steatohepatitis (NASH), which can progress to hepatic cirrhosis [1], and is associated with overall and liver-related increased mortality [2]. Two of the main risk factors for developing NAFLD are insulin resistance and obesity, in which the peripheral adipose tissue reservoir capacity is overwhelmed, allowing ectopic fat accumulation.

There is increasing awareness of the importance of the muscle as a central player in the adaptation to an excessive input of energy, as one of the main fuel consuming organs [3]. In the muscle, lipids are stored either as metabolically inert interstitial adipocyte triglycerides in the interfascicular space, extramyocellular lipids (EMCL), or droplets in the cytoplasm of myocytes, intramyocellular lipids (IMCL) [4]. IMCL accumulate in athletes, where they are in constant turnover and believed to act as fuel [5], or in association with obesity, insulin resistance/type 2 diabetes mellitus and high fat diets [6], [7], [8], [9]. In this case, lipids are either not consumed or incompletely oxidized, potentially forming dangerous active metabolites that may inhibit the insulin signaling cascade [10], [11], [12], [13], [14], thus further contributing to metabolic disturbances. In fact, IMCL may constitute the missing link between obesity and development of insulin resistance, since overweight individuals can improve their insulin sensitivity with exercise training, even in the absence of significant changes in total body adiposity [15]. In addition, interventions in obese individuals that decrease IMCL result in better glucose control [16]. Nonetheless, the accumulation of active fatty acids metabolites such as acyl CoA, ceramides and diacylglycerol, rather than the accumulation of triglycerides, may play a major role in insulin signaling impairment. In fact, the up-regulation of triglyceride synthesis was able to protect skeletal muscle from fat-induced insulin resistance in a mouse model [17].

Previous studies with indirect assessment of ectopic fat in the liver and muscle, either by computer tomography scan [18] or magnetic resonance spectroscopy [7], have suggested that fat accumulation in these two tissues may be correlated. Therefore, we aimed to evaluate skeletal muscle changes in morphology, mitochondrial function and insulin signaling, in morbidly obese patients, and correlate them with NAFLD severity.

7.2 METHODS

7.2.1 PATIENTS

A cross-sectional study was performed with prospective and consecutive recruitment of morbid obese patients submitted to bariatric surgery, at Hospital of Santa Maria, CHLN, Lisbon, Portugal, from 2006 to 2009. Inclusion criteria were age higher or equal to 18 years old and indication to bariatric surgery. This was defined as body mass index (BMI) superior or equal to 40 kg/m^2 or superior to 35 kg/m^2 if associated with significant morbidity related with obesity [19], such as arterial hypertension, diabetes mellitus type 2, obstructive sleep apnea or dyslipidemia. Exclusion criteria were: significant alcohol consumption defined as superior to 20 grams per day; positivity to hepatitis B virus surface antigen; positivity to anti-hepatitis C virus; other type of liver diseases namely primary biliary cirrhosis, autoimmune hepatitis, primary sclerosing cholangitis, Wilson's disease, hemochromatosis or α1-antitripsin deficiency; treatment with potentially steatogenic drugs such as steroids, high-dose estrogen, tamoxifen, methotrexate or amiodarone within six months of enrollment and history of gastrointestinal bypass surgery or segmental small bowel resection. The study protocol conformed to the Ethical Guidelines of the 1975 Declaration of Helsinki, revised in 2000, as reflected in an a priori approval by the Hospital de Santa Maria Human Ethics Committee and written informed consent was obtained from all participants.

7.2.2 CLINICAL ASSESSMENT AND LABORATORIAL TESTS

Patients were submitted to an interview assessing past medical history and a semi-structured questionnaire regarding alcohol consumption. BMI was defined as an individual's weight in kilograms divided by the square of height in meters (kg/m^2). Waist was measured at half way between the inferior rib and the iliac crest and hip was measured at the gluteus muscle at the level of maximum circumference. Hypertension was defined as a systolic blood pressure greater than or equal to 140 mmHg, a diastolic blood pressure greater than or equal to 90 mmHg or as being treated with antihypertensive drugs [20].

Venous blood was drawn in the morning after an overnight fast. Laboratorial assessment included liver biochemistry, plasma concentrations of cholesterol, high-density lipoprotein-cholesterol (HDL-C), triglycerides, insulin and glucose. LDL-cholesterol was calculated by the Friedewald's equation i.e. [total cholesterol – HDL-cholesterol – (triglycerides/5)]. Homeostasis model assessment of insulin resistance (HOMA-IR) was calculated using fasting glucose and insulin measurements: (fasting insulin (mU/mL)×fasting glucose (mmol/L)/22.5) [21]. Insulin resistance was considered if HOMA was greater than or equal to 3 [22]. Diabetes mellitus was defined as fasting blood glucose greater than or equal to 126 mg/dL (7 mmol/L), or by the regular use of hypoglycemic medications [23]. Metabolic syndrome was defined according to the Third Adult Treatment Panel of the National Cholesterol Education Program, as the presence of at least three of the following criteria: central obesity (waist circumference greater than 102 cm in men and 88 cm in women), hypertriglyceridemia (greater than or equal to 150 mg/dL), low HDL-cholesterol (lower than 40 mg/dL in men and 50 mg/dL in women), elevated fasting glucose (higher than 110 mg/dL) or the use of hipoglicemic drugs and high blood pressure (higher or equal to 130/85 mmHg or under antihypertensive drugs) [24].

Serum levels of adiponectin, leptin and ghrelin were assessed by enzyme-linked immunosorbent assay (ELISA) or radioimmunoassay (RIA). In order to minimize individual variations, serum levels were determined in duplicate.

7.2.3 LIVER BIOPSIES

At the time of surgery, all patients were submitted to wedge liver biopsy. All biopsies were evaluated by the same experienced hepatopathologist, blinded to the laboratorial parameters and clinical data. The specimens were fixed in formalin, embedded in paraffin and stained with hematoxylin eosin, Masson trichrome and reticulin coloration. NAFLD was defined as the presence of more than 5% of steatosis in the liver [25] and NASH was defined as any degree of steatosis along with centrilobular ballooning and/or Mallory-Denk bodies or any degree of steatosis along with centrilobular pericellular/perisinusoidal fibrosis or bridging fibrosis in the absence of another identifiable cause [26]. Steatosis severity was graded from 0 to 3 according to steatosis in less than 5% of hepatocytes, 5–33%, 33–66% and more than 66%; hepatocyte ballooning was classified from 0 to 2, namely absent, few or many; lobular inflammation was classified from 0 to 3, according to the presence of no inflammatory foci, mild or less than 2 foci per 200× field, moderate or 2–4 foci per 200× field and severe or more than 4 foci per 200× foci. Finally, fibrosis was staged from 0 to 4, according to no fibrosis, perisinuoidal or periportal, perisinusoidal and periportal, bridging fibrosis or cirrhosis, as described by the Pathology Committee of NASH Clinical Research Network [27].

7.2.4 DELTOID MUSCLE BIOPSIES

Deltoid muscle samples from 51 morbidly obese patients with NAFLD and 34 lean healthy controls were evaluated. Left deltoid muscle biopsies were obtained during surgery, with collection of three fragments, of about 10×5 mm in size, which were immediately flash frozen in 2-methylbutan cooled in liquid nitrogen and kept at −80°C. Two fragments were used for histological evaluation and biochemistry.

Histological evaluation of muscle biopsies included myocyte fibers morphology, lipid and glycogen content, inflammation and necrosis, as well as mitochondrial abnormalities. Morphological characterization of muscle fibers was performed using the ATPase technique, with pre-incubation at pH 9.4 that allows differentiation according to the intensity of the stain; light fibers were classified as type I and dark fibers as type II. To evaluate the proportion of each type of fiber, computerized counting of 400 consecutive muscle fibers was performed using informatics program Motic Images Advanced 3.1. In addition, the lower diameter of 150 consecutive muscle fibers was measured to evaluate length variation. Semi-quantitative assessment of lipid content was performed with the Oil Red stain, to differentiate intramyocellular and/or extramyocellular and interfascicular lipids overload. Glycogen content was assessed with the Periodic-Acid-Schiff (PAS) stain. The assessment of mitochondrial abnormalities included the determination of ragged red fibers (RRF) with modified Gomori Trichrome stain, which allows the identification of a peripheral reddish discoloration translating excessive mitochondrial proliferation; and cytochrome c oxidase (COX) negative fibers, through histoenzymatic evaluation with the identification of fibers with no COX activity as a result of mitochondrial DNA mutations that predominantly compromise complex IV of the mitochondrial respiratory chain.

The mitochondrial respiratory chain enzymes activities were evaluated with an enzymatic assay through spectrophotometric analysis to determine complex I (NADH-ubiquinone oxidoreductase), II (succinate-ubiquinone reductase), III (ubiquinol-cytochrome c reductase) and IV (cytochrome c oxidase), as well as citrate synthase, activities. Each complex enzymatic assay was normalizated with the citrate synthase activity of each sample. Assays were performed using cellular homogenates of 50–80 mg of muscle. Three assays for each enzyme in each sample were done using a spectrophotometer Shimadzu CPS-240A and the informatics program PC160PLS.

7.2.5 MUSCLE INSULIN SIGNALING CASCADE

Muscle samples from 26 patients were used to evaluate insulin signaling cascade through immunoblotting. Total protein extracts were subjected to SDS-PAGE electrophoresis [28]. Blots were incubated with primary rabbit polyclonal antibodies against insulin receptor, phosphorylated insulin receptor Tyr1162/1163, insulin receptor substrate-1 (IRS-1), phosphorylated IRS-1 Tyr632, or with primary mouse monoclonal antibodies reactive to Akt and phosphorylated Akt Ser473 (Santa Cruz Biotechnology, Santa Cruz, CA, USA), and finally with secondary antibodies conjugated with horseradish peroxidase (Bio-Rad Laboratories, Hercules, CA, USA). Levels of phosphorylated proteins were normalized to corresponding unphosphorylated proteins. Glyceraldehyde-3-phosphate dehydrogenase was used as loading control. Membranes were processed for protein detection using Super Signal substrate (Pierce, Rockford, IL, USA). The relative intensities of protein bands were analyzed using a densitometry analysis program (Quantity One Version 4.6; Bio-Rad Laboratories).

7.2.6 STATISTICAL ANALYSIS

Basic descriptive statistics means, standard deviation, ranges and percentages, were used to characterize the different populations. Qualitative variables were analyzed by χ^2 test and one-way ANOVA. Results are also presented as odds ratio (OR) with 95% confidence interval (CI). Quantitative variables were compared by unpaired Student's t-test and one-way ANOVA and correlations by Pearson correlation coefficient. The independence of the associations of variables with the presence of NASH (dependable

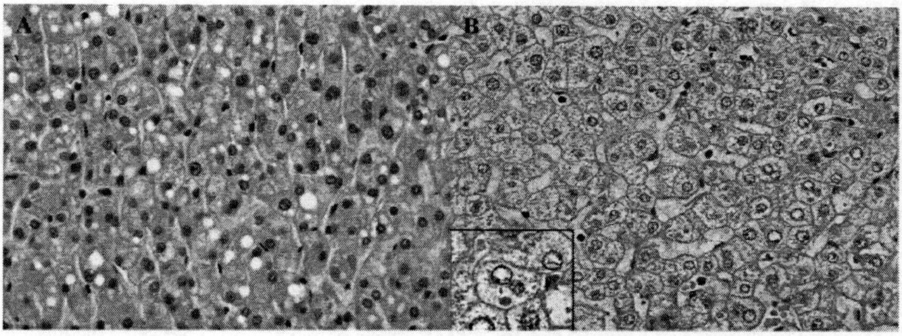

FIGURE 1: Liver histology. Slides stained with hematoxylin & eosin representing patients with simple steatosis (20×) (A) and NASH (40×) (B). Note the presence of a ballooned hepatocyte and lobular inflammatory infiltrate. Insert: ballooned hepatocyte with a Mallory-Denk body and megamitochondria.

variable) was assessed by multivariable logistic regression analysis and expressed as odds ratio (OR). The covariates included were selected by their statistical association in univariate analysis. Analyzes were run using SPSS software version 16.0 (SPSS, Chicago, IL) for Windows and GraphPad InStat version 3.00 (GraphPad Software, San Diego, CA, USA) for the analysis of variance and Bonferroni's multiple comparison tests. Two-tailed P values less than 0.05 were considered statistically significant.

7.3 RESULTS

7.3.1 PATIENTS' CHARACTERISTICS

Fifty one morbid obese patients with NAFLD were included, of whom 22 (43%) were classified as NASH (Typical case - Figure 1 B) and 29 (57%) as non-NASH (Typical case - Figure 1 A). One patient (4%) had unsuspected hepatic cirrhosis. Thirteen patients were male and mean body mass index was 45±6 kg/m^2. Insulin resistance was present in 57%, diabetes mellitus 26%, arterial hypertension 39% and metabolic syndrome 43%. Main characteristics of the patient population are showed in Table 1.

TABLE 1: Patients' main features.

Characteristic	Total (N = 51)	NASH (N = 22)	No NASH (N =29)	P*	OR [95% CI]
Age (years)	42 ± 10	45 ± 9	41 ± 11	0.105	
Male sex (%)	26	32	21	0.280	0.56 [0.16–2.00]
BMI (kg/m²)	45 ± 6	45 ± 6	46 ± 7	0.739	
Waist (cm)	132 ±13	133 ± 17	134 ± 17	0.930	
WTH ratio	0.97 ± 0.10	1.01 ± 0.10	0.96 ± 0.11	0.095	
Diabetes mellitus (%)	26	27	24	0.525	1.18 [0.33–4.18]
Insulin resistance (%)	57	79	44	**0.020**	**4.77** [1.23–18.53]
HOMA	3.9 ± 2.3	4.7 ± 2.4	3.3 ± 2.0	**0.049**	
Hypertension (%)	39	41	38	0.528	1.13 [0.36–3.52]
Smoking (%)	30	24	34	0.311	0.59 [0.17–2.10]
Sleep apnea (%)	23	23	24	0.588	0.92 [0.25–3.43]
Hypertrigliceridaemia (%)	19	25	15	0.305	1.92 [0.44–8.41]
Triglycerides (mg/dL)	119 ± 43	127 ± 49	112 ± 37	0.223	
HDL-cholesterol (mg/dL)	51 ± 13	48 ± 12	53 ± 13	0.146	
LDL-cholesterol (mg/dL)	122 ± 36	128 ± 30	117 ± 40	0.293	
Metabolic syndrome (%)	43	59	30	**0.037**	**3.43** [1.15–11.22]
AST (IU/L)	27 ± 20	31 ± 29	24 ± 9	0.272	
ALT (IU/L)	33 ± 29	41 ± 42	27 ± 12	0.141	
γ–GT (IU/L)	37 ± 45	54 ± 64	25 ± 14	**0.022**	
ALP (IU/L)	74 ± 22	73 ± 26	71 ± 14	0.306	
Total bilirubin (ng/mL)	0.7 ± 0.4	0.6 ± 0.2	0.7 ± 0.4	0.274	
Adiponectin (ng/mL)	20.7 ± 6.2	21.1 ± 7.7	20.4 ± 5.3	0.798	
Leptin (ng/mL)	19.8 ± 7.3	19.9 ± 7.3	19.7 ± 7.5	0.912	
Chrelin (pg/mL)	20.8 ± 13.1	18.8 ± 13.9	21.9 ± 12.8	0.481	
NAS score	2.7 ± 1.6	3.2 ± 1.8	2.4 ± 1.3	0.105	
Steatosis grade	1.8 ± 0.8	1.9 ± 0.8	1.7 ± 0.7	0.309	
1 (n)	21	8	13		
2 (n)	18	7	11		
3 (n)	13	7	5		
Hepatocelular ballooning (n)	3	2	1	0.379	
Lobular inflammatory grade	0.8 ± 0.8	1.1 ± 0.9	0.6 ± 0.8	0.084	

TABLE 1: *Cont.*

Characteristic	Total (N = 51)	NASH (N = 22)	No NASH (N =29)	P*	OR [95% CI]
0 (n)	23	7	16		
1 (n)	16	8	8		
2 (n)	11	6	5		
3 (n)	1	1	0		
Fibrosis stage	1.4 ± 0.8	2.1 ± 0.5	0.9 ± 0.3	<0.001	
0 (n)	4	0	4		
1 (n)	25	0	25		
2 (n)	20	20	0		
3 (n)	1	1	0		
4 (n)	1	1	0		

NASH = non alcoholic steatohepatitis, BMI = body mass index, WTH = waist to hip, AST = aspartate aminotransferase, ALT = alanine aminotransferases, γ–GT = γ–glutamyl transpeptidase, ALP = alkaline phosphatase, NAS = NAFLD activity score. P = significance level in the comparison between NASH and non NASH.*

7.3.2 METABOLIC FACTORS AND HEPATIC HISTOLOGY

Age, male:female ratio and anthropometric parameters including BMI were similar in NASH and non-NASH patients. NASH was associated with the presence of insulin resistance (OR 4.76 [1.23–18.52], p = 0.045) and metabolic syndrome (OR 3.41 [1.15–11.22], p = 0.038), as well as higher levels of gamma-glutamyl transpeptidase (γ-GT) (Table 1). In multivariate analysis, the metabolic syndrome lost statistical significance. Plasma levels of adipokines (adiponectin, leptin) and ghrelin were not associated with NASH.

Steatosis severity paralleled a progressive increase in insulin levels (p = 0.002), mean HOMA-IR (p = 0.001) and prevalence of insulin resistance (p = 0.009) (Figure 2 A). Also, steatosis severity was associated with progressively higher levels of aminotransferases serum levels, aspartate – AST (p = 0.011) and alanine aminotransferase – ALT (p = 0.001). Similarly, there was a statistical positive association between fibrosis stage and higher levels of γ-GT (p = 0.003), insulin (p = 0.006) (Figure 2) and HOMA-IR (p = 0.005) (Figure 2B), as well as progressively higher prevalence of insulin resistance ($p = 0.009$) and the metabolic syndrome ($p = 0.029$). There was also a trend to a positive association between age and fibrosis severity ($p = 0.054$). Lastly, progressive lobular inflammatory activity was not associated with HOMA-IR ($p = 0.065$) (Figure 2C) or insulin resistance ($p = 0.120$), but was associated with older age ($p = 0.001$), AST ($p<0.001$) and ALT serum levels ($p<0.001$), as well as higher prevalence of the metabolic syndrome ($p = 0.031$).

7.3.3 MUSCLE MORPHOLOGY IN MORBIDLY OBESE NAFLD PATIENTS AND NORMAL LEAN CONTROLS

Deltoid muscle morphology was evaluated in 34 lean healthy controls and 51 morbidly obese patients with NAFLD. There were no differences in number, proportion, length and length variability of type 1 and 2 fibers in controls and NAFLD patients, as well as NASH and non-NASH obese patients. However, severity of hepatic steatosis was associated with progressively higher type 1 ($p = 0.021$) and type 2 ($p = 0.007$) fiber length. No associations with fibrosis stage or lobular inflammatory grade were found.

The presence of EMCL and IMCL (Figure 3B and 3A respectively) was more frequent in obese NAFLD patients as compared to controls (70.6% vs 8.8%, $p<0.001$ and 31.4% vs 0%, $p<0.001$, respectively). Also, although the percentage of patients presenting EMCL was not different between NASH and non-NASH obese patients, the percentage of patients with IMCL was significantly higher in NASH patients (59.1 vs 10.3, $p<0.001$; OR 12.52 [2.89–54.26], $p<0.001$). Furthermore, even though there was no significant association between IMCL and steatosis severity, there was a significant tendency to a progressive increase in the prevalence of IMCL and the severity of fibrosis stage ($p = 0.010$) and lobular inflammation grade ($p = 0.029$). In turn, no association was found between EMCL and liver histology (Figure 4). Surprisingly, IMCL or EMCL were not associated with metabolic factors, namely BMI, waist to hip ratio, insulin resistance or HOMA-IR, hypertension, diabetes mellitus, dyslipidemia or the metabolic syndrome. Furthermore, IMCL or EMCL did not change in patients under treatment with anti-diabetics or statins, nor with cytokines levels, namely adiponectin, leptin or ghrelin.

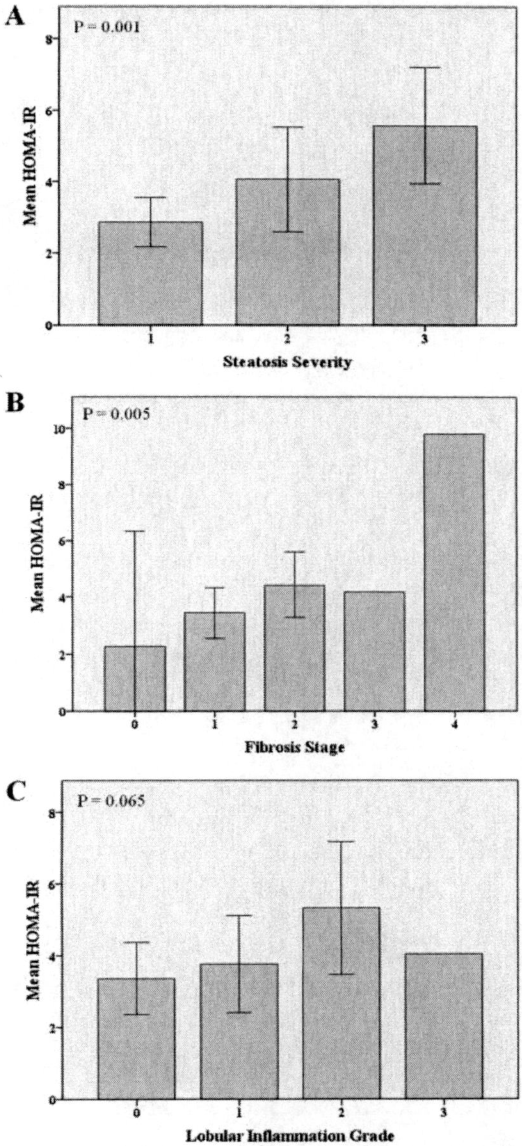

FIGURE 2: Insulin resistance according to liver histology. Differences in HOMA-IR according to the severity of steatosis (A), fibrosis stage (B) and lobular inflammatory grade (C). Error bars: 95% CI (not possible to calculate for fibrosis stage 3 or 4 or lobular inflammation grade 3, only one patient). HOMA-IR progressively increased with severity of hepatic steatosis, lobular inflammation and fibrosis.

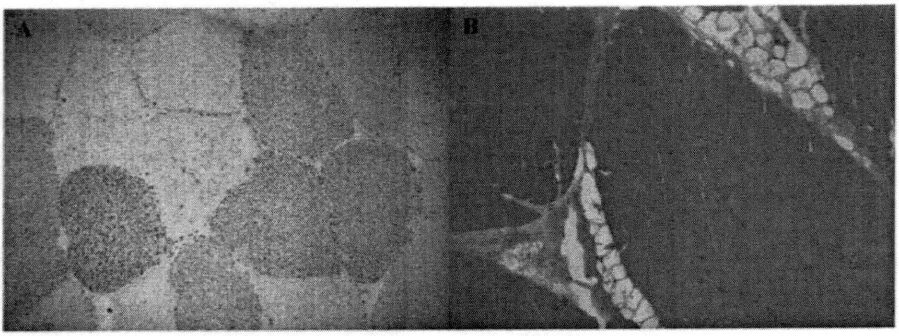

FIGURE 3: Deltoid muscle histology. Slides showing intramyocellular fat accumulation highlighted in Oil red, (40×) (A) and inter fascicular fat, stained with hematoxylin & eosin (10×) (B).

In morbidly obese patients, as well as in controls, there was no significant muscle inflammation or necrosis, irrespective of the presence of IMCL. Lean controls presented more mitochondrial aggregates, and less cytochrome c oxidase negative myocytes and glycogen overload. However, no significant differences were observed between NASH and non-NASH obese patients (Table 2). Still, there was a tendency, though with no statistical significance, to a higher percentage of glycogen overload prevalence with increasing steatosis (29% vs 39% vs 59%, p = 0.101). Also, the prevalence of cytochrome c oxidase negative fibers increased gradually with lobular inflammation activity severity (p = 0.045). No other associations, namely with steatosis, fibrosis or lobular inflammation severity were found.

7.3.4 MUSCLE MITOCHONDRIAL ENZYMES ACTIVITY IN MORBIDLY OBESE NAFLD PATIENTS AND NORMAL LEAN CONTROLS

Muscle mitochondrial activity of citrate synthase and respiratory chain complex I, II, III and IV were evaluated in 25 lean healthy controls and 42 morbidly obese patients with NAFLD. In obese patients, there was a lower citrate synthase activity compared with lean controls, translating into a decreased mitochondrial content (101±30 vs 117±34 nmol/min/mg/PNC, p = 0.047). Moreover, complex I and III activities were higher in obese NAFLD

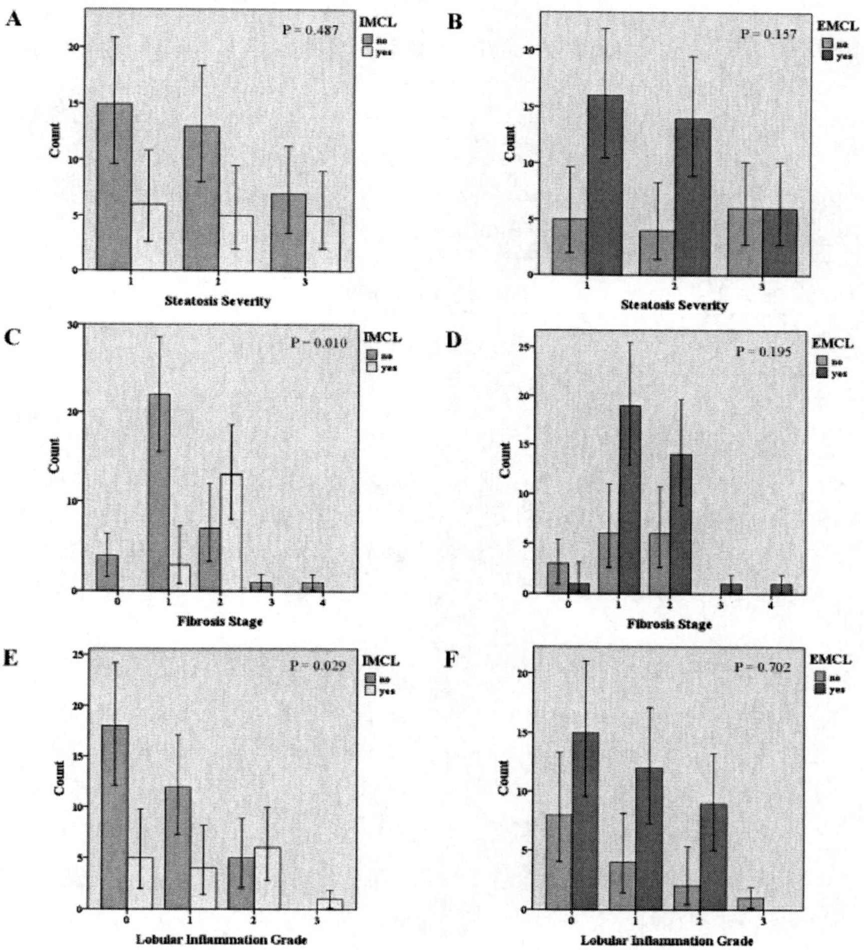

FIGURE 4: Distribution of muscle fat according to liver histology. Prevalence of IMCL and EMCL according to steatosis severity (A and B), fibrosis stage (C and D) and lobular inflammation grade (E and F). Error bars: 95% CI. IMCL was progressively more prevalent with more severe liver disease, namely fibrosis and lobular inflammation. EMCL did not associate with hepatic histology.

patients compared with controls (20±10 vs 16±5 nmol/min/mg/PNC and 87±46 vs 68±36 nmol/min/mg/PNC, $p<0.05$ respectively). There were no differences in enzymatic activities between obese groups (Table 3).

There were also no differences in enzymatic activities regarding the presence of IMCL. On the contrary, the presence of EMCL was globally associated with lower citrate synthase (99±16 vs 115±32 nmol/min/mg/PNC, p = 0.047) and complex II (15±6 vs 18±5 nmol/min/mg/PNC, p = 0.026) activities, and higher complex III activities (91±50 vs 69±31 nmol/min/mg/PNC, p = 0.043). However, differences were lost when analyzing obese patients with NAFLD alone.

TABLE 2: Muscle morphology in morbidly obese patients with NAFLD and lean controls

Feature	Controls (N = 35)	Obese (N = 51)	P*	NASH (N = 22)	Non-NASH (N = 29)	P**
T1F (N)	200 ± 37	215 ± 38	0.102	215 ± 37	214 ± 40	0.894
T1F proportion (%)	50 ± 9	54 ± 10	0.102	54 ± 9	53 ± 10	0.894
T1F length (μm)	52.5 ± 8.3	55.6 ± 10.0	0.154	55.1 ± 8.6	55.9 ± 11.1	0.792
T1F Δ coefficient	172.1 ± 27.7	182.4 ± 20.8	0.069	185.7 ± 20.9	179.9 ± 20.8	0.378
T2F (N)	202 ± 44	185 ± 38	0.076	184 ± 37	186 ± 40	0.894
T2F proportion (%)	50 ± 11	46 ± 10	0.076	46 ± 9	47 ± 10	0.894
T2F length (μm)	52.5 ± 10.2	52.8 ± 11.6	0.911	52.0 ± 8.5	53.3 ± 13.7	0.708
T2F Δ coefficient	219 ± 103.1	215.3 ± 31.0	0.783	217.4 ± 35.1	213.6 ± 28.3	0.698
EMCL (%)	8.8	70.6	**<0.001**	72.7	69.0	0.510
IMCL (%)	0	31.4	**<0.001**	59.1	10.3	**<0.001**
RRF (%)	8.8	21.6	0.103	18.2	24.1	0.437
Mitochondrial aggregates	79.4	51	**0.007**	45.5	55.5	0.689
COX (%)	5.9	39.2	**<0.001**	45.5	34.5	0.306
Inflammation	0	2.0	0.600	0	3.4	0.569
Necrosis	2.9	7.8	0.331	9.1	6.9	0.814
Glycogen overload	0	39.2	**<0.001**	40.9	37.9	0.528

NASH = non alcoholic steatohepatitis, T1F = type 1 fibers, Δ coefficient = variability coefficient, T2F = type 2 fibers, EMCL = extramyocellular lipids, EMCL = intramyocellular lipids, RRF = ragged red fibers presence, COX = presence of cytochrome oxidase negative fibers. P = significance level in the comparison between controls and obese patients; P** = significance level in the comparison between NASH and non-NASH*

TABLE 3: Muscle mitochondrial respiratory chain enzymes activity in morbidly obese patients with NAFLD and lean controls.

Feature	Controls (N = 25)	Obese (N = 42)	P*	NASH (N = 18)	Non-NASH (N = 24)	P**
Citrate Synthase	117.3 ± 34.0	101.3 ± 29.7	**0.047**	109.2 ± 32.7	95.3 ± 26.5	0.138
Comple I	16.2 ± 5.3	20.3 ± 10.5	**0.040**	22.6 ± 12.1	18.6 ± 9.0	0.223
Complex II	17.0 ± 3.8	15.6 ± 6.3	0.242	16.6 ± 5.4	14.8 ± 6.9	0.364
Complex III	67.7 ± 35.7	87.4 ± 46.3	**0.036**	83.0 ± 43.7	90.6 ± 48.8	0.604
Complex IV	18.2 ± 5.3	17.7 ± 7.7	0.755	17. 2 ± 7.0	18.0 ± 8.4	0.738

NASH = non alcoholic steatohepatitis. All enzymatic activities expressed in nmol/min/mg PNC. P = significance level in the comparison between controls and obese patients. P** = significance level in the comaprison between NASH and non-NASH*

In addition, in patients with insulin resistance, complex I activity was higher (24±11 vs 16±18 nmol/min/mg/PNC, p = 0.023) whereas complex IV (15±4 vs 21±9 nmol/min/mg/PNC, p = 0.036) was lower. Also, complex I activity positively correlated with glucose (r = 0.38, p = 0.029) and insulin (r = 0.40, p = 0.018) plasma levels, although there were no differences regarding the presence of diabetes mellitus or metabolic syndrome. Surprisingly, adiponectin and complex III activity presented a negative correlation (r = −0.41, p = 0.014).

Concerning liver lesion, complex III activity was positively correlated with ALT levels (r = 0.35, p = 0.024) whereas complex IV negatively correlated with AST (r = −0.41, p = 0.008) and ALT (r = −0.33, p = 0.031) levels. Complex I activity gradually increased with progressive steatosis (p = 0.049) and fibrosis severity (p = 0.056). No other associations were found between enzymatic activities and steatosis, fibrosis or lobular inflammation severity (Figures 5, 6 and 7).

7.3.5 MUSCLE INSULIN SIGNALING CASCADE IN MORBIDLY OBESE NAFLD PATIENTS AND ITS RELATION WITH MUSCLE AND HEPATIC MORPHOLOGY

The insulin signaling cascade in the muscle was evaluated in 26 morbid obese patients with NAFLD, of whom 43% had NASH, 59% insulin resistance and

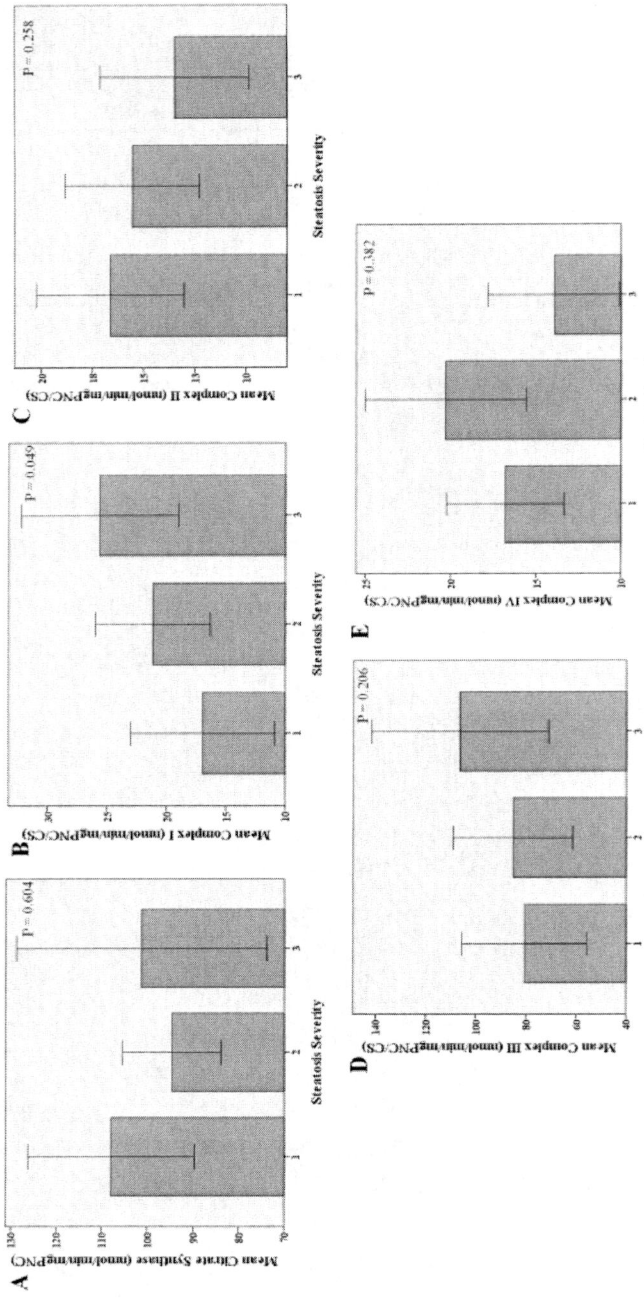

FIGURE 5: Muscle mitochondrial enzymatic activities according to hepatic steatosis degree. Differences in mean mitochondrial enzymatic activities, citrate synthase (A), complex I (B), complex II (C), complex III (D) and complex IV (E) with steatosis severity. Error bars: 95% CI. Complex I activity progressively increased with hepatic steatosis severity.

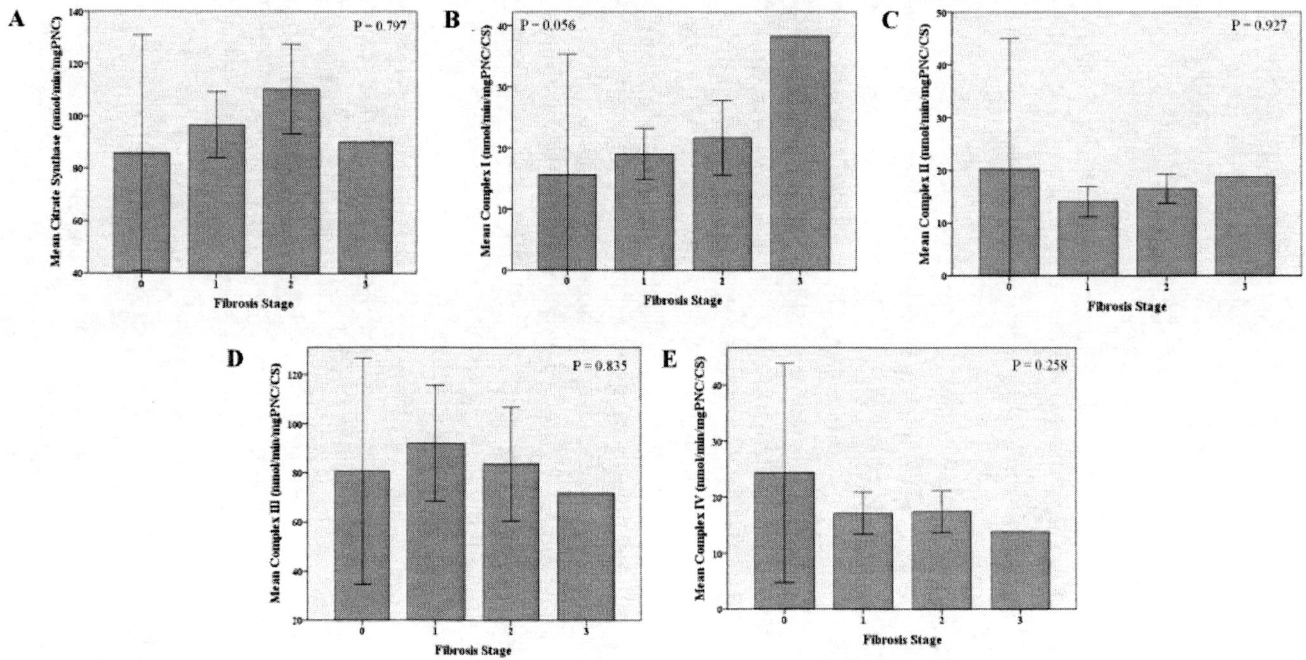

FIGURE 6: Muscle mitochondrial enzymatic activities according to hepatic fibrosis severity. Differences in mean mitochondrial enzymatic activities, citrate synthase (A), complex I (B), complex II (C), complex III (D) and complex IV (E) with fibrosis severity. Error bars: 95% CI. There was a trend to a progressive increase in complex I activity according to fibrosis stage.

26% type 2 diabetes mellitus. No differences were found between insulin cascade proteins and the presence of insulin resistance assessed by HOMA-IR, diabetes mellitus or the metabolic syndrome. However, there was a trend to a positive correlation between glucose plasma levels and phosphorylated IRS-1 ($r = 0.480$, $p = 0.0913$) and a negative correlation with HDL-cholesterol plasma levels ($r = -0.393$, $p = 0.057$). Regarding BMI, there was a positive correlation with increased phosphorylated IRS-1 ($r = 0.388$, $p = 0.043$) and a trend towards a negative correlation with total Akt levels ($r = -0.336$, $p = 0.093$). Surprisingly, no correlations were found with adiponectin. However, phosphorylated IRS-1 was positively correlated with leptin ($r = 0.393$, $p = 0.047$), while the insulin receptor protein levels were positively correlated with ghrelin levels ($r = 0.447$, $p = 0.042$).

Although there were no differences regarding the presence of EMCL and the insulin cascade, IMCL was associated with a 1.5 fold decrease in phosphorylated Akt levels ($p = 0.059$). The only correlations found with respiratory chain enzymes activities were a positive correlation between complex I and phosphorylated insulin receptor ($r = 0.537$, $p = 0.007$) and a trend to a negative correlation between complex III and phosphorylated Akt levels ($r = -0.378$, $p = 0.069$).

Concerning hepatic histology, patients with at least moderate steatosis presented a 2.4-fold increase in phosphorylated insulin receptor ($p = 0.005$), a trend to a 1.4-fold increase in phosphorylated IRS-1 ($p = 0.052$), a 2.7-fold increase in total Akt ($p = 0.015$), and a 2.4-fold decrease in phosphorylated Akt levels ($p = 0.004$). In addition, there was a gradual increase of phosphorylated insulin receptor ($p = 0.014$) and a gradual decrease of phosphorylated Akt ($p<0.001$), with increased steatosis severity (Figure 8). Similarly, the presence of at least moderate lobular inflammation associated with a 2.1-fold decrease in total Akt ($p = 0.043$) and a 1.9-fold decrease in phosphorylated Akt ($p = 0.005$). Finally, lobular inflammation severity was associated with progressive decrease in phosphorylated Akt ($p = 0.013$), while the presence of fibrosis was only associated with a 2-fold increase in phosphorylated insulin receptor levels ($p = 0.008$).

Changes in phosphorylated insulin receptor and Akt in muscle tissue with hepatic steatosis severity (A). Insulin receptor phosphorylation in the muscle increases with hepatic steatosis severity (B) and Akt phosphorylation decreases with steatosis (C). Changes in phosphorylated Akt in muscle

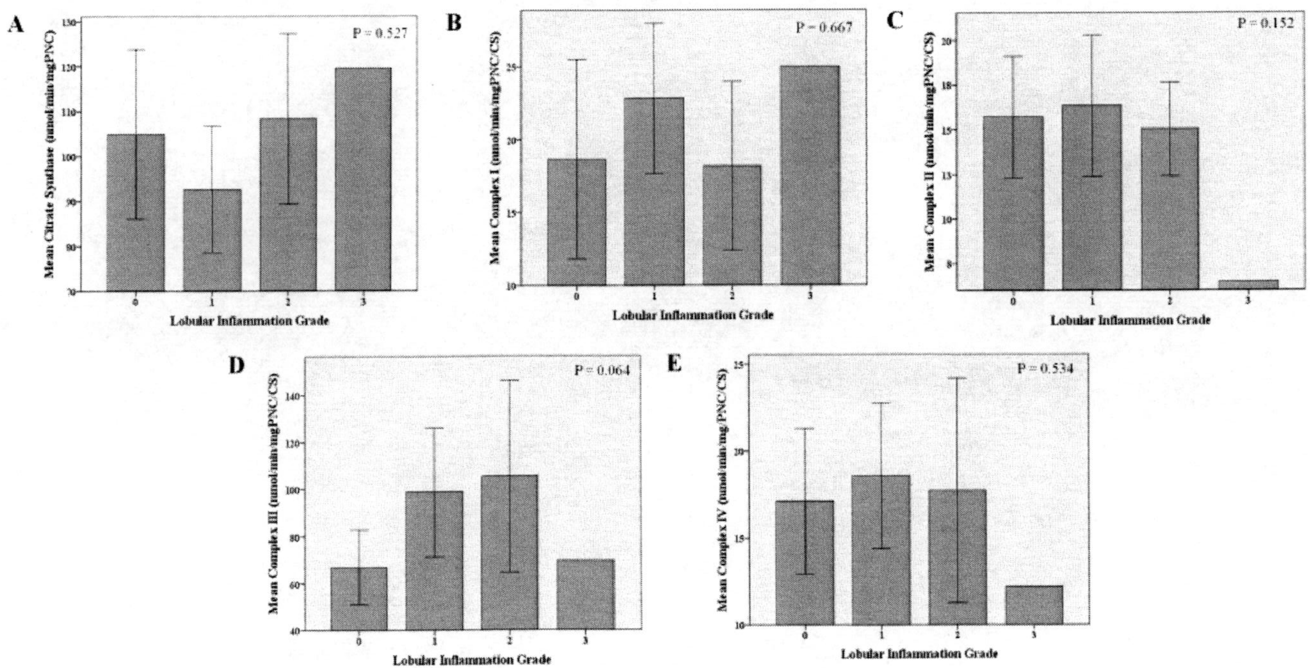

FIGURE 7: Muscle mitochondrial enzymatic activities according to hepatic inflammation severity. Differences in mean mitochondrial enzymatic activities, citrate synthase (A), complex I (B), complex II (C), complex III (D) and complex IV (E) with lobular inflammation severity. Error bars: 95% CI. There was a trend to a progressive increase in complex III activity according to lobular inflammation grade.

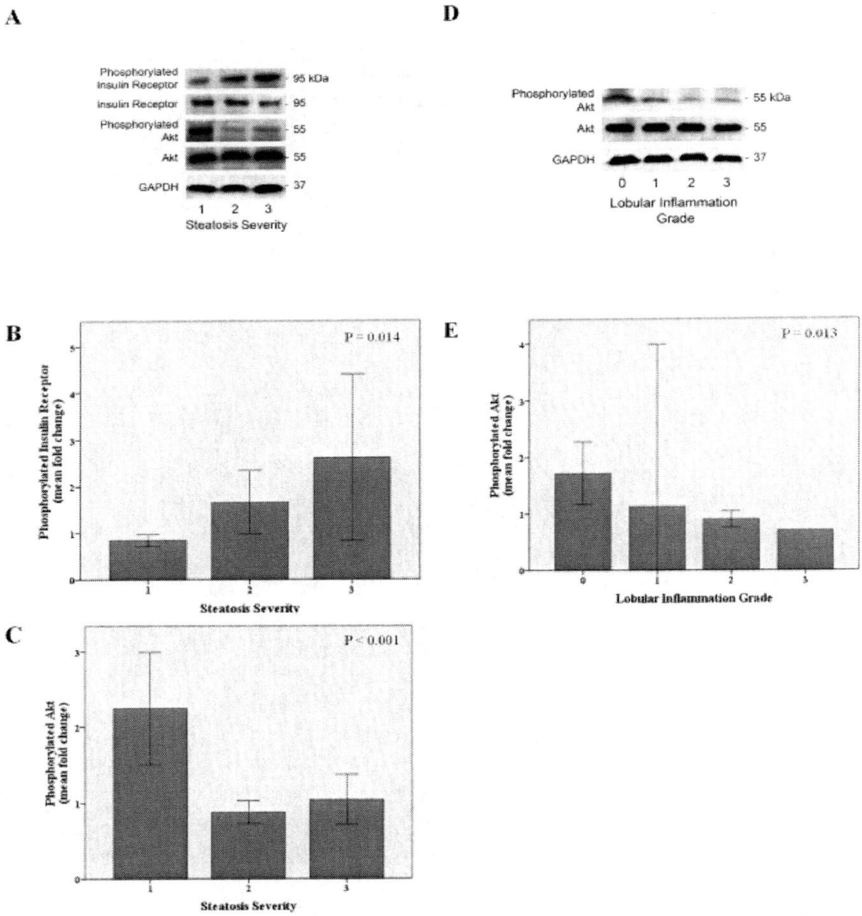

FIGURE 8: Muscle insulin receptor pathway according to hepatic histology.

tissue with hepatic lobular inflammation grade (D). Akt phosphorylation in the muscle decreases with lobular inflammation grade (E). Total proteins were extracted for immunoblot analysis as described. Representative immunoblots for insulin receptor, phosphorylated insulin recptor, Akt, and phosphorylated Akt are shown. Tissue blots of phosphorylated proteins were normalized to corresponding unphosphorylated proteins. Glyceraldehyde-3-phosphate dehydrogenase (GAPDH) was used as loading control. Error bars: 95% CI.

7.4 DISCUSSION

To our knowledge, this is the first study that evaluates the interplay between muscle and hepatic histology in morbid obese patients. As expected, morbid obese patients presented a higher prevalence of fatty muscle than lean controls. However, unlike the liver, in which ectopic fat may be associated with necroinflammation and fibrosis progression our results suggest that ectopic fat in the muscle does not seem to exhibit a predominant toxic role. In fact, no evidence of muscle inflammation or cellular necrosis was found in histology assessment. Previous studies had shown an association between IMCL and hepatic steatosis [7], [18]. In the present study, we further demonstrated that IMCL associates with a more than 12-fold risk for NASH in morbid obese patients, as well as with hepatic inflammation and advanced fibrosis. Indeed, IMCL may translate into a higher susceptibility to lipotoxicity and a decreased ability to keep lipids in inert reservoirs. It would be interesting to understand if there is a temporal sequence between IMCL and NASH development with one favoring the other or if both are parallel phenomena that share the same risk factors. For that, sequential biopsies would be necessary, and hence only possible to study in animal models. Although IMCL was not associated with increased HOMA-IR or overt diabetes mellitus, it was associated with impairment in muscle insulin signaling cascade. Therefore, IMCL may constitute a more sensitive and earlier marker of glucose metabolism disturbance. Finally, IMCL did not associate with muscle mitochondrial dysfunction, thus suggesting ectopic fat accumulation to be a result of an excess of fatty acids supply rather than an impairment in mitochondrial fatty acids oxidation [29].

Our findings also show a decrease in muscle mitochondrial content, as assessed by citrate synthase activity in obese patients as compared to controls. However, we did not find any signs of mitochondrial dysfunction. On the opposite, obese patients presented increased complex I and III activities. Previous studies had shown that mitochondrial content and fatty acids oxidation are decreased in obesity [30], [31]. This may be explained by lipid-derived oxidative mitochondrial damage [32], [33]. Alternatively, mitochondrial content may decrease as a result of sedentary lifestyle rather than obesity itself [34], [35], [36], [37]. However, it has also been previously described that isolated mitochondria from obese subjects maintain its ability to oxidize fatty acids [32]. There may be, indeed, a compensatory increase in mitochondrial enzymes activity in response to fat overload [38]. In fact, both obesity and high fat diets are associated with increased protein expression of transcriptional coactivator peroxisome proliferator-activated receptor gamma coactivator 1-alpha (PGC-1α) [39], the main transcription factor regulating mitochondrial biogenesis and oxidative phosphorylation enzymes expression [40]. However, we found no associations between IMCL and mitochondrial enzymes activity. In this group of obese patients, insulin resistance appears to be associated with higher complex I activity, which is not the case with diabetes mellitus. Also, insulin resistance negatively correlated with complex IV activity. Mitochondrial dysfunction may not be a cause, but rather a consequence of insulin resistance. In accordance, in a chronological model of diet induced obesity in rats, mitochondrial oxidative capacity first presented a compensatory increase, whereas mitochondrial dysfunction was a late event, only appearing after changes in lipid metabolism and insulin sensitivity had occurred [41]. Regarding hepatic lesion, steatosis and fibrosis severity were progressively associated with higher complex I activity, which may suggest a muscle compensatory mechanism to a higher fat overload. Although NASH was not associated with mitochondrial enzymes activity changes, aminotransferases levels were correlated negatively with complex IV activity, which may be translated into a higher hepatic necroinflammatory activity in patients with sustained metabolic disturbance.

Regarding the insulin signaling cascade, activation of the first steps, namely insulin receptor and IRS-1, correlated with BMI, glucose levels and plasma lipids disturbance. However, in the following step, Akt phosphorylation rather presented a negative correlation with the above mentioned metabolic factors. Similar correlations were found, regarding leptin and ghrelin levels, mitochondrial enzymes activities (complex I and III), IMCL accumulation, and degree of hepatic steatosis, inflammation and fibrosis. These data suggest a more intense metabolic disturbance, with compensatory hyperinsulinism and insulin receptor stimulation in the muscle during NAFLD progression in obese patients. Also, in this set, insulin resistance in muscle seems to occur distally in insulin signaling cascade. This is corroborated by the data of Cusi et al. that described muscle resistance in the phosphoinositide-3-kinase (Pi3K)/Akt signaling pathway, with an intact stimulation of mitogen-activated protein kinase (MAPK) translating into normal insulin receptor function in obese individuals [42]. In fact, skeletal muscle ceramide content, which is increased in obese patients [43], is known to inhibit insulin signaling via inhibition at Akt levels [44]. Strong evidence suggests that muscle accumulation of diacylglycerol and long chain acyl-CoA leads to insulin resistance through the activation of serine protein kinase C, which impairs insulin receptor and IRS-1 tyrosine phosphorylation [45], [46]. In fact, muscle diacylglycerol accumulation seems to be more related with an increased supply of fatty acids in the diet, while ceramide accumulation is associated with physical inactivity [47]. Interestingly, physical inactivity may be a major factor contributing to the development of insulin resistance in morbid obesity, where an increase in diacylglycerol content may not occur [43]. However, previous studies from our group [48] showed a decrease in insulin receptor and IRS-1 tyrosine phosphorylation in morbid obese patients with severe NASH, which suggests that at some point in the progression of NAFLD, a continuous overstimulation of insulin receptor may lead to impairment in insulin signaling more proximally in the cascade.

A possible link between increased lipid IMCL and disturbances in insulin pathway signaling could be tumor necrosis factor-alpha (TNF-α). Recently, it has been shown that local generation of TNF-α in skeletal muscle acts paracrinally or autocrinally, inducing insulin resistance [49]. Locally produced pro-TNF-α is a membrane-bound protein that is then processed and released from the cell surface by the action of TNF-α converting enzyme (TACE). Tissue inhibitor of matrix metalloproteinase 3

(TIMP3) is TACE's natural inhibitor [49]. In vitro studies, as well as in vivo, in mice and humans, had shown that fatty acids and high fat diet inhibits TIMP3 expression leading to an increase in TACE activity, in the muscle and in the liver [49], [50]. In the muscle, TACE/TIMP3 deregulation associates with insulin resistance [49], and in the liver with NASH development [50], [51].

One unexpected finding was the lack of association between adiponectin levels and presence of NASH or lipid accumulation in the liver. It is produced mainly by adipocytes, however it is inversely proportional to the adipose mass and visceral obesity, most likely through a negative loop from down-regulation by tumor necrosis factor-α (TNF-α) derived from adipose tissue infiltrating macrophages. Adiponectin has favorable metabolic effects, acting as an insulin sensitizer as well as an anti-inflammatory and TNF-α antagonist [52]. It is known to decrease hepatic fat content in animal models [53] and it is believed to inversely relate with NAFLD in human; however, not all studies are consensual and a meta-analysis using liver biopsy data failed to demonstrate it [54]. Also, differences in adiponectin levels between patients with simple steatosis and NASH are still not clear [55]. The failure to show an association between adiponectin and hepatic or muscle histology, as well as with deregulation in insulin signaling may be due to lack of power to detect them. However, we can speculate that in a population of morbid obese patients, where adiponectin levels are already extremely low and associated with NAFLD, the correlation with more severe disease such as NASH is weakened.

Our study has some limitations, mainly in respect to the normal control group. When evaluating muscle morphology and muscle mitochondrial function, anthropometric, laboratorial and liver biopsy data were not collected. Also, when assessing muscle insulin cascade signaling, a comparison with a healthy lean control group was not possible. However, the main goal of the study was to assess the muscle morphology and metabolism according to liver injury in a homogenous group of patients, with similar metabolic risk factors, namely BMI.

In conclusion, obesity is associated with IMCL in a similar and parallel fashion with NAFLD. However, in opposite to the liver in which ectopic fat seems to be associated with a risk of liver disease progression with necroinflammatory and fibrogenic responses, in the muscle, ectopic fat does not lead to inflammation or myocyte necrosis. Moreover, IMCL is associated with a higher risk of NASH and advanced fibrosis. Also, muscle mitochondrial dysfunction does not appear to be a major driving mechanism to IMCL accumulation, insulin resistance and liver disease in obese patients. Skeletal muscle insulin resistance occurs at a late point in the insulin signaling cascade and is associated with IMCL and NAFLD severity.

REFERENCES

1. Argo CK, Northup PG, Al-Osaimi AM, Caldwell SH (2009) Systematic review of risk factors for fibrosis progression in non-alcoholic steatohepatitis. J Hepatol 51: 371–379. doi: 10.1016/j.jhep.2009.03.019.
2. Ekstedt M, Franzen LE, Mathiesen UL, Thorelius L, Holmqvist M, et al. (2006) Long-term follow-up of patients with NAFLD and elevated liver enzymes. Hepatology 44: 865–873. doi: 10.1002/hep.21327.
3. Defronzo RA (2009) Banting Lecture. From the triumvirate to the ominous octet: a new paradigm for the treatment of type 2 diabetes mellitus. Diabetes 58: 773–795. doi: 10.2337/db09-9028.
4. Kuhlmann J, Neumann-Haefelin C, Belz U, Kalisch J, Juretschke HP, et al. (2003) Intramyocellular lipid and insulin resistance: a longitudinal in vivo 1H-spectroscopic study in Zucker diabetic fatty rats. Diabetes 52: 138–144. doi: 10.2337/diabetes.52.1.138.
5. van Herpen NA, Schrauwen-Hinderling VB (2008) Lipid accumulation in non-adipose tissue and lipotoxicity. Physiol Behav 94: 231–241. doi: 10.1016/j.physbeh.2007.11.049.
6. Goodpaster BH, Theriault R, Watkins SC, Kelley DE (2000) Intramuscular lipid content is increased in obesity and decreased by weight loss. Metabolism 49: 467–472. doi: 10.1016/S0026-0495(00)80010-4.
7. Sinha R, Dufour S, Petersen KF, LeBon V, Enoksson S, et al. (2002) Assessment of skeletal muscle triglyceride content by (1)H nuclear magnetic resonance spectroscopy in lean and obese adolescents: relationships to insulin sensitivity, total body fat, and central adiposity. Diabetes 51: 1022–1027. doi: 10.2337/diabetes.51.4.1022.
8. Thamer C, Machann J, Bachmann O, Haap M, Dahl D, et al. (2003) Intramyocellular lipids: anthropometric determinants and relationships with maximal aerobic capacity and insulin sensitivity. J Clin Endocrinol Metab 88: 1785–1791. doi: 10.1210/jc.2002-021674.
9. Bachmann OP, Dahl DB, Brechtel K, Machann J, Haap M, et al. (2001) Effects of intravenous and dietary lipid challenge on intramyocellular lipid content and the relation with insulin sensitivity in humans. Diabetes 50: 2579–2584. doi: 10.2337/diabetes.50.11.2579.

10. Hulver MW, Berggren JR, Cortright RN, Dudek RW, Thompson RP, et al. (2003) Skeletal muscle lipid metabolism with obesity. Am J Physiol Endocrinol Metab 284: E741–747.
11. Hajduch E, Balendran A, Batty IH, Litherland GJ, Blair AS, et al. (2001) Ceramide impairs the insulin-dependent membrane recruitment of protein kinase B leading to a loss in downstream signalling in L6 skeletal muscle cells. Diabetologia 44: 173–183. doi: 10.1007/s001250051596.
12. Ellis BA, Poynten A, Lowy AJ, Furler SM, Chisholm DJ, et al. (2000) Long-chain acyl-CoA esters as indicators of lipid metabolism and insulin sensitivity in rat and human muscle. Am J Physiol Endocrinol Metab 279: E554–560.
13. Holland WL, Knotts TA, Chavez JA, Wang LP, Hoehn KL, et al. (2007) Lipid mediators of insulin resistance. Nutr Rev 65: S39–46. doi: 10.1111/j.1753-4887.2007.tb00327.x.
14. Eckardt K, Taube A, Eckel J (2011) Obesity-associated insulin resistance in skeletal muscle: Role of lipid accumulation and physical inactivity. Rev Endocr Metab Disord 12: 163–172. doi: 10.1007/s11154-011-9168-2.
15. Dengel DR, Pratley RE, Hagberg JM, Rogus EM, Goldberg AP (1996) Distinct effects of aerobic exercise training and weight loss on glucose homeostasis in obese sedentary men. J Appl Physiol 81: 318–325. doi: 10.1097/00005768-199605001-00474.
16. Perseghin G, Scifo P, Danna M, Battezzati A, Benedini S, et al. (2002) Normal insulin sensitivity and IMCL content in overweight humans are associated with higher fasting lipid oxidation. Am J Physiol Endocrinol Metab 283: E556–564.
17. Liu L, Zhang Y, Chen N, Shi X, Tsang B, et al. (2007) Upregulation of myocellular DGAT1 augments triglyceride synthesis in skeletal muscle and protects against fat-induced insulin resistance. J Clin Invest 117: 1679–1689. doi: 10.1172/JCI30565.
18. Kitajima Y, Eguchi Y, Ishibashi E, Nakashita S, Aoki S, et al. (2010) Age-related fat deposition in multifidus muscle could be a marker for nonalcoholic fatty liver disease. J Gastroenterol 45: 218–224. doi: 10.1007/s00535-009-0147-2.
19. (1992) Gastrointestinal surgery for severe obesity: National Institutes of Health Consensus Development Conference Statement. Am J Clin Nutr 55: 615S–619S.
20. Group NHBPEPW (1993) Report on primary prevention of hypertension. Arch Intern Med 153: 325–334. doi: 10.1001/archinte.1993.00410020042003.
21. Matthews DR, Hosker JP, Rudenski AS, Naylor BA, Treacher DF, et al. (1985) Homeostasis model assessment: insulin resistance and beta-cell function from fasting plasma glucose and insulin concentrations in man. Diabetologia 28: 412–419. doi: 10.1007/BF00280883.
22. Marchesini G, Bugianesi E, Forlani G, Cerrelli F, Lenzi M, et al. (2003) Nonalcoholic fatty liver, steatohepatitis, and the metabolic syndrome. Hepatology 37: 917–923. doi: 10.1053/jhep.2003.50161.
23. Genuth S, Alberti KG, Bennett P, Buse J, Defronzo R, et al. (2003) Follow-up report on the diagnosis of diabetes mellitus. Diabetes Care 26: 3160–3167. doi: 10.2337/diacare.26.11.3160.
24. (2002) Third Report of the National Cholesterol Education Program (NCEP) Expert Panel on Detection, Evaluation, and Treatment of High Blood Cholesterol in Adults

(Adult Treatment Panel III) final report. Circulation 106: 3143–3421. doi: 10.1001/jama.285.19.2486.
25. Ratziu V, Bellentani S, Cortez-Pinto H, Day C, Marchesini G (2010) A position statement on NAFLD/NASH based on the EASL 2009 special conference. J Hepatol 53: 372–384. doi: 10.1016/j.jhep.2010.04.008.
26. Younossi Z, Stepanova M, Rafiq N, Makhlouf H, Younoszai Z, et al. (2011) Pathologic criteria for non-alcoholic steatohepatitis (NASH): Inter-protocol agreement and ability to predict liver-related mortality. Hepatology 53: 1874–1882. doi: 10.1002/hep.24268.
27. Kleiner DE, Brunt EM, Van Natta M, Behling C, Contos MJ, et al. (2005) Design and validation of a histological scoring system for nonalcoholic fatty liver disease. Hepatology 41: 1313–1321. doi: 10.1002/hep.20701.
28. Ramalho RM, Cortez-Pinto H, Castro RE, Sola S, Costa A, et al. (2006) Apoptosis and Bcl-2 expression in the livers of patients with steatohepatitis. Eur J Gastroenterol Hepatol 18: 21–29. doi: 10.1097/00042737-200601000-00005.
29. Kraegen EW, Cooney GJ, Turner N (2008) Muscle insulin resistance: a case of fat overconsumption, not mitochondrial dysfunction. Proc Natl Acad Sci U S A 105: 7627–7628. doi: 10.1073/pnas.0803901105.
30. Kim JY, Hickner RC, Cortright RL, Dohm GL, Houmard JA (2000) Lipid oxidation is reduced in obese human skeletal muscle. Am J Physiol Endocrinol Metab 279: E1039–1044.
31. Kelley DE, He J, Menshikova EV, Ritov VB (2002) Dysfunction of mitochondria in human skeletal muscle in type 2 diabetes. Diabetes 51: 2944–2950. doi: 10.2337/diabetes.51.10.2944.
32. Holloway GP, Bonen A, Spriet LL (2009) Regulation of skeletal muscle mitochondrial fatty acid metabolism in lean and obese individuals. Am J Clin Nutr 89: 455S–462S. doi: 10.3945/ajcn.2008.26717B.
33. Abdul-Ghani MA, DeFronzo RA (2010) Pathogenesis of insulin resistance in skeletal muscle. J Biomed Biotechnol 2010: 476279. doi: 10.1155/2010/476279.
34. Hawley JA, Lessard SJ (2007) Mitochondrial function: use it or lose it. Diabetologia 50: 699–702. doi: 10.1007/s00125-007-0595-2.
35. Alves RM, Vitorino R, Figueiredo P, Duarte JA, Ferreira R, et al. (2010) Lifelong physical activity modulation of the skeletal muscle mitochondrial proteome in mice. J Gerontol A Biol Sci Med Sci 65: 832–842. doi: 10.1093/gerona/glq081.
36. Safdar A, Hamadeh MJ, Kaczor JJ, Raha S, Debeer J, et al. (2010) Aberrant mitochondrial homeostasis in the skeletal muscle of sedentary older adults. PLoS One 5: e10778. doi: 10.1371/journal.pone.0010778.
37. Rimbert V, Boirie Y, Bedu M, Hocquette JF, Ritz P, et al. (2004) Muscle fat oxidative capacity is not impaired by age but by physical inactivity: association with insulin sensitivity. Faseb J 18: 737–739. doi: 10.1096/fj.03-1104fje.
38. Turner N, Bruce CR, Beale SM, Hoehn KL, So T, et al. (2007) Excess lipid availability increases mitochondrial fatty acid oxidative capacity in muscle: evidence against a role for reduced fatty acid oxidation in lipid-induced insulin resistance in rodents. Diabetes 56: 2085–2092. doi: 10.2337/db07-0093.

39. Hancock CR, Han DH, Chen M, Terada S, Yasuda T, et al. (2008) High-fat diets cause insulin resistance despite an increase in muscle mitochondria. Proc Natl Acad Sci U S A 105: 7815–7820. doi: 10.1073/pnas.0802057105.
40. Benton CR, Wright DC, Bonen A (2008) PGC-1alpha-mediated regulation of gene expression and metabolism: implications for nutrition and exercise prescriptions. Appl Physiol Nutr Metab 33: 843–862. doi: 10.1139/H08-074.
41. Chanseaume E, Tardy AL, Salles J, Giraudet C, Rousset P, et al. (2007) Chronological approach of diet-induced alterations in muscle mitochondrial functions in rats. Obesity (Silver Spring) 15: 50–59. doi: 10.1038/oby.2007.511.
42. Cusi K, Maezono K, Osman A, Pendergrass M, Patti ME, et al. (2000) Insulin resistance differentially affects the PI 3-kinase- and MAP kinase-mediated signaling in human muscle. J Clin Invest 105: 311–320. doi: 10.1172/JCI7535.
43. Thrush AB, Brindley DN, Chabowski A, Heigenhauser GJ, Dyck DJ (2009) Skeletal muscle lipogenic protein expression is not different between lean and obese individuals: a potential factor in ceramide accumulation. J Clin Endocrinol Metab 94: 5053–5061. doi: 10.1210/jc.2008-2565.
44. Adams JM 2nd, Pratipanawatr T, Berria R, Wang E, DeFronzo RA, et al. (2004) Ceramide content is increased in skeletal muscle from obese insulin-resistant humans. Diabetes 53: 25–31. doi: 10.2337/diabetes.53.1.25.
45. Yu C, Chen Y, Cline GW, Zhang D, Zong H, et al. (2002) Mechanism by which fatty acids inhibit insulin activation of insulin receptor substrate-1 (IRS-1)-associated phosphatidylinositol 3-kinase activity in muscle. J Biol Chem 277: 50230–50236. doi: 10.1074/jbc.M200958200.
46. Samuel VT, Petersen KF, Shulman GI (2010) Lipid-induced insulin resistance: unravelling the mechanism. Lancet 375: 2267–2277. doi: 10.1016/S0140-6736(10)60408-4.
47. Dube JJ, Amati F, Toledo FG, Stefanovic-Racic M, Rossi A, et al. (2011) Effects of weight loss and exercise on insulin resistance, and intramyocellular triacylglycerol, diacylglycerol and ceramide. Diabetologia 54: 1147–1156. doi: 10.1007/s00125-011-2065-0.
48. Ferreira DM, Castro RE, Machado MV, Evangelista T, Silvestre A, et al. (2011) Apoptosis and insulin resistance in liver and peripheral tissues of morbidly obese patients is associated with different stages of non-alcoholic fatty liver disease. Diabetologia 54: 1788–1798. doi: 10.1007/s00125-011-2130-8.
49. Monroy A, Kamath S, Chavez AO, Centonze VE, Veerasamy M, et al. (2009) Impaired regulation of the TNF-alpha converting enzyme/tissue inhibitor of metalloproteinase 3 proteolytic system in skeletal muscle of obese type 2 diabetic patients: a new mechanism of insulin resistance in humans. Diabetologia 52: 2169–2181. doi: 10.1007/s00125-009-1451-3.
50. Fiorentino L, Vivanti A, Cavalera M, Marzano V, Ronci M, et al. (2010) Increased tumor necrosis factor alpha-converting enzyme activity induces insulin resistance and hepatosteatosis in mice. Hepatology 51: 103–110. doi: 10.1002/hep.23250.
51. Menghini R, Menini S, Amoruso R, Fiorentino L, Casagrande V, et al. (2009) Tissue inhibitor of metalloproteinase 3 deficiency causes hepatic steatosis and adipose tissue inflammation in mice. Gastroenterology 136: 663–672 e664. doi: 10.1053/j.gastro.2008.10.079.

52. Polyzos SA, Kountouras J, Zavos C, Tsiaousi E (2010) The role of adiponectin in the pathogenesis and treatment of non-alcoholic fatty liver disease. Diabetes Obes Metab 12: 365–383. doi: 10.1111/j.1463-1326.2009.01176.x.
53. Xu A, Wang Y, Keshal H, Xu LY, Lam KS, et al. (2003) The fat-derived hormone adiponectin alleviates alcoholic and nonalcoholic fatty liver diseases in mice. J Clin Invest 112: 91–100. doi: 10.1172/jci200317797.
54. Polyzos SA, Toulis KA, Goulis DG, Zavos C, Kountouras J (2011) Serum total adiponectin in nonalcoholic fatty liver disease: a systematic review and meta-analysis. Metabolism 60: 313–326. doi: 10.1016/j.metabol.2010.09.003.
55. Bugianesi E, Pagotto U, Manini R, Vanni E, Gastaldelli A, et al. (2005) Plasma adiponectin in nonalcoholic fatty liver is related to hepatic insulin resistance and hepatic fat content, not to liver disease severity. J Clin Endocrinol Metab 90: 3498–3504. doi: 10.1210/jc.2004-2240.

CHAPTER 8

SARCOPENIA EXACERBATES OBESITY-ASSOCIATED INSULIN RESISTANCE AND DYSGLYCEMIA: FINDINGS FROM THE NATIONAL HEALTH AND NUTRITION EXAMINATION SURVEY II

PREETHI SRIKANTHAN, ANDREA L. HEVENER, and ARUN S. KARLAMANGLA

8.1 INTRODUCTION

Obesity and type 2 diabetes constitute a significant health care concern in the United States and other developing and developed nations, especially since their incidence is on the rise in children and young adults. Sarcopenic obesity, the co-existence of sarcopenia and obesity, [1] is seen in 5–10% of healthy, ambulatory, community-dwelling Americans in their sixties, rising to over 50% in those over age eighty [2]. Studies indicate that up to 50% of muscle may be lost by the age of 90 years[3]. Since muscle is the primary tissue contributing to whole-body insulin-mediated glucose

This chapter was originally published under the Creative Commons Attribution License. Srikanthan P, Hevener AL, and Karlamangla AS. Sarcopenia Exacerbates Obesity-Associated Insulin Resistance and Dysglycemia: Findings from the National Health and Nutrition Examination Survey III. PLoS ONE *5,5 (2010), doi:10.1371/journal.pone.0010805.*

disposal, sarcopenia may be an important causal factor in age-induced insulin resistance and type 2 diabetes susceptibility.

Inflammation is a central underpinning in the pathogenesis of insulin resistance and is also seen in both obesity and sarcopenia. Inflammation may be an important mediator in restraining myogenesis and/or accelerating muscle protein degradation. In addition, intramyocellular lipid accumulation, seen in obesity, results in the formation of bioactive lipid intermediates and lipid peroxides, which are known to activate pro-inflammatory cascades [4]. Furthermore, myokines secreted by skeletal muscle [5] have been found to prevent inflammation and insulin resistance, thus counteracting the pro-inflammatory and metabolic effects of adipokines produced in adipose tissue; the relative paucity of myokines relative to adipokines in sarcopenic obesity may increase the risk of metabolic and cardiovascular disease[6].

Recent studies in rodents suggest a strong inverse association between muscle mass and disease risk. Even a modest increase in muscle mass can prevent diet-induced obesity and insulin resistance as well as atherogenesis in prone mice[5],[7]. Consistent with this, Stephen et al. found a positive association between sarcopenic obesity and cardiovascular disease in the older adults from the Cardiovascular Health Study [8]. However, since type II muscle fibers, described as glycolytic and insulin resistant [9], are lost to a greater extent than type I fibers [10] in age-related muscle atrophy, sarcopenia could theoretically also increase insulin sensitivity and cause some beneficial alterations in glucose metabolism in older adults [11].

Accordingly, we hypothesize that sarcopenic obese individuals have more insulin resistance and higher prevalence of dysglycemia (i.e., impaired glucose tolerance and diabetes), than individuals with neither sarcopenia nor obesity, those with obesity alone (without sarcopenia), and those with sarcopenia alone (without obesity). We further hypothesize that this association will be stronger in young and middle aged adults than in older adults, in whom sarcopenia may mean a preferential reduction in insulin-resistant fibers.

To test this hypothesis, we assessed the level of insulin resistance and dysglycemia in sarcopenic obese individuals, obese individuals without sarcopenia, sarcopenic individuals without obesity, and in those with neither sarcopenia nor obesity, in a nationally representative sample, and tested for effect modification by age.

8.2 METHODS

8.2.1 ETHICS STATEMENT

Written informed consent was obtained from all participants, and the protocol was approved by the institutional review board of the National Center for Health Statistics, and the study procedures were carried out in accordance with the principles of the Declaration of Helsinki.

8.2.2 DESIGN AND METHODS

The National Health and Nutrition Examination Survey (NHANES) III was a national survey conducted from 1988 through 1994, using a stratified, multistage, probability cluster design. The total sample included 33,199 persons[12] of whom, 17,756 were older than 20 years and non-pregnant. The full evaluation included a standardized home interview (with a medication review), a physical examination in a mobile examination center, and a fasting blood draw.

Our analytic sample (N = 14,528) was restricted to those who were 20 years or older and non-pregnant, and had measurements of bioelectrical impedance (BI), height, and body weight, the three variables we utilized to indirectly estimate the presence of sarcopenic obesity. Participants who had cardiac pacemakers or had previously undergone limb amputation were excluded from the measurement of BI [13].The analytic sample included 2370 women and 2284 men who were 60 years of age or older.

8.2.3 MEASUREMENTS: EXPOSURES

Body height and weight were measured, and converted to body mass index (BMI) in units of kg/meter-squared. Obesity was defined as BMI >30 kg/m^2. Waist size and hip size were measured by standard protocols and waist-to-hip circumference ratio was created. BI was measured using the Valhalla Scientific Body Composition Analyzer 1990 B [14], and used to estimate skeletal muscle mass (in kg) via the BI analysis equation of Janssen et al [15].

$$\text{Skeletal muscle mass} = [0.401 \text{ x } (\text{height}^2/\text{BI}) + 3.825 \text{ x sex}) + (0.071 \text{ x age})] + 5.102$$

with height measured in cm, BI measured in ohms, sex coded 1 for men and 0 for women, and age measured in years. Muscle mass (in kg) was divided by body mass (in kg) and multiplied by 100% to create skeletal muscle index (SMI). Similar to the approach used to identify osteoporosis from bone mineral density [16], sarcopenia is defined as SMI more than two standard deviations below the sex-specific, young adult (ages, 18-39) means: 31.0% in men and 22.0% in women [17].

8.2.4 MEASUREMENTS: OUTCOMES

Serum insulin and plasma glucose were measured from fasting blood samples (if fasted 6 hours or more) using radioimmunoassay and a hexokinase enzymatic method, respectively [13], and used to calculate insulin resistance by the Homeostasis model assessment of insulin resistance (HOMA-IR) which is approximated using the formula below:

$$\text{HOMA} - \text{IR} = \text{fasting glucose x fasting insulin}/22.5$$

with glucose in mmol/L and insulin in μU/ml, for participants whose fasting plasma glucose ranged from 3.0 to 25.0 mmol/l and fasting insulin ranged from 3 to 55 μU/ml[18]. HOMA-IR data were available for 12,046 subjects. Glycosylated hemoglobin (HbA1c) was measured using an ion-exchange high-performance liquid chromatography method using the Diamat Analyzer System, and used to define dysglycemia based on standard HbA1C thresholds [19]. Specifically, diabetes (DM) was defined as one or more of 1) HbA1C ≥6.5% 2) Fasting glucose ≥7 mmol/L (126 mg/dl), 3) self report of DM and /or 4) use of DM medication (oral hypoglycemic agents and /or insulin), and pre-diabetes was defined by 1) HbA1C ≥6% but <6.5% OR fasting ≥5.5 mmol/L(100 mg/dL) but <7.0 mmol/L(126 mg/dL), 2) no self-reported DM, and 3) absence of DM medications.

8.2.5 MEASUREMENTS: COVARIATES

Age, race/ethnicity (non-Hispanic white, non-Hispanic black, Mexican American, and other), and completed years of education and sex were obtained from self reports. Serum C-reactive protein (CRP) concentration was measured using latex-enhanced nephelometry with a Behring Nephelometer Analyzer System (Behring Diagnostics Inc)[20]. Details about the laboratory procedures and quality control have been published [20]. Serum CRP levels greater than 10 mg/dL were set to missing to avoid capturing acute elevations in CRP due to infectious causes.

8.2.6 STATISTICAL ANALYSES

To study the association between sarcopenic obesity and insulin resistance/dysglycemia, we examined four outcomes (HOMA-IR, HbA1C, prevalence of pre-diabetes, prevalence of diabetes mellitus) in sarcopenic obese individuals, sarcopenic non-obese individuals, obese non-sarcopenic individuals, and those with neither sarcopenia nor obesity (the reference group). To control for confounders (namely age, sex, education, and race/ethnicity), we used multivariable logistic regression for the two prevalence outcomes (diabetes and pre-diabetes) and multivariable linear regression for the continuous outcomes: HbA1C and HOMA-IR; these variables were log-transformed before model fitting. To minimize residual confounding by age, we included age both as a continuous and a categorical variable (20–29 y, 30–39 y, 40–49 y, 50–59 y, 60–74 y, and ≥75 y). We similarly, included years of education both as a continuous and a categorical variable (<12 y, 12–14 y, 15–17 y, and >17 y, intended to capture the effect of credentialing at high school and college). We also repeated the analyses after excluding diabetics to minimize confounding by reverse causation (i.e., diabetes leading to sarcopenia and/or obesity).

We tested for effect modification by age (dichotomized: <60 years vs. > = 60 years) and gender by including interaction terms in the models for each of the four dependent variables. Based on the results of the interaction testing, we conducted further stratified analyses. In supplementary analyses, to test if sarcopenia/obesity associations with inflammation are consistent with their dysglycemia associations, we also examined serum CRP level (after log-transformation) as a continuous outcome in multivariable linear regression.We used SAS, release 9.2 (SAS Institute Inc, Cary, NC) for all the analyses.

8.3 RESULTS

The study sample was representative of the complete NHANES sample that was non pregnant and 20 years or older (Table 1), except that the study participants were younger, less frequently male, non-Hispanic White, and diabetic than those excluded from the study. Those excluded had similar BMI, HOMA-IR, and HbA1C as those in the study sample. The average age of participants in the study sample was 45 years, 51.7% were female and 42.2% were non-Hispanic Whites.

Sarcopenia was more prevalent in obese than non-obese participants (4.5% vs. 1.14%), and this was true both in those under 60 years of age (3.4% vs. 0.2%) and in those 60 years and older (6.9% vs. 3.2%). Comparing participants under 60 years of age with those 60 years or older in the study sample, the older group had lower SMI and more sarcopenia without obesity but less obesity without sarcopenia. Yet, the older adults had more insulin resistance and dysglycemia than the younger group:

Median HbA1C, HOMA IR, and prevalence of pre-diabetes and DM were all higher in older adults.

TABLE 1: Descriptive statistics (median with inter-quartile range, or percentage).

	Study Sample			
	Complete sample (N = 14,528)	Under 60 years (N = 9,892)	60 years or older (N = 4,636)	*Excluded** (N = 3,228)
Age (years)	45.0 (32.0–64.0)	37.0 (29.0 – 45.0)	71.0 (65.0 – 78.0)	66.0 (41.0 – 80.0)
Body mass index (kg/m²)	26.3 (23.2 – 30.0)	26.2 (23.0 –30.2)	26.5 (23.6 – 29.8)	26.3 (22.6 – 30.4)
Skeletal muscle index (%)	33.9 (27.9 – 39.4)	35.0 (29.2 – 40.5)	31.0 (25.8 – 36.9)	---
Glycosylated hemoglobin (%)	5.40 (5.00 – 5.7) (n = 14026)	5.20 (4.90 – 5.60) (n = 9527)	5.60 (5.30 – 6.10) (n = 4489)	5.50 (5.10 – 5.90) (n = 1622)
HOMA-IR (mg/dl x μU/ml)	2.12 (1.45 – 3,30) (n = 12046)	2.00 (1.38 – 3.10) (n = 8173)	2.38 (1.61 – 3.67) (n = 3873)	2.25 (1.46 – 3.46) (n = 1031)
Gender: Male	48.3%	47.9%	49.2%	50.3%
NH White	42.2%	34.6%	58.2%	51.2%
NH Black	27.3%	31.0%	19.6%	24.9%
Hispanic	26.4%	29.8%	19.0%	21.8%
Other	4.18%	4.60%	3.28%	2.23%
Sarcopenic without obesity	1.14%	0.18%	3.17%	---
Obese without sarcopenia	21.0%	22.9%	17.1%	---
Sarcopenic obesity	4.50%	3.39%	6.9%	---
Pre-diabetes	25.6%	20.6%	35.8%	22.9%
Diabetes	13.9%	8.7%	24.4%	35.0%

Those in the NHANES III sample who were older than 20 years and not pregnant, but were excluded because they were missing bioelectrical impedance of body index measurement.

In the complete sample, adjusted for age, sex, educational level (both as a continuous and categorical variable) and race/ethnicity, sarcopenia (without obesity) was significantly associated with increased HOMA-IR and pre-diabetes, but not with dysglycemia or diabetes outcomes, and in particular there was a marginally significant association with decreased risk of DM (Table 2). In contrast, obesity with and without sarcopenia was associated positively with all four outcomes. However, consistent with our

TABLE 2: Associations of insulin resistance and dysglycemia with sarcopenia, obesity, and sarcopenic obesity, adjusted for age, sex, race, and education.

Outcomes: Effect size	Insulin resistance HOMA-IR ratio[1] (95% CI) p value	Glycosylated hemoglobin HbA1C ratio[2] (95% CI) p value	Pre-diabetes odds ratio[3] (95% CI) p value	Diabetes odds ratio (95% CI) p value
Sarcopenia without obesity	1.39 (1.26 – 1.52) $p < 0.0001$	1.00 (0.97 – 1.02) $p = 0.7$	1.43 (1.02 – 2.01) $p = 0.04$	0.78 (0.50 – 1.23) $p = 0.3$
Obesity without sarcopenia	1.84 (1.80 – 1.89) $p < 0.0001$	1.054 (1.048 – 1.061) $p < 0.0001$	1.44 (1.30 – 1.59) $p < 0.0001$	2.44 (2.16 – 2.76 $p < 0.0001$
Sarcopenic obesity	2.13 (2.02 – 2.23) $p < 0.0001$	1.075 (1.061 – 1.088) $p < 0.0001$	1.46 (1.21 – 1.75) $p < 0.0001$	2.81 (2.30 – 3.43) $p < 0.0001$
Sarcopenia without opesity—diabetics excluded	1.37 (1.26 – 1.50) $p < 0.0001$	1.00 (0.99 – 1.02) $p = 0.6$		
Obesity without sarcopenia—diabetics excluded	1.75 (1.71 – 1.79) $p < 0.0001$	1.025 (1.021 – 1.029) $p < 0.0001$		
Sarcopenic obesity—diabetics excluded	1.99 (1.89 – 2.08) $p < 0.0001$	1.035 (1.027 – 1.044) $p < 0.0001$		

[1]*Ratio of HOMA IR in sarcopenic obese group to HOMA IR in reference group (neither sarcopenic nor obese) where HOMA IR is the Homeostatic Model Assessment of Insulin Resistence.*

[2]*Ratio of HbA1C in sacropenic obese group to HbA1C in reference group (neither sarcopenic nor obese) where HbA1C is the blood level of glycosylated hemoglobin.*

[3]*Pre-diabetes is defined as 1) HbA1C $\geq$ 6% but $<$ 6.5%, OR fasting glucose $\geq$ 5.5 but $<$7 mmol/L, 2) no self-reported DM, and 3) absence of DM medications*

main hypothesis, participants with sarcopenic obesity had significantly higher index of insulin resistance (HOMA-IR ratio 1.16, 95% CI 1.12 to 1.18, $p<0.001$) and chronic hyperglycemia (HbA1C ratio 1.021, 95%% CI 1.011 to 1.043, $p = 0.002$) than obese, non-sarcopenic participants, but they did not have higher prevalence of pre-diabetes and DM. This pattern of associations was essentially unchanged when diabetics were excluded to reduce confounding by reverse causation (i.e. diabetes leading to sarcopenia or obesity)—See Table 2.

In interaction testing, age (dichotomized at 60 years) modified effects of sarcopenia and obesity (Table 3). All interactions between gender and sarcopenia/obesity were non significant at the 0.1 level (data not shown).

TABLE 3: P values for interactions of age (<60 years vs. ≥60 years) with sarcopenia, obesity, and sarcopenic obesity in models adjusted for age, sex, race, and education.

Outcomes: Effect size	Insulin resistance HOMA-IR ratio	Glycosylated hemoglobin HbA1C ratio	Pre-diabetes odds ratio	Diabetes odds ratio
Sarcopenia without obesity	0.13	0.01	0.4	0.07
Obesity without sarcopenia	<0.0001	0.3	0.003	0.04
Sarcopenic obesity	<0.0001	<0.0001	0.04	0.0005
Sarcopenia without opesity—diabetics excluded	0.2	0.3		
Obesity without sarcopenia—diabetics excluded	<0.0001	0.6		
Sarcopenic obesity—diabetics excluded	<0.0001	<0.0001		

In age-stratified analyses, associations with insulin resistance and dysglycemia were stronger in the younger group (See Tables 4 and 5). In those under 60 years of age, sarcopenia without obesity was associated with higher HOMA-IR and HbA1C, but not with pre-diabetes and DM prevalence (see Table 4). However, the odds ratio confidence intervals for the latter two outcomes were unusually wide, which may reflect reduced power due to the small number of sarcopenic non-obese participants in the younger age group. In comparison to obese, non-sarcopenic participants, younger participants with sarcopenic obesity had significantly higher HOMA-IR (HOMA-IR (ratio 1.26, 95% CI 1.22 to 1.31, $p = <.0001$), higher HbA1C (ratio 1.054, 95% CI 1.032 to 1.062, $p <.0001$), and higher prevalence of DM (odds ratio 1.54, 95% CI 1.44 to 1.65, $p = <.0001$).

TABLE 4: Associations of insulin resistance and dysglycemia with sarcopenia, obesity, and sarcopenic obesity, in adults younger than 60 years, adjusted for age, sex, race, and education.

Outcomes: Effect size	Insulin resistance HOMA-IR ratio[1] (95% CI) p value	Glycosylated hemo-globin HbA1C ratio[2] (95% CI) p value	Pre-diabetes odds ratio[3] (95% CI) p value	Diabetes odds ratio (95% CI) p value
Sarcopenia without obesity	1.67 (1.27 – 2.20) $p = 0.0003$	1.086 (1.024 – 1.155) $p = 0.02$	0.77 (0.21 – 2.79) $p = 0.7$	2.39 (0.64 – 8.96) $p = 0.2$
Obesity without sarcopenia	1.90 (1.84 – 1.95) $p < 0.0001$	1.053 (1.045 – 1.060) $p < 0.0001$	1.62 (1.43 – 1.84) $p < 0.0001$	2.73 (2.30 – 3.24 $p < 0.0001$
Sarcopenic obesity	2.39 (2.24 – 2.55) $p < 0.0001$	1.10 (1.09 – 1.12) $p < 0.0001$	1.81 (1.39 – 2.36) $p < 0.0001$	4.20 (3.31 – 5.34) $p < 0.0001$
Sarcopenia without opesity—diabetics excluded	1.58 (1.20 – 2.06) $p < 0.001$	1.033 (0.983 – 1.081) $p = 0.2$		
Obesity without sarcopenia—diabetics excluded	1.80 (1.75 – 1.85) $p < 0.0001$	1.026 (1.021 – 1.030) $p < 0.0001$		
Sarcopenic obesity—diabetics excluded	2.20 (2.06 – 2.35) $p < 0.0001$	1.051 (1.039 – 1.063) $p < 0.0001$		

[1]*Ratio of HOMA IR in sarcopenic obese group to HOMA IR in reference group (neither sarcopenic nor obese) where HOMA IR is the Homeostatic Model Assessment of Insulin Resistence.*

[2]*Ratio of HbA1C in sacropenic obese group to HbA1C in reference group (neither sarcopenic nor obese) where HbA1C is the blood level of glycosylated hemoglobin.*

[3]*Pre-diabetes is defined as 1) HbA1C ≥ 6% but < 6.5%, OR fasting glucose ≥ 5.5 but < 7 mmol/L, 2) no self-reported DM, and 3) absence of DM medications*

Table 5. Associations of insulin resistance and dysglycemia with sarcopenia, obesity, and sarcopenic obesity, in adults 60 years or older, adjusted for age, sex, race, and education.

Outcomes: Effect size	Insulin resistance HOMA-IR ratio[1] (95% CI) p value	Glycosylated hemoglobin HbA1C ratio[2] (95% CI) p value	Pre-diabetes odds ratio[3] (95% CI) p value	Diabetes odds ratio (95% CI) p value
Sarcopenia without obesity	1.34 (1.20 – 1.49) $p < 0.0001$	0.99 (0.96 – 1.02) $p = 0.3$	1.50 (1.05 – 2.14) $p = 0.03$	0.71 (0.44 – 1.16) $p = 0.2$
Obesity without sarcopenia	1.70 (1.61 – 1.79) $p < 0.0001$	1.062 (1.041 – 1.073) $p < 0.0001$	1.12 (0.94 – 1.33) $p = 0.2$	2.09 (1.74 – 2.51) $p < 0.0001$
Sarcopenic obesity	1.86 (1.73 – 2.00) $p < 0.0001$	1.042 (1.021 – 1.054) $p < 0.0001$	1.16 (0.90 – 1.49) $p = 0.25$	2.10 (1.62 – 2.73) $p < 0.0001$
Sarcopenia without opesity—diabetics excluded	1.33 (1.21 – 1.46) $p < 0.0001$	1.00 (0.99 – 1.02) $p = 0.96$		
Obesity without sarcopenia—diabetics excluded	1.60 (1.52 – 1.67) $p < 0.0001$	1.021 (1.011 – 1.034) $p < 0.0001$		
Sarcopenic obesity—diabetics excluded	1.74 (1.67 – 1.87) $p < 0.0001$	1.012 (1.001 – 1.033) $p < 0.001$		

[1]*Ratio of HOMA IR in sarcopenic obese group to HOMA IR in reference group (neither sarcopenic nor obese) where HOMA IR is the Homeostatic Model Assessment of Insulin Resistence.*

[2]*Ratio of HbA1C in sacropenic obese group to HbA1C in reference group (neither sarcopenic nor obese) where HbA1C is the blood level of glycosylated hemoglobin.*

[3]*Pre-diabetes is defined as 1) HbA1C ≥ 6% but < 6.5%, OR fasting glucose ≥ 5.5 but <7 mmol/L, 2) no self-reported DM, and 3) absence of DM medications*

In contrast, in those 60 years and older, sarcopenia without obesity was associated with higher HOMA-IR and higher prevalence of pre-diabetes but not with HbA1c or prevalence of DM (see Table 5). Moreover, although sarcopenic obesity (compared to the non-sarcopenic, non-obese referent) was significantly associated with HOMA-IR, HBA1C, and DM outcomes, older sarcopenic obese individuals did not significantly differ in any of the outcomes from older obese, non-sarcopenic individuals.

To determine whether sarcopenia/obesity associations with inflammation in the two age groups are in concordance with their associations with insulin resistance and dysglycemia, we examined log CRP as outcome in parallel linear regression models. In those under 60 years of age, sarcopenia was independently associated with increased CRP in both non-obese (CRP ratio 1.13, 95% CI 1.01 to 1.30, $p = 0.02$) and obese individuals (CRP ratio 1.093, 95% CI 1.041 to 1.143, $p = 0.002$). In those 60 years or older, sarcopenia was not independently associated with increased CRP in either obese individuals (CRP ratio 1.052, 95% CI 0.991 to 1.111, $p = 0.1$) or in non-obese older adults (CRP ratio 1.00, 95% CI 0.92 to 1.08, $p = 0.99$), mirroring the pattern of sarcopenia associations with pre-diabetes and diabetes.

8.4 DISCUSSION

As hypothesized, sarcopenic obesity was strongly associated with increased insulin resistance and dysglycemia. In addition, sarcopenia was associated with increased insulin resistance in both non-obese and obese individuals, and also associated with higher levels of HbA1C in obese individuals. Thus, sarcopenic obese individuals had significantly higher HOMA-IR and HbA1C levels than obese individuals without sarcopenia, confirming our hypothesis that the combination of sarcopenia and obesity leads to more severe insulin resistance and dysglycemia.

However, there were important differences in the effect of combined sarcopenia and obesity, by age. In those under 60 years of age, sarcopenia was strongly associated with more insulin resistance and higher HbA1C levels in both non-obese and obese individuals, and also associated with higher prevalence of diabetes in obese individuals. Thus, the younger sarcopenic obese individuals had significantly and markedly higher HOMA-IR and HbA1C levels and diabetes prevalence than younger obese individuals without sarcopenia. On the other hand, in those 60 years or older, although sarcopenia was associated with increased insulin resistance in both non-obese and obese individuals, sarcopenia did not add to the risk of insulin resistance or dysglycemia in obese older adults.

This marked age difference in the metabolic effect of sarcopenia is likely to be the result of differences in the etiology of sarcopenia in young compared with old individuals. While sarcopenia in young and middle-aged adults likely reflects reduced accumulation of skeletal muscle mass over the life course, in older individuals sarcopenia results from a combination of inadequate muscle mass accumulation when younger and reduction in muscle mass from peak levels when older. Skeletal muscle is a primary tissue responsible for insulin-mediated glucose disposal; thus in sarcopenia, the lower total mass of muscle should cause diminished insulin-mediated glucose disposal, independent of obesity. However, type II muscle fibers, which are less responsive to the metabolic actions of insulin [21], are lost to a greater extent than type I fibers in age-related muscle atrophy [10]. Thus sarcopenia due to age-related muscle atrophy could mean increased insulin sensitivity and more efficient glucose disposal [11]. This might explain the observed lack of association between sarcopenia and diabetes in non-obese older adults. However, decrease in type II muscle fibers has not been shown to improve overall myocellular insulin action in post-menopausal women [11] and to the contrary, recent reports show that increased type II fiber population improves glucose disposal in mice [7]. The role of fiber type distribution in age-induced insulin resistance remains controversial. In obese older adults however, there is greater lipid content within skeletal muscle [22], which is associated with diminished muscle insulin sensitivity [23]; this might in part, explain why sarcopenia did not confer protection from dysglycemia and diabetes in obese older adults (unlike in non-obese older adults). Further work is needed to illuminate the roles of fiber type distribution and intramyocellular lipid accumulation in age-related insulin resistance and diabetes.

Chronic low-grade inflammation is now recognized as a central mediator of obesity-associated insulin resistance [24]. Genetic and pharmacologic inhibition of inflammatory mediators is shown to prevent diet- and obesity-induced insulin resistance as well as prevent accelerated loss of muscle mass with age [25]. Our data also suggest that in young and middle-aged individuals (both obese and non-obese) sarcopenia is associated with greater inflammation (higher levels of serum CRP). This association was not seen in non-obese older adults. This pattern mirrors the strong association of sarcopenia with insulin resistance and dysglycemia in young adults, in contrast to the weaker association in older adults, suggesting that inflammation may have a role in the development of metabolic complications from sarcopenia.

Our study had some important limitations. The cross-sectional nature of the study limits our ability to draw causal inferences from the relationships observed. For instance, it is possible that diabetes and dysglycemia lead to sarcopenia and sarcopenic obesity. However, the strength of the observed associations and their persistence after exclusion of individuals with type 2 diabetes, bolster the case for sarcopenia and sarcopenic obesity causing insulin resistance and dysglycemia. Secondly, as NHANES III was conducted among the non-institutionalized U.S. population, and because participants who were physically unable to attend the mobile examination center were not included in our analysis, we may have underestimated the prevalence of sarcopenia. Finally, we used BI to estimate muscle mass, which may have led to some individuals being erroneously classified in or out of the sarcopenic obese category. However, such misclassification errors would only have weakened associations between sarcopenic obesity and insulin resistance or dysglycemia.

In conclusion, this large national study found that sarcopenic obesity, to a greater extent than sarcopenia or obesity alone, is strongly associated with insulin resistance in both young and old adults, underscoring the important role of low muscle mass as an independent risk factor for metabolic disease. In those under 60 years of age, sarcopenia also increased the risk of dysglycemia, in both non-obese and obese individuals. In young as well as in old adults, sarcopenia was also much more prevalent in obese than in non-obese individuals. With the ongoing obesity epidemic in the U.S. and the disturbing increases in the incidence of obesity in children and young adults, our data suggest that we can expect to see sharp increases in sarcopenia and diabetes in the coming years. In this environment, interventions aimed at increasing muscle mass in younger ages and preventing loss of muscle mass in older ages may have the potential to reduce type 2 diabetes risk. Further research is required to understand the pathophysiology and metabolic basis of the associations documented here, as well as to develop effective means of preventing sarcopenic obesity and its metabolic consequences.

REFERENCES

1. Davison KK, Ford ES, Cogswell ME, Dietz WH (2002) Percentage of body fat and body mass index are associated with mobility limitations in people aged 70 and older from NHANES III. J Am Geriatr Soc 50: 1802–1809. doi: 10.1046/j.1532-5415.2002.50508.x.
2. Baumgartner RN, Stauber PM, Koehler KM, Romero L, Garry PJ (1996) Associations of fat and muscle masses with bone mineral in elderly men and women. Am J Clin Nutr 63: 365–372.
3. Roubenoff R (2001) Origins and clinical relevance of sarcopenia. Can J Appl Physiol 26: 78–89. doi: 10.1139/h01-006.
4. Guo ZK (2007) Intramyocellular lipid kinetics and insulin resistance. Lipids Health Dis 6: 18. doi: 10.1186/1476-511X-6-18.
5. Walsh K (2009) Adipokines, myokines and cardiovascular disease. Circ J 73: 13–18. doi: 10.1253/circj.CJ-08-0961.
6. Pedersen BK (2010) Muscle-to-fat interaction: a two-way street? J Physiol 588 (Pt 1): 21. doi: 10.1113/jphysiol.2009.184747.
7. Izumiya Y, Hopkins T, Morris C, Sato K, Zeng L, et al. (2008) Fast/Glycolytic muscle fiber growth reduces fat mass and improves metabolic parameters in obese mice. Cell Metab 7: 159–172. doi: 10.1016/j.cmet.2007.11.003.
8. Stephen WC, Janssen I (2009) Sarcopenic-obesity and cardiovascular disease risk in the elderly. J Nutr Health Aging 13: 460–466. doi: 10.1007/s12603-009-0084-z.
9. Tanner CJ, Barakat HA, Dohm GL, Pories WJ, MacDonald KG, et al. (2002) Muscle fiber type is associated with obesity and weight loss. Am J Physiol Endocrinol Metab 282: E1191–1196.
10. Doherty TJ (2003) Invited review: Aging and sarcopenia. J Appl Physiol 95: 1717–1727.
11. Aubertin-Leheudre M, Lord C, Goulet ED, Khalil A, Dionne IJ (2006) Effect of sarcopenia on cardiovascular disease risk factors in obese postmenopausal women. Obesity (Silver Spring) 14: 2277–2283. doi: 10.1038/oby.2006.267.
12. Nagi S (1976) An epidemiology of disability among adults in the United States. Milbank Memorial Fund Quarterly 6: 493–508. doi: 10.2307/3349677.

13. NCHS (National Center for Health Statistics) (1996) Third National Health and Nutrition Examination Survey (NHANES III), 1988-1994: NHANES III Examination Data File Documentation. Hyattsville MD: US Department of Health and Human services Press.
14. Chumlea WC, Guo SS, Kuczmarski RJ, Flegal KM, Johnson CL, et al. (2002) Body composition estimates from NHANES III bioelectrical impedance data. Int J Obes Relat Metab Disord 26: 1596–1609. doi: 10.1038/sj.ijo.0802167.
15. Janssen I, Heymsfield SB, Baumgartner RN, Ross R (2000) Estimation of skeletal muscle mass by bioelectrical impedance analysis. J Appl Physiol 89: 465–471.
16. WHO Study Group (1994) Assessment of fracture risk and its application to screening for postmenopausal osteoporosis. World Health Organ Tech Rep Ser 843: 1–129.
17. Janssen I, Heymsfield SB, Ross R (2002) Low relative skeletal muscle mass (sarcopenia) in older persons is associated with functional impairment and physical disability. J Am Geriatr Soc 50: 889–896. doi: 10.1046/j.1532-5415.2002.50216.x.
18. Wallace TM, Levy JC, Matthews DR (2004) Use and abuse of HOMA modeling. Diabetes Care 27: 1487–1495. doi: 10.2337/diacare.27.6.1487.
19. Carson AP, Reynolds K, Fonseca VA, Muntner P (2009) Comparison of A1C and Fasting Glucose Criteria to Diagnose Diabetes among U.S. Adults. Diabetes Care 33(1): 95–7. doi: 10.2337/dc09-1227.
20. National Center for Health Statistics (1994) Plan and Operation of the Third National Health and Nutrition Examination Survey, 1988–94. Bethesda, MD: Centers for Disease Control and Prevention Press.
21. Nader GA, Esser KA (2001) Intracellular signaling specificity in skeletal muscle in response to different modes of exercise. J Appl Physiol 90: 1936–1942.
22. Goodpaster BH, Theriault R, Watkins SC, Kelley DE (2000) Intramuscular lipid content is increased in obesity and decreased by weight loss. Metabolism 49: 467–472. doi: 10.1016/S0026-0495(00)80010-4.
23. Petersen KF, Befroy D, Dufour S, Dziura J, Ariyan C, et al. (2003) Mitochondrial dysfunction in the elderly: possible role in insulin resistance. Science 300: 1140–1142. doi: 10.1126/science.1082889.
24. Theuma P, Fonseca VA (2004) Inflammation, insulin resistance, and atherosclerosis. Metab Syndr Relat Disord 2: 105–113.
25. Novak ML, Billich W, Smith SM, Sukhija KB, McLoughlin TJ, et al. (2009) COX-2 inhibitor reduces skeletal muscle hypertrophy in mice. Am J Physiol Regul Integr Comp Physiol 296: R1132–1139. doi: 10.1152/ajpregu.90874.2008.

CHAPTER 9

PREVALENCE OF OBESITY AND ASSOCIATED CARDIOVASCULAR RISK: THE DARIOS STUDY

FRANCISCO JAVIER FÉLIX-REDONDO, MARHA GRAU, JOSÉ MIGUEL BAENA-DHEZ, IRENE R. DÉGANO, ANTONIO CABRERA DE LEÓN, MARIA JESÚS GUEMBE, MARHA TERESA ALZAMORA, TOMÁS VEGA-ALONSO, NICOLÁS R ROBLES, HONORATO ORTIZ, FERNANDO RIGO, EDUARDO MAYORAL-SANCHEZ, MARIA JOSÉ TORMO, ANTONIO SEGURA-FRAGOSO, AND DANIEL FERNÁNDEZ-BERGÉS

9.1 BACKGROUND

Cardiovascular diseases are the leading cause of death worldwide [1]. However, the decreasing trend observed in population cardiovascular mortality in recent years has been explained by changes in the prevention and control of cardiovascular risk factors and by the use of more effective medical and surgical treatments [2]. The increasing prevalence of obesity recently observed in Spain may have diluted to some extent the effect of other cardiovascular risk factors control to decrease coronary disease deaths [3-6].

The available evidence indicates that general obesity, measured with body mass index, and abdominal obesity, whether measured with waist circumference only or waist circumference corrected with height, are associated with coronary disease risk and mortality [7-10].

The prevalence of general and abdominal obesity has been recently studied in a national sample of Spanish general (>18 years) and elderly (≥65 years) population [11,12] and in regional samples [13-18]. However, the association of both types of obesity with the 10-year coronary disease risk estimated with the Framingham-REGICOR risk functions validated for the Spanish population [19] has not been studied in depth. The knowledge of this association may help to elucidate the excess risk presented by the population with overweight, general and abdominal obesity compared with the general population. This association may be particularly important in individuals aged 35 to 74 years, in whom the strategies of primary prevention of cardiovascular disease seem to be more effective [20].

The aims of this study are: (1) to estimate in the Spanish population aged 35 to 74 years the prevalence of overweight, general and abdominal obesity and (2) to estimate their association with cardiovascular risk factors and 10-year coronary disease risk as measured with the Framingham-REGICOR risk functions.

9.2 METHODS

9.2.1 STUDY POPULATION

Pooled analysis with individual data from 11 population-based studies conducted in 10 geographical areas of Spain since 2000 with similar methodological designs. The methodology has been described elsewhere [21]. Briefly, participants were 35 to 74 years old and gave written informed consent to take part in the component studies. The DARIOS study (Dyslipemia, Atherosclerotic Risk, Increased high sensitivity C-reactive protein, and inflammatory and Oxidative status in Spanish population) was approved by the Municipal Healthcare Institute's Clinical Research Ethics Committee (authorization nº 2009/3640).

9.2.2 ANTHROPOMETRIC MEASUREMENTS

Waist circumference (WC), weight and height were measured with participants in underwear and barefoot. Body mass index (BMI) was determined as weight divided by squared height (kg/m^2) and waist-to-height ratio (WHtR) as waist circumference (cm) divided by height (cm). All participants were classified according to BMI: (1) normal weight, BMI <25 kg/m^2; (2) overweight, BMI 25–29.9 kg/m^2; and (3) general obesity, BMI ≥30 kg/m^2; according to WC: (1) optimal, WC<94 cm in men and <80 cm in women(2) suboptimal, WC 94–102 cm in men and WC 80–88 cm in women; and (3) abdominal obesity, WC ≥102 cm in men and WC ≥88 cm in women [22,23]; and according to WHtR: (1) <0.5 and (2) ≥0.5 [24,25].

9.2.3 OTHER MEASUREMENTS

Standardized questionnaires were used to collect sociodemographic and lifestyle variables, and the previous history of cardiovascular disease (coronary artery disease and stroke) and treatments for diabetes, hypertension and hypercholesterolemia. Current smoking was defined as actively smoking within the preceding year.

Prevalence of hypertension, diabetes and hypercholesterolemia was considered if the participant had been diagnosed, was treated for these disorders or presented with systolic blood pressure ≥140 mmHg or diastolic blood pressure ≥90 mmHg, glycaemia≥126 mg/dl or total cholesterol ≥240 mg/dl, respectively.

Blood pressure was measured with a periodically calibrated sphygmomanometer. A cuff adapted to upper arm perimeter (young, adult, obese) was selected for each participant. Measurements were performed in a seated position after a 5-minute rest. Two measurements were taken and the mean value was recorded for the study.

Blood samples were taken following >10 h fast. Analysis was performed in local laboratories on fresh blood or aliquots of serum stored at −80°C in samples not previously thawed. Triglycerides, glucose, total and high-density lipoprotein (HDL) cholesterol were measured using standard methods. When triglycerides were <300 mg/dL, low density lipoprotein (LDL) cholesterol was calculated using the Friedewald formula. Analysis of concordance of lipid profile results using a reference laboratory was performed to correct the few deviations observed [21].

Cardiovascular risk in all participants aged 35 to 74 years with no history of cardiovascular disease was calculated with the REGICOR function adapted from the original Framingham function and validated for the Spanish population [19].

9.2.4 STATISTICAL ANALYSIS

The mean value of BMI, WC and WHtR and the prevalence of the corresponding categories were calculated by sex, standardized for the European age distribution [26] and accompanied by the 95% confidence interval.

We summarized the baseline characteristics in three groups based on categories of BMI (i.e. normal weight, overweight and general obesity), WC (optimal, suboptimal and abdominal obesity) and WHtR (<0.5 and ≥0.5), using percentages for categorical data, means and standard deviations for normally distributed data, and median and interquartile range when the distribution departed from normal (e.g., glycaemia and triglycerides). We tested for differences and linear trend using Student t test, U-Mann Whitney and χ^2 as appropriate.

To determine whether the associations found between BMI, WC and WHtR categories, and between cardiovascular risk factors and coronary risk were independent of age, we fitted multinomial logistic regression models adjusted for age.

Statistical analysis was done with R Statistical Package (R Foundation for Statistical Computing, Vienna, Austria; Version 2.15.0).

9.3 RESULTS

The study enrolled 28,887 participants from 11 epidemiological studies from 10 autonomous communities. Table 1 presents the mean BMI, WC and WHtR and the prevalence of general and abdominal obesity standardized to the European population. The prevalence in each component study of DARIOS is shown in Additional file 1: Tables S1 and S2.

The prevalence of cardiovascular risk factors significantly increased with BMI category (normal weight, overweight, general obesity), except for smoking and HDL cholesterol, which significantly decreased in both men and women (Table 2). Similar results were found when we compared the prevalence of risk factors in different WC categories (Table 3) and WHtR (Additional file 1: Table S3).

Overweight, suboptimal WC, general and abdominal obesity and high WHtR were associated with diabetes, hypertension, hypercholesterolemia and coronary risk independently of age in both sexes. The magnitude of these associations was higher in women than in men in all instances, except for hypercholesterolemia and the suboptimal WC category, which were higher in men (Tables 4, 5 and 6).

TABLE 1: Mean and distribution by categories of body mass index and waist circumference for men and women, standardized to the European population

	Men N=13,425	Women N=15,462
BMI (kg/m^2), mean (95% CI)	28.1 (28.0-28.1)	27.5 (27.5-27.6)
BMI categories, summarized,% (95% CI)		
Normal weight (<25)	21.3 (20.6-22.1)	36.1 (35.4-36.8)
Overweight (25–29.9)	50.7 (49.8-51.5)	35.6 (34.9-36.4)
General obesity (≥30)	28.0 (27.2-28.8)	28.3 (27.6-29)
Waist circumference (cm), mean	98.2 (98.0-98.4)	90.2 (90.0-90.4)
Waist circumference categories, summarized, % (95% CI)		
Men <94 cm; Women <80 cm	33.8 (32.9-34.7)	23.5 (22.8-24.2)
Men ≥94 and <102 cm; Women ≥80 and <88 cm	30.4 (29.6-31.3)	21.9 (21.2-22.6)
Men ≥102 cm; Women ≥88 cm	35.8 (34.9-36.7)	54.6 (53.8-55.4)
Waist-to-height ratio, mean	0.59 (0.58-0.60)	0.57 (0.57-0.58)
Waist-to-height ratio ≥0.5,% (95% CI)	89.1 (88.5-89.7)	77.3 (76.6-78.0)

ATPIII, Adult Treatment Panel III, BMI body mass index, CI confidence interval.

TABLE 2: Population baseline characteristics by sex and body mass index category

Men	Normal weight N=2,760	Overweight N=6,810	Obesity N=3,801	p-value	p for linear trend
Age, years, mean (SD)	51 (12)	54 (11)	55 (11)	<0.001	<0.001
Current smoker	1138 (41.2%)	2089 (30.7%)	1094 (28.8%)	<0.001	<0.001
Systolic blood pressure, mean (SD)	127 (18)	134 (18)	139 (18)	<0.001	<0.001
Diastolic blood pressure, mean (SD)	77 (10)	81 (10)	84 (11)	<0.001	<0.001
Hypertension	861 (31.4%)	3389 (50.0%)	2594 (68.4%)	<0.001	<0.001
Glycaemia, median [IQR]	93 [87–101]	98 [90–108]	103 [94–118]	<0.001	<0.001
Diabetes	239 (8.7%)	1066 (15.7%)	965 (25.5%)	<0.001	<0.001
Total cholesterol, mean (SD)	210 (38)	215 (39)	215 (40)	<0.001	<0.001
HDL cholesterol, mean (SD)	53 (12)	49 (11)	46 (10)	<0.001	<0.001
LDL cholesterol, mean (SD)	135 (34)	140 (35)	138 (34)	<0.001	0.004
Triglycerides, median [IQR]	96 [74–131]	114 [86–158]	134 [99–192]	<0.001	<0.001
Hypercholesterolemia	1016 (37.1%)	3204 (47.4%)	1975 (52.3%)	<0.001	<0.001
History of CV disease	121 (4.5%)	446 (6.8%)	338 (9.2%)	<0.001	<0.001
Waist circumference, mean (SD)	87 (7)	97 (7)	110 (9)	<0.001	<0.001
Waist-to-height ratio, mean (SD)	0.51 (0.05)	0.57 (0.04)	0.65 (0.05)	<0.001	<0.001
10-year CAD risk, median [IQR]	2.8 [1.5-5.2]	4.0 [2.3-7.1]	5.2 [3.0-8.3]	<0.001	<0.001
10-year CAD risk ≥10%	166 (6.6%)	716 (11.9%)	551 (16.7%)	<0.001	<0.001

TABLE 2: *Cont.*

Women	Normal weight N=5,244	Overweight N=5,557	Obesity N=4,571	p-value	p for linear trend
Age, years, mean (SD)	48 (10)	55 (11)	57 (10)	<0.001	<0.001
Current smoker	1546 (29.5%)	955 (17.2%)	481 (10.5%)	<0.001	<0.001
Systolic blood pressure, mean (SD)	117 (18)	128 (20)	137 (20)	<0.001	<0.001
Diastolic blood pressure, mean (SD)	73 (10)	78 (10)	82 (10)	<0.001	<0.001
Hypertension, (%)	1001 (19.2%)	2391 (43.3%)	3035 (66.6)	<0.001	<0.001
Glycaemia, median [IQR]	89 [83–95]	92 [86–101]	98 [90–111]	<0.001	<0.001
Diabetes	242 (4.6%)	572 (10.3%)	982 (21.6%)	<0.001	<0.001
Total cholesterol, mean (SD)	209 (38)	218 (39)	218 (38)	<0.001	<0.001
HDL cholesterol, mean (SD)	61 (13)	57 (13)	54 (12)	<0.001	<0.001
LDL cholesterol, mean (SD)	131 (34)	140 (34)	139 (34)	<0.001	<0.001
Triglycerides, median [IQR]	78 [62–101]	96 [73–128]	117 [88–157]	<0.001	<0.001
Hypercholesterolemia	1821 (35.0%)	2610 (47.3%)	2383 (52.5%)	<0.001	<0.001
History of CV disease	108 (2.1%)	211 (4.0%)	239 (5.4%)	<0.001	<0.001
Waist circumference, mean (SD)	79 (9)	90 (8)	104 (10)	<0.001	<0.001
Waist-to-height ratio, mean (SD)	0.49 (0.06)	0.58 (0.06)	0.67 (0.07)	<0.001	<0.001
10-year CAD risk, median [IQR]	1.2 [0.5-2.3]	2.4 [1.3-3.9]	3.5 [2.1-5.3]	<0.001	<0.001
10-year CAD risk ≥10%	24 (0.5%)	83 (1.6%)	185 (4.5%)	<0.001	<0.001

CAD Coronary artery disease, CV Cardiovascular, HDL High-density Lipoprotein, IQR Interquartile Range, LDL Low-density lipoprotein, SD Standard Deviation.

TABLE 3: Baseline characteristics by sex and categories of waist circumference

Men	Waist circumference				
	<94 cm N=3,702	≥94 and <102 cm N=3,473	≥102 cm N=4,215	p-value	p for linear trend
Age, mean (SD)	50 (11)	54 (11)	56 (11)	<0.001	<0.001
Current smoker	1406 (38.0%)	1035 (29.8%)	1280 (30.4%)	<0.001	<0.001
Systolic blood pressure, mean (SD)	128 (17)	134 (18)	140 (18)	<0.001	<0.001
Diastolic blood pressure, mean (SD)	78 (10)	81 (10)	84 (11)	<0.001	<0.001
Hypertension	1219 (33.1%)	1764 (51.0%)	2894 (68.8%)	<0.001	<0.001
Glycaemia (mg/dl), median [IQR]	94 [88–102]	99 [91–109]	103 [93–117]	<0.001	<0.001
Diabetes	330 (8.9%)	539 (15.6%)	1038 (24.8%)	<0.001	<0.001
Total cholesterol (mg/dl), mean (SD)	212 (38)	217 (39)	214 (40)	<0.001	0.021
HDL cholesterol (mg/dl), mean (SD)	51 (12)	49 (10)	47 (10)	<0.001	<0.001
LDL cholesterol (mg/dl), mean (SD)	138 (34)	141 (34)	138 (34)	<0.001	0.884
Triglycerides (mg/dl), median [IQR]	102 [78–139]	120 [88–165]	132 [97–188]	<0.001	<0.001
Hypercholesterolemia	1438 (39.1%)	1710 (49.7%)	2181 (52.0%)	<0.001	<0.001
History of CV disease	150 (4.2%)	192 (5.8%)	402 (10.0%)	<0.001	<0.001
Body mass index (kg/m2), mean (SD)	24.7 (2.4)	27.7 (2.1)	31.7 (3.5)	<0.001	<0.001
Waist-to-height ratio, mean (SD)	0.51 (0.04)	0.58 (0.03)	0.65 (0.05)	<0.001	<0.001
10-year CAD risk, median [IQR]	2.8 [1.6-4.9]	4.1 [2.3-7.1]	5.4 [3.2-8.6]	<0.001	<0.001
10-year CAD risk ≥10%	184 (5.4%)	352 (11.4%)	650 (18.2%)	<0.001	<0.001
Women	<80 cm N=2,900	≥80 cm and <88 N=2,800	≥88 cm N=7,434	p-value	p for linear trend
Age, mean (SD)	46 (9)	51 (10)	57 (11)	<0.001	<0.001
Current smoker	918 (31.7%)	671 (24.0%)	1019 (13.7%)	<0.001	<0.001
Systolic blood pressure, mean (SD)	115 (16)	122 (19)	134 (20)	<0.001	<0.001

TABLE 3: *Cont.*

Women	<80 cm N=2,900	≥80 cm and <88 N=2,800	≥88 cm N=7,434	p-value	p for linear trend
Diastolic blood pressure, mean (SD)	72 (10)	75 (10)	80 (10)	<0.001	<0.001
Hypertension	465 (16.1%)	808 (29.0%)	4289 (57.9%)	<0.001	<0.001
Glycaemia (mg/dl), median [IQR]	88 [83–94]	90 [85–97]	96 [88–107]	<0.001	<0.001
Diabetes	87 (3.0%)	151 (5.4%)	1312 (17.8%)	<0.001	<0.001
Total cholesterol (mg/dl), mean (SD)	206 (36)	215 (37)	219 (38)	<0.001	<0.001
HDL cholesterol (mg/dl), mean (SD)	61 (13)	59 (12)	55 (12)	<0.001	<0.001
LDL cholesterol (mg/dl), mean (SD)	129 (32)	137 (33)	139 (34)	<0.001	<0.001
Triglycerides (mg/dl), median [IQR]	75 [60–95]	86 [68–114]	109 [82–149]	<0.001	<0.001
Hypercholesterolemia	881 (30.5%)	1163 (42.0%)	3807 (51.5%)	<0.001	<0.001
History of CV disease	69 (2.5%)	86 (3.2%)	326 (4.6%)	<0.001	<0.001
Body mass index (kg/m2), mean (SD)	22.7 (2.4)	25.3 (2.5)	30.9 (4.8)	<0.001	<0.001
Waist-to-height ratio, mean (SD)	0.46 (0.03)	0.53 (0.03)	0.64 (0.07)	<0.001	<0.001
10-year CAD risk, median [IQR]	0.9 [0.5-1.9]	1.7 [0.8-3.1]	3.1 [1.7-4.9]	<0.001	<0.001
10-year CAD risk ≥10%	9 (0.3%)	17 (0.7%)	229 (3.4%)	<0.001	<0.001

Abbreviation: CAD Coronary artery disease, CV Cardiovascular, HDL High-density Llipoprotein, IQR Interquartile range, LDL low-density lipoprotein, SD Standard deviation.

TABLE 4: Age-adjusted odds ratio of overweight and general obesity for cardiovascular risk factors by sex

	Overweight (BMI ≥25 and <30)				General obesity (BMI ≥30)			
	Men		Women		Men		Women	
	OR (CI 95%)	p-value	OR (CI 95%)	p-value	OR (CI 95%)	p-value	OR (CI 95%)	p-value
Age (1 year)	1.02 (1.02-1.03)	<0.001	1.06 (1.06-1.06)	<0.001	1.03 (1.03-1.04)	<0.001	1.09 (1.08-1.09)	<0.001
Diabetes	1.71 (1.47-1.99)	<0.001	2.53 (2.28-2.81)	<0.001	3.08 (2.64-3.60)	<0.001	2.95 (2.56-3.40)	<0.001
Hypertension	1.99 (1.81-2.21)	<0.001	2.10 (1.91-2.31)	<0.001	4.50 (4.02-5.04)	<0.001	5.20 (4.70-5.75)	<0.001
Hypercholesterolemia	1.45 (1.32-1.58)	<0.001	1.14 (1.05-1.24)	0.002	1.73 (1.57-1.92)	<0.001	1.22 (1.17-1.34)	<0.001
Coronary risk (1 percentage point)	1.11 (1.08-1.13)	<0.001	1.34 (1.30-1.39)	<0.001	1.18 (1.16-1.20)	<0.001	1.58 (1.53-1.63)	<0.001

Prevalence of hypertension, diabetes and hypercholesterolemia was considered if the participant was diagnosed, treated for these disorders or presented with systolic blood pressure ≥140 mmHg or diastolic blood pressure ≥90 mmHg, glycaemia≥126 mg/dl or total cholesterol ≥240 mg/dl, respectively.

TABLE 5: Age-adjusted odds ratio of suboptimal waist circumference and abdominal obesity for cardiovascular risk factors by sex

	Waist circumference							
	≥94 and <102 in men, and ≥80 and <88 in women				≥102 in men, and ≥88 in women			
	Men		Women		Men		Women	
	OR (CI 95%)	p-value	OR (CI 95%)	p-value	OR (CI 95%)	p-value	OR (CI 95%)	p-value
Age (1 year)	1.03 (1.03-1.04)	<0.001	1.05 (1.04-1.06)	<0.001	1.05 (1.05-1.06)	<0.001	1.10 (1.10-1.11)	<0.001
Diabetes	1.54 (1.32-1.79)	<0.001	1.36 (1.04-1.80)	<0.001	2.48 (2.17-2.85)	<0.001	3.86 (3.09-4.89)	<0.001
Hypertension	1.78 (1.60-1.97)	<0.001	1.45 (1.26-1.66)	<0.001	3.51 (3.18-3.88)	<0.001	3.61 (3.21-4.07)	<0.001
Hypercholesterolemia	1.42 (1.29-1.56)	<0.001	1.22 (1.08-1.37)	<0.001	1.50 (1.37-1.65)	<0.001	1.30 (1.17-1.44)	<0.001
Coronary risk (1 percentage point)	1.10 (1.07-1.12)	<0.001	1.34 (1.27-1.42)	<0.001	1.17 (1.15-1.19)	<0.001	1.71 (1.62-1.79)	<0.001

Prevalence of hypertension, diabetes and hypercholesterolemia was considered if the participant has been already diagnosed, was treated for these disorders or presented with systolic blood pressure ≥140 mmHg or diastolic blood pressure ≥90 mmHg, glycaemia ≥126 mg/dl or total cholesterol ≥240 mg/dl, respectively.

TABLE 6: Age-adjusted odds ratio of waist-to-height ratio ≥0.5 for cardiovascular risk factors by sex

	Waist-to-height ratio ≥0.5			
	Men		Women	
	OR (CI 95%)	p-value	OR (CI 95%)	p-value
Age (1 year)	1.08 (1.07-1.09)	<0.001	1.10 (1.10-1.11)	<0.001
Diabetes	2.72 (2.04-3.62)	<0.001	2.73 (2.16-3.44)	<0.001
Hypertension	2.94 (2.52-3.43)	<0.001	3.02 (2.66-3.42)	<0.001
Hypercholesterolemia	1.81 (1.58-2.08)	<0.001	1.36 (1.23-1.51)	<0.001
Coronary risk (1 percentage point)	1.27 (1.22-1.32)	<0.001	1.68 (1.59-1.77)	<0.001

Reference value: Waist-to-height ratio <0.5. Model adjusted for age.
Prevalence of hypertension, diabetes and hypercholesterolemia was considered if the participant had been diagnosed, was treated for these disorders or presented with systolic blood pressure ≥140 mmHg or diastolic blood pressure ≥90 mmHg, glycaemia≥126 mg/dl or total cholesterol ≥240 mg/dl, respectively.

In men, coronary risk was directly related to increased BMI in the WC<94 category but increased in parallel with WC for all BMI categories. Notably, the highest mean coronary risk (7.6%) was identified in men with abdominal obesity and normal weight; however, only 0.2% of the sample presented this phenotype. In women, coronary risk increased with both WC and BMI. On the other hand, the risk of all individuals with WHtR ≥0.5 increased in parallel with BMI. Those with WHtR <0.5 presented minimal differences in coronary risk across BMI categories (Figure 1).

9.4 DISCUSSION

The present study showed that almost 80% and 65% of Spanish men and women, respectively, weigh more than the recommended values for their height. Indeed, 28% of men and women presented general obesity, 36% of men and 55% of women presented abdominal obesity, and 89% of men and 77% of women have a WHtR ≥0.5. Our results also showed a significant association independent of age between the obesity measures and cardiovascular risk factors (e.g., diabetes, hypertension and hypercholesterolemia).

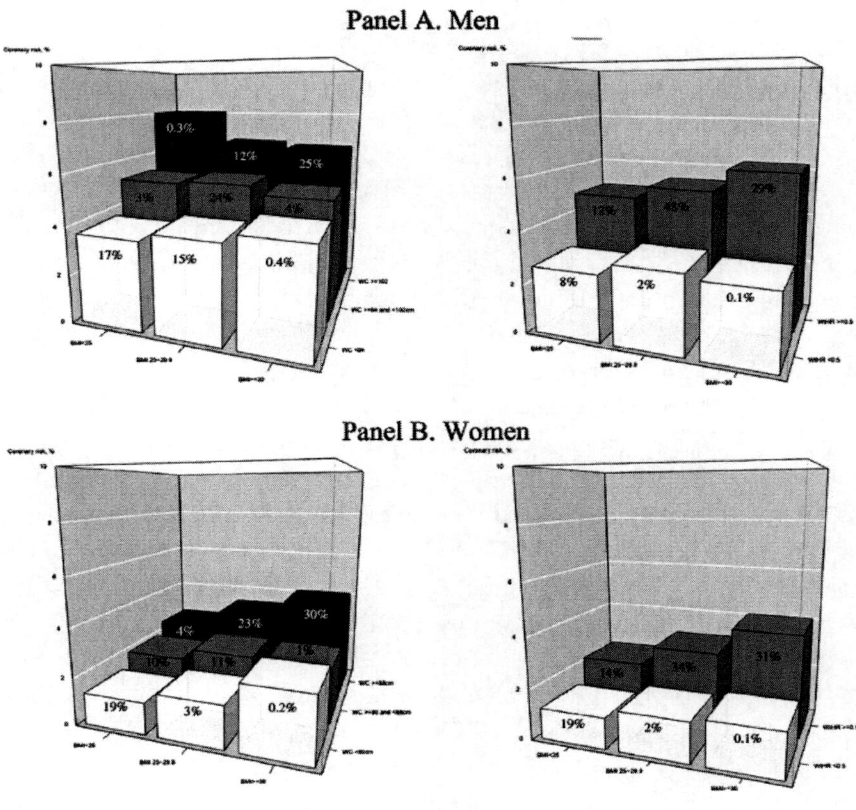

FIGURE 1: Coronary risk according to body mass index and waist circumference (left) and waist-to-height ratio (right) categories in men (Panel A) and in women (Panel B).

As a result, 10-year coronary disease risk significantly increased with the categories of BMI, WC and WHtR, which could indicate an important disease burden in coming years.

9.4.1 COMPARISON WITH PREVIOUS STUDIES

The main Spanish study on cardiovascular risk factors (DORICA study) conducted between 1990 and 2000 in individuals aged 25–60 years reported a general obesity prevalence of 13% in men and 18% in women [27], lower than the DARIOS results in data collected since 2000. This supports the increasing trend in the prevalence of obesity evidenced in other studies [2-5]. On the other hand, the prevalence of general and abdominal obesity was lower in the nationwide ENRICA Study conducted between 2008 and 2010 than in DARIOS. The age ranges of the populations studied (>18 years in ENRICA and 35–74 years in DARIOS) may account for these differences [11]. However, since 2004 two studies have reported age-specific prevalence of general obesity in the Spanish elderly population [28,29] that is similar to DARIOS results. Since age is one of the main determinants of obesity, the prevalence is likely to increase as the population ages dramatically in coming years. The high prevalence of WHtR ≥0.5 observed could be related to the threshold chosen, which has been internationally recommended [25]. However, a higher threshold (0.55) better discriminated cardiovascular risk in a population with high prevalence of obesity [18].

An international study by Doak et al. showed that Romanian men and Bulgarian women aged 25–64 years presented the lowest prevalence of obesity among European countries (10%). On the contrary, Scottish men and women presented the highest prevalence (28% and 26%, respectively) [30], similar to the DARIOS results. Finally, analysis of National Health and Nutrition Examination Survey (NHANES) data showed that the prevalence in the US is around 32% [31]. The authors attributed the differences to the socioeconomic context of the countries studied [30].

9.4.2 CARDIOVASCULAR RISK FACTORS, OBESITY AND SEX

Obesity is key in the development of hypertension and diabetes [32,33]. Indeed, both diseases were associated with general and abdominal obesity in the DARIOS data, independently of age. Hypercholesterolemia also showed a significant but weaker association, even though obese individuals in our sample presented the classical lipid disorder of hypertriglyceridemia and low HDL cholesterol [34].

In several population-based studies and a meta-analysis, the different measures of obesity were better discriminators and had a stronger association with cardiometabolic risk factors in women [10,18,24,25,35].

The sedentary lifestyle could be a possible cause, which is more prevalent in Spanish women than in men [36]. In addition, sex-related differences in fat distribution [37] and in eating behaviours [38] may play a key role. Further cohort studies are needed to ascertain sex-related differences in the use of these variables as predictors of cardiovascular events.

9.4.3 CARDIOVASCULAR RISK AND OBESITY

A recent study has shown improved coronary risk prediction in men if a general obesity diagnosis is included [39], and higher mortality has been associated with overweight, general and abdominal obesity in men [40]. In DARIOS results, the baseline coronary risk was higher in men, although 10-year coronary disease risk was strongly associated with overweight, general and abdominal obesity in women as well. Previous studies in Spain report that obesity did not increase the incidence of cardiovascular events; however, further cohort studies with longer follow-up are needed [41,42]. In the Framingham Heart Study, for instance, obesity was associated with increased relative risk for development of cardiovascular disease in a population aged 35–75 and followed for 44 years [43].

9.4.4 CORONARY RISK AND OBESITY TYPES

Finally, there is some controversy about the obesity measurement (i.e., general or abdominal) that better correlates to cardiovascular risk [18,24,25,35,44,45]. The abdominal obesity measures were significant predictors of cardiovascular events and death; BMI was not [10].

In our results, increased WC and WHtR implied higher coronary risk independently of BMI category. Surprisingly, men with WC ≥102 cm and BMI <25 kg/m^2 presented the highest 10-year coronary disease risk. This finding could be explained by the sparse number of individuals included in this category. However, the subcutaneous fat storage in patients with high BMI seems to diminish cardiovascular risk compared to individuals with higher perivisceral fat storage [46]. Another possible explanation may be the presence of sarcopenic obesity (i.e., age-related body composition changes characterized by decreased skeletal muscle mass and increased body fat mass) [47] that is more associated with cardiometabolic risk [48] and mortality in individuals with coronary heart disease [49]. Both explanations may show the incapacity of the subcutaneous fat storage in these individuals due to genetics, ageing, sedentary lifestyle or unknown causes that result in ectopic fat storage with higher cardiometabolic risk [50,51]. In women, on the other hand, a risk gradient was found between BMI and both WC and WHtR. Therefore, we believe that both types of obesity should now be measured in the clinical setting.

9.4.5 STRENGTHS AND LIMITATIONS

The DARIOS Study includes 11 studies conducted in different regions of Spain in the first decade of the 21st century. All these studies used standardized methodology. The DARIOS data is drawn from 10 Autonomous Communities that comprise approximately 70% of the total Spanish population aged 35–74 years. In addition, the sample size (>28,000 individuals) and response rate (>70% in 8 out of 11 studies) ensure that our results accurately reflect the prevalence of obesity in Spain. The response rate was estimated according to the cooperation rate in the 2011 guidelines of The American Association for Public Opinion Research [52].

The cross-sectional design of the study limits the causal interpretation of the associations described. Therefore, cohort studies are needed to ascertain the role of obesity in the incidence of coronary events, particularly in our society, where the prevalence of this cardiovascular risk factor has dramatically increased in recent years [3]. Notably, the cut-off point 0.55 for WHtR has shown higher predictive value for assessing the risk of diabetes and cardiovascular events [10,53].

9.5 CONCLUSION

The prevalence of general and abdominal obesity in Spain was high: 28% of men and women presented weight values above those recommended for their height. On the other hand, the prevalence of increased WC was 36% and 55% in men and women, respectively. Diabetes, hypertension, hypercholesterolemia and 10-year coronary risk were significantly associated with all categories of general and abdominal obesity. Therefore, these lower cut-off points for both BMI and particularly WC could be used to identify the population at risk and effective preventive measures.

REFERENCES

1. World Health Statistics: World Health Organization. Geneva; 2011. http://www.who.int/ncd_surveillance/infobase/web/InfoBaseCommon/ webcite
2. Flores-Mateo G, Grau M, O'Flaherty M, Ramos R, Elosua R, Violan-Fors C, Quesada M, Martí R, Sala J, Marrugat J, Capewell S: Analyzing the coronary heart disease mortality decline in a Mediterranean population: Spain 1988–2005. Rev Esp Cardiol 2011, 64(11):988-996.
3. Grau M, Subirana I, Elosua R, Solanas P, Ramos R, Masiá R, Cordón F, Sala J, Juvinyà D, Cerezo C, Fitó M, Vila J, Covas MI, Marrugat J: Trends in cardiovascular risk factor prevalence (1995-2000-2005) in northeastern Spain. Eur J Cardiovasc Prev Rehabil 2007, 14(5):653-659.
4. Schröder H, Elosua R, Vila J, Marti H, Covas MI, Marrugat J: Secular trends of obesity and cardiovascular risk factors in a Mediterranean population. Obesity (Silver Spring) 2007, 15(3):557-562.

5. García-Alvarez A, Serra-Majem L, Ribas-Barba L, Castell C, Foz M, Uauy R, Plasencia A, Salleras L: Obesity and overweight trends in Catalonia, Spain (1992–2003): gender and socio-economic determinants. Public Health Nutr 2007, 10(11A):1368-1378.
6. Divisón Garrote JA, Massó Orozco J, Carrión Valero L, López Abril J, Carbayo Herencia JA, Artigao Rodenas LM, Gil Guillén V, Grupo de Enfermedades Vasculares de Albacete (GEVA): Trends in prevalence of risk factors and global cardiovascular risk in general population of Albacete, Spain (1992–94 a 2004–06). Rev Esp Salud Publica 2011, 85(3):275-284.
7. Prospective Studies Collaboration: Body-mass index and cause-specific mortality in 900 000 adults: collaborative analisys of 57 prospective studies. Lancet 2009, 373:1083-1096.
8. Yusuf S, Hawken S, Ounpuu S, Bautista L, Franzosi MG, Commerford P, INTERHEART study investigators, et al.: Obesity and the risk of myocardial infarction in 27,000 participants from 52 countries: a case–control study. Lancet 2005, 366(9497):1540-1549.
9. Donini LM, Savina C, Gennaro E, De Felice MR, Rosano A, Pandolfo MM, Del Balzo V, Cannella C, Ritz P, Chumlea WC: A systematic review of the literature concerning the relationship between obesity and mortality in the elderly. J Nutr Health Aging 2012, 16(1):89-98.
10. Schneider HJ, Friedrich N, Klotsche J, Pieper L, Nauck M, John U, Dörr M, Felix S, Lehnert H, Pittrow D, Silber S, Völzke H, Stalla GK, Wallaschofski H, Wittchen HU: The predictive value of different measures of obesity for incident cardiovascular events and mortality. J Clin Endocrinol Metab 2010, 95(4):1777-1785.
11. Gutiérrez-Fisac JL, Guallar-Castillón P, León-Muñoz LM, Graciani A, Banegas JR, Rodríguez-Artalejo F: Prevalence of general and central obesity in the adult population of Spain, 2008–2010: the ENRICA study. Obes Rev 2012, 13(4):388-392.
12. Gomez-Cabello A, Pedrero-Chamizo R, Olivares PR, Luzardo L, Juez-Bengoechea A, Mata E, Albers U, Aznar S, Villa G, Espino L, Gusi N, Gonzalez-Gross M, Casajus JA, Ara I, EXERNET Study Group: Prevalence of overweight and obesity in non-institutionalized people aged 65 or over from Spain: the elderly EXERNET multi-centre study. Obes Rev 2011, 12(8):583-592.
13. Gomez-Huelgas R, Mancera-Romero J, Bernal-Lopez MR, Jansen-Chaparro S, Baca-Osorio AJ, Toledo E, Perez-Gonzalez R, Guijarro-Merino R, Tinahones FJ, Martinez-Gonzalez MA: Prevalence of cardiovascular risk factors in an urban adult population from southern Spain. IMAP Study. Int J Clin Pract 2011, 65(1):35-40.
14. Escribano García S, Vega Alonso AT, Lozano Alonso J, Alamo Sanz R, Lleras Muñoz S, Castrodeza Sanz J, Gil Costa M, Study of Cardiovascular Risk in Castile and Leon, Spain: Obesity in Castile and Leon, Spain: epidemiology and association with other cardiovascular risk factors. Rev Esp Cardiol 2011, 64(1):63-66.
15. Aguilera-Zubizarreta E, Ugarte-Miota T, Muñoz Cacho P, Vara-González L, Sanz de Castro S, Grupo CANHTABRIA: Prevalence of overweight and obesity in Cantabria [Spain]. Gac Sanit 2008, 22(5):461-464.
16. López Suárez A, Elvira González J, Beltrán Robles M, Alwakil M, Saucedo JM, Bascuñana Quirell A, Barón Ramos MA, Fernández PF: Prevalence of obesity, dia-

betes, hypertension, hypercholesterolemia and metabolic syndrome in over 50-year-olds in Sanlúcar de Barrameda. Spain. Rev Esp Cardiol 2008, 61(11):1150-1158.
17. Félix-Redondo FJ, Baena-Díez JM, Grau M, Tormo MÁ, Fernández-Bergés D: Prevalence of obesity and cardiovascular risk in the general population of a health area in Extremadura (Spain): the Hermex study. Endocrinol Nutr 2012, 59(3):160-168.
18. Cristo Rodríguez Pérez MD, Cabrera De León A, Aguirre-Jaime A, Domínguez Coello S, Brito Díaz B, Almeida González D, Borges Alamo C, Castillo Rodríguez JC, Carrillo Fernández L, González Hernández A, Alemán Sánchez JJ: The waist to height ratio as an index of cardiovascular risk and diabetes. Med Clin (Barc) 2010, 134(9):386-391.
19. Marrugat J, Subirana I, Comín E, Cabezas C, Vila J, Elosua R, Nam BH, Ramos R, Sala J, Solanas P, Cordón F, Gené-Badia J, D'Agostino RB, VERIFICA Investigators: Validity of an adaptation of the Framingham cardiovascular risk function: the VERIFICA Study. J Epidemiol Community Health 2007, 61(7):40-47.
20. Perk J, De Backer G, Gohlke H, Graham I, Reiner Z, Verschuren M, Albus C, Benlian P, Boysen G, Cifkova R, Deaton C, Ebrahim S, Fisher M, Germano G, Hobbs R, Hoes A, Karadeniz S, Mezzani A, Prescott E, Ryden L, Scherer M, Syvänne M, Scholte op Reimer WJ, Vrints C, Wood C, Zamorano JL, Zannad F: European Guidelines on cardiovascular disease prevention in clinical practice (version 2012). The Fifth Joint Task Force of the European Society of Cardiology and Other Societies on Cardiovascular Disease Prevention in Clinical Practice. Eur Heart J 2012, 33(13):1635-1701.
21. Grau M, Elosua R, Cabrera De León A, Guembe MJ, Baena-Díez JM, Vega Alonso T, Javier Félix F, Zorrilla B, Rigo F, Lapetra J, Gavrila D, Segura A, Sanz H, Fernández-Bergés D, Fitó M, Marrugat J: Cardiovascular risk factors in Spain in the first decade of the 21st Century, a pooled analysis with individual data from 11 population-based studies: the DARIOS study. Rev Esp Cardiol 2011, 64(4):295-304.
22. Alberti KG, Eckel RH, Grundy SM, Zimmet PZ, Cleeman JI, Donato KA, Fruchart JC, James WP, Loria CM, Smith SC Jr, International Diabetes Federation Task Force on Epidemiology and Prevention: Harmonizing the metabolic syndrome: a joint interim statement of the International Diabetes Federation Task Force on Epidemiology and Prevention; National Heart, Lung, and Blood Institute; American Heart Association; World Heart Federation; International Atherosclerosis Society; and International Association for the Study of Obesity. Circulation 2009, 120(16):1640-1645.
23. Alberti KG, Zimmet P, Shaw J, IDF Epidemiology Task Force Consensus Group: The metabolic syndrome–a new worldwide definition. Lancet 2005, 366(9491):1059-1062.
24. Lee CMY, Huxley RR, Wildman RP, Woodward M: Indices of abdominal obesity are better discrimantors of cardiovascular risk factors than BMI: a meta-analysis. J Clin Epidemiol 2008, 61(7):646-653.
25. Ashwell M, Hsieh SD: Six reasons why the waist-to-height ratio is a rapid and effective global indicator for health risks of obesity and how its use could simplify the international public health message on obesity. Int J Food Sci Nutr 2005, 56(5):303-307.

26. Ahmad OE, Boschi-Pinto C, López AD, Murray CJL, Lozano R, Inoue M: Age standardization of rates: a new WHO standard GPE. Discussion Paper Series: No. 31. Geneva: World Health Organization; 2000.
27. Aranceta-Bartrina J, Serra-Majem L, Foz-Sala M, Moreno-Esteban B, Grupo Colaborativo SEEDO: Prevalence of obesity in Spain. Med Clin (Barc) 2005, 125(12):460-466.
28. Gutiérrez-Fisac JL, López E, Banegas JR, Graciani A, Rodríguez-Artalejo F: Prevalence of overweight and obesity in elderly people in Spain. Obes Res 2004, 12(4):710-715.
29. Cea-Calvo L, Moreno B, Monereo S, Gil-Guillén V, Lozano JV, Martí-Canales JC, Llisterri JL, Aznar J, González-Esteban J, Redón J, PREV-ICTUS Study: Prevalence and related factors of overweight and obesity in Spanish population aged 60 years-old or older. The PREV-ICTUS study. Med Clin (Barc). 2008, 131(6):205-210.
30. Doak CM, Wijnhoven TM, Schokker DF, Visscher TL, Seidell JC: Age standardization in mapping adult overweight and obesity trends in the WHO European Region. Obes Rev 2012, 13(2):174-191.
31. Wang Y, Beydoun MA: The obesity epidemic in the United States–gender, age, socioeconomic, racial/ethnic, and geographic characteristics: a systematic review and meta-regression analysis. Epidemiol Rev 2007, 29:6-28.
32. Nolan CJ, Damm P, Prentki M: Type 2 diabetes across generations: from pathophysiology to prevention and management. Lancet 2011, 378(9786):169-181.
33. Zalesin KC, Franklin BA, Miller WM, Peterson ED, McCullough PA: Impact of obesity on cardiovascular disease. Endocrinol Metab Clin North Am 2008, 37(3):663-684.
34. Bamba V, Rader DJ: Obesity and atherogenic dyslipidemia. Gastroenterology 2007, 132(6):2181-2190.
35. Meisinger C, Döring A, Thorand B, Heier M, Löwel H: Body fat distribution and risk of type 2 diabetes in the general population: are there differences between men and women? The MONICA/KORA Augsburg cohort study. Am J Clin Nutr 2006, 84(3):483-489.
36. Cabrera De León A, Rodríguez-Pérez Mdel C, Rodríguez-Benjumeda LM, Anía-Lafuente B, Brito-Díaz B, Muros De Fuentes M, Almeida-González D, Batista-Medina M, Aguirre-Jaime A: Sedentary lifestyle: physical activity duration versus percentage of energy expenditure. Rev Esp Cardiol 2007, 60(3):244-250.
37. Power ML, Schulkin J: Sex differences in fat storage, fat metabolism, and the health risks from obesity: possible evolutionary origins. Br J Nutr 2008, 99(5):931-940.
38. Provencher V, Drapeau V, Tremblay A, Després JP, Lemieux S: Eating behaviors and indexes of body composition in men and women from the Québec family study. Obes Res 2003, 11(6):783-792.
39. Van Dis I, Geleijnse JM, Kromhout D, Boer JM, Boshuizen H, Verschuren WM: Do obesity and parental history of myocardial infarction improve cardiovascular risk prediction? Eur J Prev Cardiol. in press
40. Pischon T, Boeing H, Hoffmann K, Bergmann M, Schulze MB, Overvad K, van der Schouw YT, Spencer E, Moons KG, Tjønneland A, Halkjaer J, Jensen MK, Stegger J, Clavel-Chapelon F, Boutron-Ruault MC, Chajes V, Linseisen J, Kaaks R, Trichopoulou A, Trichopoulos D, Bamia C, Sieri S, Palli D, Tumino R, Vineis P, Panico

S, Peeters PH, May AM, Bueno-de-Mesquita HB, van Duijnhoven FJ, Hallmans G, Weinehall L, Manjer J, Hedblad B, Lund E, Agudo A, Arriola L, Barricarte A, Navarro C, Martinez C, Quirós JR, Key T, Bingham S, Khaw KT, Boffetta P, Jenab M, Ferrari P, Riboli E: General and abdominal adiposity and risk of death in Europe. N Engl J Med 2008, 359(20):2105-20.
41. Grau M, Subirana I, Elosua R, Fitó M, Covas MI, Sala J, Masiá R, Ramos R, Solanas P, Cordon F, Nieto FJ, Marrugat J, REGICOR Investigators: Why should population attributable fractions be periodically recalculated? An example from cardiovascular risk estimation in southern Europe. Prev Med 2010, 51(1):78-84.
42. Huerta JM, Tormo MJ, Gavrila D, Navarro C: Cardiovascular risk estimated after 13 years of follow-up in a low-incidence Mediterranean region with high-prevalence of cardiovascular risk factors. BMC Public Health 2010, 10:640.
43. Wilson PW, D'Agostino RB, Sullivan L, Parise H, Kannel WB: Overweight and obesity as determinants of cardiovascular risk: the Framingham experience. Arch Intern Med 2002, 162(16):1867-72.
44. Lemieux I, Poirier P, Bergeron J, Alméras N, Lamarche B, Cantin B, Dagenais GR, Després JP: Hypertriglyceridemic waist: a useful screening phenotype in preventive cardiology? Can J Cardiol 2007, 23(Suppl B):23B-31B.
45. Qiao Q, Nyamdorj R: Is the association of type II diabetes with waist circumference or waist-to-hip ratio stronger than that with body mass index? Eur J Clin Nutr 2010, 64(1):30-4.
46. Porter SA, Massaro JM, Hoffmann U, Vasan RS, O'Donnel CJ, Fox CS: Abdominal subcutaneous adipose tissue: a protective fat depot? Diabetes Care 2009, 32(6):1068-75.
47. Zamboni M, Mazzali G, Fantin F, Rossi A, Di Francesco V: Sarcopenic obesity: a new category of obesity in the elderly. Nutr Metab Cardiovasc Dis 2008, 18(5):388-95.
48. Chung JY, Kang HT, Lee DC, Lee HR, Lee YJ: Body composition and its association with cardiometabolic risk factors in the elderly: A focus on sarcopenic obesity. Arch Gerontol Geriatr 2013, 56(1):270-8.
49. Coutinho T, Goel K, Corrêa de Sá D, Carter RE, Hodge DO, Kragelund C, Kanaya AM, Zeller M, Park JS, Kober L, Torp-Pedersen C, Cottin Y, Lorgis L, Lee SH, Kim YJ, Thomas R, Roger VL, Somers VK, Lopez-Jimenez F: Combining body mass index with measures of central obesity in the assessment of mortality in subjects with coronary disease: role of "normal weight central obesity". J Am Coll Cardiol 2013, 61(5):553-60.
50. Després JP, Lemieux I, Bergeron J, Pibarot P, Mathieu P, Larose E, Rodés-Cabau J, Bertrand OF, Poirier P: Abdominal obesity and the metabolic syndrome: contribution to global cardiometabolic risk. Arterioscler Thromb Vasc Biol 2008, 28(6):1039-49.
51. Britton KA, Fox CS: Ectopic fat depots and cardiovascular disease. Circulation 2011, 124(24):e837-41.
52. The American Association for Public Opinion Research: Standard Definitions: Final dispositions of case codes and outcomes rates for surveys. 7th edition. 2011. Available at: http://www.aapor.org/Home.htm

53. de León AC, Coello SD, González DA, Díaz BB, Rodríguez JC, Hernández AG, Aguirre-Jaime A, Pérez M del C: Impaired fasting glucose, ancestry and waist-to-height ratio: main predictors of incident diagnosed diabetes in the Canary Islands.

CHAPTER 10

OBSTRUCTIVE SLEEP APNEA IS A PREDICTOR OF ABNORMAL GLUCOSE METABOLISM IN CHRONICALLY SLEEP DEPRIVED OBESE ADULTS

GIOVANNI CIZZA, PAOLO PIAGGI, ELIANE A. LUCASSEN, LILIAN DE JONGE, MARY WALTER, MEGAN S. MATTINGLY, HEATHER KALISH, GYORGY CSAKO, AND KRISTINA I. ROTHER, FOR THE SLEEP EXTENSION STUDY GROUP

10.1 INTRODUCTION

Several epidemiological studies have shown that people who report sleeping less than 6.5 h are at greater risk of gaining weight over time [1]. Furthermore, obesity and obstructive sleep apnea (OSA) frequently coexist: about 40% of obese individuals have OSA; conversely approximately 70% of individuals with OSA are obese [2], [3]. Similar to diabetes, OSA frequently goes undiagnosed [4]. Sleep duration and OSA may affect insulin resistance independently of body mass index (BMI) [5]. In addition, OSA is associated with decreased insulin sensitivity in lean, male subjects,

This chapter was originally published under the Creative Commons Attribution License. Cizza G, Piaggi P, Lucassen EA, de Jonge L, Walter M, Mattingly MS, Kalish H, Csako G, and Rother KI. Obstructive Sleep Apnea Is a Predictor of Abnormal Glucose Metabolism in Chronically Sleep Deprived Obese Adults. PLoS ONE ***8**,5 (2013), doi:10.1371/journal.pone.0065400.*

suggesting that OSA per se may induce insulin resistance, independent of adiposity [6]. Several ongoing studies currently listed in Clinical Trials.gov and other similar web sites are addressing the relationship between OSA and glucose metabolism in obese subjects.

Seminal studies conducted by Van Cauter et al. demonstrated that acute sleep deprivation can induce insulin resistance in lean volunteers [7], [8]. Similarly, experimentally induced sleep fragmentation caused insulin resistance in healthy volunteers [9]. However, the effects of real life conditions, such as chronic sleep deprivation, on glucose metabolism have not been well characterized. The goal of the present report was to determine the relationship between short sleep, and OSA on glucose metabolism in a cohort of obese subjects reporting less than 6.5 h of nightly sleep.

10.2 METHODS

This analysis pertains to the Sleep Extension Study, a randomized, prospective, intervention trial of obese (BMI 30–55 kg/m^2) men and premenopausal women 18 to 50 years old, who reported sleeping less than 6.5 h per night on average [10]. Subject recruitment took place between January 22, 2007, and June 28, 2011. All analyses presented here include data obtained at baseline prior to sleep intervention. Type 2 diabetes treated with insulin, a diagnosis of sleep disorders other than treated OSA, chronic use of sleep medications, chronic excess caffeine use, shift work and nocturnal occupations or current DSM-IV diagnoses, including anxiety, eating- or severe mood disorders, were exclusion criteria. Subjects taking oral hypoglycemic agents were allowed in the study.

10.2.1 ETHICS STATEMENT

The study was conducted at the NIH Clinical Center in Bethesda, MD, USA after obtaining approval from the NIDDK Institutional Review Board (ClinicalTrials.gov identifier: NCT00261898). Each subject signed an approved written informed consent.

10.2.2 ANTHROPOMETRIC MEASUREMENTS

Height was measured to the nearest centimeter using a wall-mounted stadiometer (SECA 242, SECA North America East, Hanover, MD, USA) and weight was measured using a stand-on-scale in a hospital gown to the nearest 1/10th of a kg (SR555 SR Scales, SR Instruments, INC, Tonawanda, NY, USA). Waist circumference was measured at the midpoint between the inferior tip of the ribcage and the superior aspect of the iliac crest. Neck circumference was measured at the minimal circumference with the subjects' head in the Frankfort Horizontal Plane.

10.2.3 BODY COMPOSITION MEASUREMENTS

Dual-energy X-ray absorptiometry (DXA) for body composition assessment was performed with a Hologic DXA QDR 4500 (Hologic Inc., Bedford, MA, USA). Abdominal fat content and distribution was measured at the level of both L2–3 and L4–5, using a HiSpeed Advantage CT/I scanner (GE Medical Systems, Milwaukee, WI, USA) and analyzed on a SUN workstation using the MEDx image analysis software package (Sensor System, Sterling, VA, USA). Conventional (non-helical) 10 mm thick X-ray abdominal computed tomography images limited to the L2-3 and L4-5 levels were obtained at 120 kVp, with mAs adjusted according to patient size. Fully automatic processing of these images according to the method of Yao [11] resulted in measurements at these levels of visceral and subcutaneous adipose tissue areas, which were then summed and normalized by the imaged volume to estimate subcutaneous and visceral abdominal fat.

10.2.4 SLEEP MEASURES

Sleep was assessed by a combination of different methods. Subjects were instructed to wear a wrist activity monitor continuously for two weeks

(Actiwatch-64, Mini Mitter/Respironics/Philips, Bend, OR, USA). Additional information on these instruments and data analysis was reported previously [12]. Sleep duration and sleep efficiency (percent of time asleep of total time spent in bed) were obtained from actigraphy. Self-reported sleep duration was derived from sleep diaries kept for two weeks, concurrent with the actigraphy measurements and from Question Four of the Pittsburgh Sleep Quality Index (PSQI), asking: "During the past month, how many hours of actual sleep did you get at night?". The PSQI is a validated 21-item questionnaire that assesses subjective sleep quality over the past month [13]. PSQI scores range from 0 to 21, with higher scores indicating worse sleep quality. A score over 5 is considered the threshold for poor sleep quality. Each morning subjects were required to record the amount of sleep during the previous night in the sleep diaries. Daytime sleepiness was assessed by the Epworth Sleepiness Scale (ESS), a validated 8-item questionnaire [14]. ESS scores range from 0 to 24, with higher scores representing greater daytime sleepiness. A score greater than 10 indicates excessive daytime sleepiness.

The presence of sleep disordered breathing was evaluated over one night using a portable screening device (Apnea Risk Evaluation System, Advanced Brain Monitoring Inc., Carlsbad, CA, USA). This device provides an estimate of the respiratory disturbance index (RDI), which is the number of apneas and hypopneas per hour of sleep. An episode of apnea was defined as the complete cessation of airflow for at least 10 seconds. Hypopnea events were defined as at least 10 seconds with the airflow decreasing by more than 50% and with more than 3.5% oxygen desaturation, or more than 1% desaturation accompanied by at least one surrogate arousal indicator (head movement, changes in snoring, or changes in pulse rate) [15]. This device has demonstrated high sensitivity and specificity when validated against polysomnography [16].

10.2.5 GLUCOSE METABOLISM ASSESSMENTS

Fasting serum glucose and insulin were measured after a 10-h overnight fast. Each subject underwent a 75g oral glucose tolerance test (oGTT) during which plasma glucose and serum insulin levels were determined at 0,

30, 60, 90 and 120 min. Glucose levels ≥100 mg/dL at baseline and ≥140 mg/dL at 120 min of the OGTT were defined as abnormal, and the diagnosis of diabetes was made if glucose levels were ≥126 mg/dL at baseline and ≥200 mg/dL at 120 min. Insulin resistance was determined using the homeostasis model assessment for insulin resistance (HOMA): (fasting insulin (mU/L) * fasting plasma glucose (mg/dL))/405. The insulinogenic index was calculated with the following equation: (30 min insulin –0 min insulin)/(30 min glucose –0 min glucose). The AUC for glucose and insulin was calculated using the trapezoidal rule: 15 * (0 min plasma levels) +2 * (30 min, 60 min and 90 min plasma levels) +120 min plasma levels.

10.2.6 CLINICAL LABORATORY ANALYSIS

Plasma glucose was determined with an enzymatic method. Plasma adrenocorticotropic hormone (ACTH), (total) serum cortisol, insulin, and growth hormone (GH) levels were measured with chemiluminescence immunoassays (Immulite 2000 and/or 2500 analyzers, Siemens). Urinary free cortisol (UFC) and catecholamines were collected in 24 h urine collection and measured using liquid chromatography-tandem mass spectrometry (LC-MS/MS) and high-performance liquid chromatography (HPLC), respectively.

Sixteen cytokines/chemokines were measured with an ELISA that uses the Quansys multiplex system (Quansys Biosciences, Logan, Utah, USA). All samples were run in duplicate. Values are reported in pg per mL after normalization to 1 μg total protein per mL of sample, to account for variations in the total protein content of the samples. CRP concentrations were measured in 87 subjects with a high sensitivity chemiluminescent immunometric assay with a detection limit of 0.1 mg/L (Immulite 2000, Siemens/DPC, Los Angeles, California, USA).

10.2.7 STATISTICAL ANALYSIS

Descriptive statistics for each variable were calculated based on the presence of OSA according to a RDI cutoff value of 5 and on glucose status (i.e. normal and abnormal oGTT results). Statistical tests included Student's t test and ANOVA for difference in means, Mann-Whitney U test for skewed variables, Fisher exact test and Pearson Chi-square test for difference in counts and frequency, respectively. The Kolmogorov-Smirnov test was used to assess normality of data; logarithmic transformations were applied for skewed variables before parametric statistical analyses (e.g. RDI and HOMA values). Pearson (r) and Spearman (ρ) correlation coefficients were used for Gaussian and skewed variables, respectively. The effect of OSA on the relationship between hormones and anthropometric parameters was assessed by analysis of covariance (ANCOVA). Multivariate regression models were also carried out. Data are presented as mean values ± standard deviation (SD) or median with interquartile range (IQR), as indicated. Analyses were performed using SAS (version 9.1.3, SAS Institute Inc., Cary, NC, USA), JMP (version 8.0, SAS Institute Inc., Cary, NC, USA) and SPSS (version 19. IBM SPSS North America. Chicago, IL, USA).

10.3 RESULTS

10.3.1 DEMOGRAPHIC AND ANTHROPOMETRIC CHARACTERISTICS ACCORDING TO FASTING GLUCOSE AND OGTT

Of the 125 randomized into the study, six subjects were excluded due to the use of oral hypoglycemic agents and 96 subjects had measurements of OSA available at the Randomization Visit. Demographic, anthropometric and life-style characteristics of these 96 subjects are shown in Table 1. Based on a RDI cut-off of 5, we divided subjects into two groups, with or without OSA. Approximately 40% of subjects had an RDI less than 5. Subjects with OSA were more often men, had higher body weight, waist and neck circumferences, similar subcutaneous fat but approximately twice as much visceral fat by CT.

TABLE 1: Demographic and anthropometric characteristics of the study subjects.

	No sleep apnea (RDI < 5) (N = 38)	Sleep apnea (RDI ≥ 5) (N = 58)	p-value
Age (years)	3.9.9 ± 6.6	42.5 ± 5.9	**0.049**
Female	89.5%	69.5%	**0.041**
Race			0.646
Black	60.5%	50.8%	
White	34.2%	42.4%	
Other	5.3%	6.8%	
Years of Education	16.5 ± 2.4	15.8 ± 2.5	0.162
Weight (kg)	99.7 ± 16.6	110.4 ± 19.8	**0.007**
Current or past smoking status			
Smoking history	13.1%	20.7%	0.496
Currently smoking	2.6%	10.3%	0.308
Medications			
Psychotropics (Prozac, Zoloft)	18.4%	5.2%	0.084
Hormonal conttraceptives	18.4%	3.4%	**0.035**
Antihypertensives	10.5%	13.8%	0.871
Statins	5.3%	6.9%	0.909
Anti-asthma/allergy (Advair, Allegra)	5.3%	12.1%	0.448
Synthroid	2.6%	5.2%	0.919
BMI (kg/m^2)	36.5 ± 5.8	38.9 ± 6.2	0.058
Body fat (%)	42.4 ± 5.6	40.5 ± 7.9	0.213
Body lean (%)	55.2 ± 5.5	57.1 ± 7.7	0.191
Waist circumference (cm)	108.7 ± 12.3	116.4 ± 12.4	**0.003**
Neck circumference (cm)	36.9 ± 2.7	40.2 ± 3.8	**<0.001**
Visceral fat by CT (cm^3)	250.8 ± 122.9	416.2 ± 168.7	**<0.001**
Subcutaneous fat by CT (cm^3)	921.6 ± 294.8	88.3 ± 296.1	0.606
Abdominal fat by CT (cm^3)	1172.4 ± 319.8	1172.4 ± 319.8	0.060

Values in each cell are reported as mean ± SD or as percentage.

Subjects with OSA had also significantly higher fasting glucose, fasting insulin, HOMA index and HbA1C (Table 2). More precisely, 42% of the subjects with OSA had abnormal HOMA, 14% had abnormal fasting glucose, and 7.8% had abnormal HbA1c. Of the 58 subjects with OSA, 8 had a fasting glucose ≥126 mg/dL, 24 had glucose levels ≥140 mg/dL and 4 had glucose levels ≥200 mg/dL at 120 min of the OGTT test. None of the individuals without sleep apnea (SA) had either a fasting glucose ≥126 mg/dL or glucose levels ≥200 mg/dL at 120 min, however eight subjects had a 120 min glucose level ≥140 mg/dL.

Fig. 1 depicts glucose (upper panels A–C) and insulin (lower panels B-D) concentrations and AUC during the oGTT in subjects with and without OSA. Subjects with OSA had significantly higher plasma glucose levels at each time point, and higher insulin at baseline, 60, 90 and 120 min; they had also approximately 10% higher glucose and insulin AUCs.

TABLE 2: Glucose characteristics for study subjects during fasting conditions and the oral glucose tolerance test.

	No sleep apnea (RDI < 5) (N=38)	Sleep apnea (RDI ≥ 5) (N = 58)	p-value
Fasting glucose (mg/dL)	84.9 ± 6.7	91.3 ± 11.5	**0.003**
% subjects with abnormal fasting glucose (≥ 100 mg/dL)	2.6%	13.6%	0.144
Fasting insulin (mU/L)	8.8 ± 6.4	11.7 ± 6.7	**0.037**
% subjects with abnormal oGTT	21.1%	44.1%	**0.036**
HOMA index[1]	1.4 (0.8–2.4)	2.4 (1.5–3.8)	**0.003**
% subjects with abnormal HOMA (≥ 2.5)	23.7%	42.4%	0.097
HBA_1c (%)	5.5 ± 0.5	5.8 ± 0.6	**0.019**
% subjects with abnormal HBA_1c (> 6.4%)	2.6%	6.8%	0.661

Unless otherwise stated, values in each cell are reported as mean ± SD or as percentage.

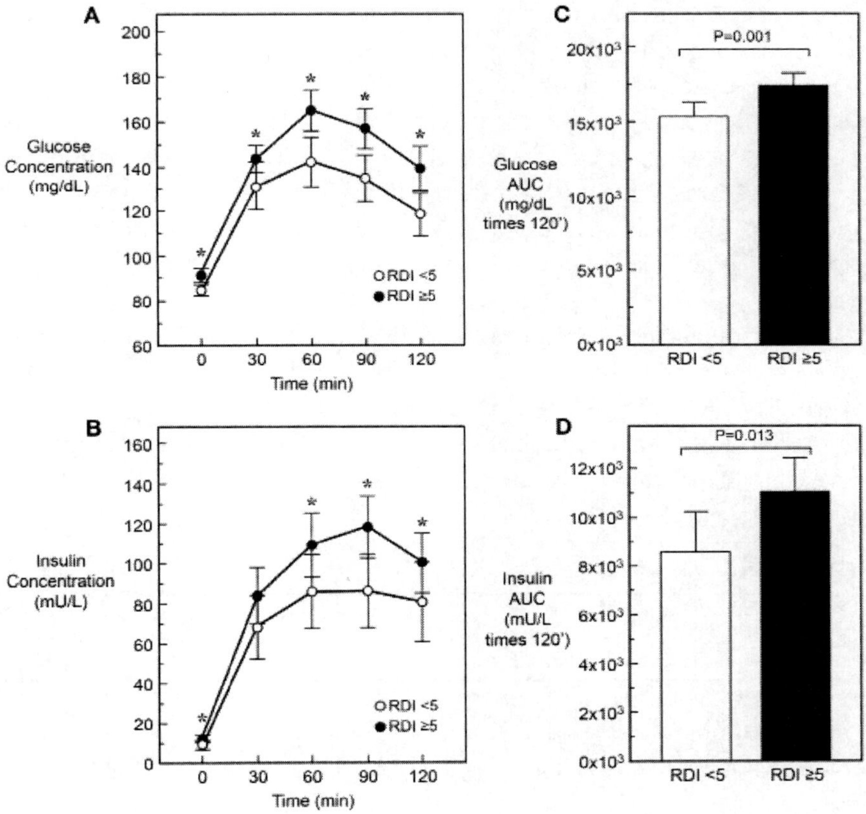

FIGURE 1: Oral glucose tolerance test. Glucose (Panel A) and insulin (Panel B) concentrations during 120-min OGTT in patients with a sleep apnea diagnosis (RDI ≥5, white circles, N = 58) and without a sleep apnea diagnosis (RDI<5, black circles, N = 38). The time-integrated area under the curve (AUC) for glucose and insulin are shown in panel C and D, respectively.

[1] *Values are reported as median with interquartile range due to skewed distribution.*

10.3.2 SLEEP CHARACTERISTICS

Because of the inclusion criteria, subjects in both groups had short sleep duration, approximately 6.5h by sleep diary and 6h by actigraphy (Table 3). Average sleep efficiency was poor, 80%, approximately 80% of subjects had low sleep quality as indicated by a score greater than 5 on the PSQI scale, and 25% experienced sleepiness during the day, as indicated by a score greater than 10 on the ESS scale. Subjects with OSA had a median of 13 episodes of OSA per hour and slightly lower oxygen saturation than subjects without OSA. There were no group differences in sleep efficiency and sleepiness scores.

Fig. 2 depicts average fasting glucose concentrations with increasing classes of severity of OSA. Fasting glucose concentrations rose progressively from subjects without OSA to those with mild, moderate and severe OSA. Subjects with moderate to severe OSA (RDI>15) had higher glucose levels at 120 min than subjects without OSA ($p = 0.017$).

TABLE 3: Sleep characteristics of study subjects.

	No sleep apnea (RDI < 5) (N = 38)	Sleep apnea (RDI ≥ 5) (N = 58)	p-value
Self-reported sleep duration (min/night)	385 ± 54	387 ± 42	0.868
Actigraphy sleep duration (min/night)	365 ± 48	350 ± 49	0.171
Actigraphy sleep efficiency (%)	80.8 ± 4.9	80.0 ± 6.8	0.559
PSQI global score	7.8 ± 2.3	7.9 ± 2.7	0.836
PSQI abnormal (>5) score	81.1%	84.5%	0.876
ESS score	8.7 ± 4.7	8.1 ± 4.4	0.504
ESS abnormal (> 10) score	34.3%	26.3%	0.541
RDI (events/h)[1]	2 (1–4)	13 (8–20)	**<0.001**
Normal (RDI < 5)	100%	0%	**<0.001**
Mild sleep apnea (RDI: 5–15)	0%	66.1%	**<0.001**
Moderate sleep apnea (RDI: 16–30)	0%	22.0%	**<0.001**
Severe sleep apnea (RDI > 30)	0%	11.9%	**<0.001**
Saturation of peripheral oxygen (%)	96.8 ± 0.9	95.6 ± 2.3	**0.002**

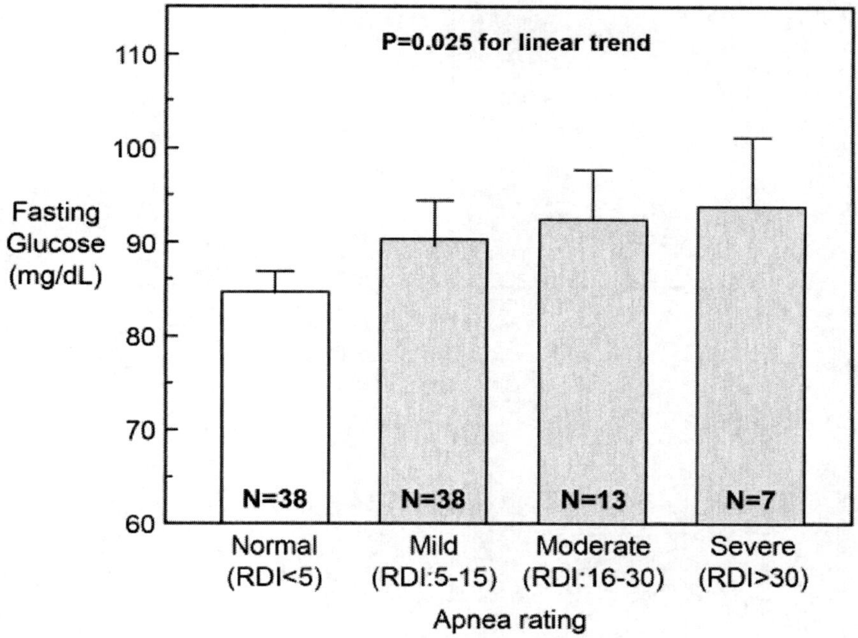

FIGURE 2: Fasting glucose concentration increases with sleep apnea severity as quantified by the RDI score. Fasting glucose concentrations rose progressively from subjects without sleep apnea (84.9±6.7 mg/dL; mean±SD) to those with mild (90.4±12.9 mg/dL), moderate (92.5±8.9 mg/dL), and severe (93.9±17.9 mg/dL) sleep apnea (test for trend: p = 0.025). Data are presented as mean with 95% CI.

Unless otherwise stated, values in each cell are reported as mean ± SD or as percentage.
[1]RDI values are reported as median with interquartile range due to its skewed distribution.

Fig. 3 illustrates the relationship of log RDI and fasting glucose and insulin concentrations, HOMA, and 120 min glucose: log RDI was directly related in a significant fashion to each one of these parameters.

10.3.3 INFLAMMATORY/IMMUNE CHARACTERISTICS

Subjects with OSA had higher levels of IL-2, IL-4, IL-5, IL-6, IL-8, IL-13, and IFN-gamma and tended to have higher levels of IL-15 and TNF-beta (Table 4). No significant differences between the two groups were observed in the remaining cytokines, as well as in CRP concentrations. CRP

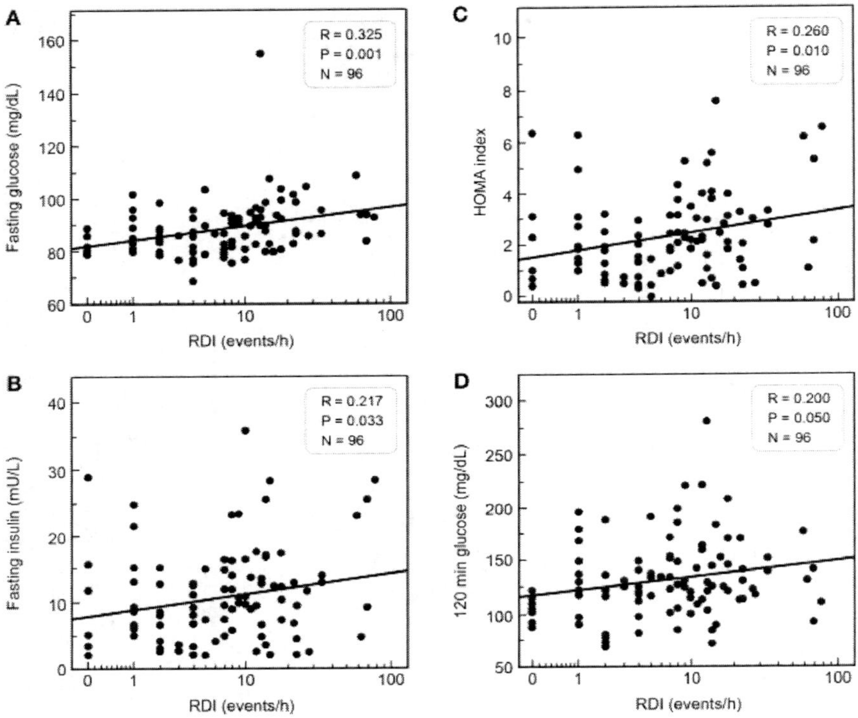

FIGURE 3: Relationship between RDI and fasting glucose (Panel A), fasting insulin (Panel B), HOMA index (Panel C), and 120-min glucose (Panel D). RDI is reported on a safe-logarithmic scale, namely, LOG10(1+ RDI).

concentrations for the whole sample were: 4.78 mg/L (1.75–8.65) median and interquartile range.

10.3.4 HORMONAL CHARACTERISTICS

Subjects with OSA had approximately 36% higher plasma ACTH levels in the setting of similar serum cortisol and UFC (Table 5). In addition, they had 16% higher 24 h urinary norepinephrine levels. GH concentrations were significantly lower in subjects with OSA while no differences were observed in IGF-1 plasma concentrations.

TABLE 4: Inflammatory/immune characteristics of study subjects.

	No sleep apnea (RDI < 5) (N = 38)	Sleep apnea (RDI ≥ 5) (N = 58)	p-value
IL-1a (pg/mL)	14.1 (9.5 – 18.9)	13.6 (0.3 – 20.7)	0.803
IL-1b (pg/mL)	30.1 (22.5 – 39.7)	32.4 (24.6 – 47.3)	0.418
IL-2 (pg/mL)	7.4 (4.5 – 12.3)	10.1 (7.5 – 15.7)	**0.047**
IL-4 (pg/mL)	3.2 (2.3 – 4.6)	4.1 (3.1 – 6.4)	**0.038**
IL-5 (pg/mL)	6.9 (4.2 – 9.0)	8.2 (5.3 – 10.7)	**0.033**
IL-6 (pg/mL)	4.5 (2.6 – 9.0)	5.8 (4.4 – 9.3)	**0.041**
IL-8 (pg/mL)	10.8 (4.7 – 15.4)	12.2 (7.7 – 21.8)	**0.050**
IL-10 (pg/mL)	7.8 (4.6 – 12.0)	8.0 (5.8 – 11.3)	0.615
IL-12 (pg/mL)	10.6 (5.0 – 12.8)	11.5 (7.8 – 14.1)	0.391
IL-13 (pg/mL)	13.2 (10.2 – 15.0)	14.3 (11.8 – 17.5)	**0.039**
IL-15 (pg/mL)	12.4 (9.9 – 14.7)	13.3 (11.3 – 15.5)	0.102
IL-17 (pg/mL)	13.9 (10.6 – 17.8)	14.3 (12.2 – 17.5)	0.358
IL-23 (pg/mL)	134.7 (95.2 – 204.2)	145.7 (123.9 – 187.2)	0.268
IFN-gamma (pg/mL)	27.0 (23.4 – 33.1)	34.0 (27.6 – 40.4)	**<0.001**
TNF-alfa (pg/mL)	16.6 (13.1 – 22.0)	19.9 (14.5 – 24.8)	0.135
TNF-beta (mg/mL)	14.1 (11.2 – 16.7)	15.5 (12.8 – 18.6)	0.095
C-reactive Protein* (mg/L)	3.81 (1.09 – 8.65)	5.27 (2.06 – 8.46)	0.584
Logarithimic values (mean ± SD)	0.53 ± 0.54	0.61 ± 0.45	0.448
<3.00 mg/L	1.20 (0.70 – 1.75)	1.77 (0.76 – 2.27)	0.339
3.00–9.99 mg/L	6.01 (4.59 – 7.49)	6.40 (5.30 – 8.44)	0.582
≥ 10.00 mg/L	16.40 (13.45 – 22.35)	14.90 (11.40 – 16.10)	0.114

Values are reported as median with interquartile range due to skewed distribution.
**N = 87*

10.3.5 MULTIVARIATE ANALYSES OF DETERMINANTS OF FASTING GLUCOSE

In a simple regression model, approximately 11% of the variability in fasting glucose was explained by RDI (Table 6). Incremental adjustments for visceral fat (Step 1), visceral fat and age (Step 2), as well as visceral fat, age, gender and sleep duration (Step 3) in multivariate models, increased the variability accounted for by the model from 11% to 16%. Based on this regression analysis, 10 episodes of OSA would increase fasting glucose by 2.01 mg/dL and a 10% increase in visceral fat would increase fasting glucose by 0.86 mg/dL. Similar results were obtained when BMI was used instead of visceral fat (data not shown).

TABLE 5: Hormonal characteristics of study subjects.

	No sleep apnea (RDI < 5) (N = 38)	Sleep apnea (RDI ≥ 5) (N = 58)	p-value
Plasma morning ACTH (pg/mL)[1]	15.2 (11.7 – 21.5)	20.0 (14.5 – 27.4)	**0.009**
Serum morning cortisol (μg/dL)	9.1 ± 4.3	10.0 ± 4.6	0.361
UFC (μg/24 h)	18.0 ± 10.6	20.7 ± 14.6	0.322
Urinary norepinephrine (μg/24 h)	39.1 ± 18.0	45.6 ± 17.9	0.093
Urinary epinephrine (μg/24 h)	4.4 ± 2.9	4.2 ± 3.0	0.807
Urinary dopamine (μg/24 h)	249.0 ± 87.8	259.3 ± 98.4	0.614
Serum GH (ng/mL)[1]	0.70 (0.20 – 2.30)	0.20 (0.10 – 0.45)	**0.002**
IGF-1 (ng/mL)	141.2 ± 52.6	135.0 ± 43.6	0.530

[1] *Values are reported as median with interquartile range due to skewed distribution.*
[a] *To convert gravimetric units for hormones to SI units, use the following conversion factors: cortisol, mg/dl * 27.59 = nmol/l; epinephrine, mg/24 h * 5.46 = nmol/24 h; NE, mg/24 h * 5.91 = nmol/24 h; corticotropin (ACTH), pg/ml * 0.22 = pmol/l; and dopamine, mg/24 h * 6.58 = nmol/24 h; IGF-1, ng/mL * 0.131 = nmol/L*

10.4 DISCUSSION

In this cohort of middle aged, obese men and premenopausal women who reported sleeping less than 6.5h on a regular basis, approximately 60% had OSA and 40% had abnormal glucose metabolisms. Prior to enrollment, the majority of subjects were unaware of having SA. SA is associated with worse glycemia and insulin resistance, known predictors of diabetes and cardiovascular disease.

The mechanisms of the relationship between abnormal glucose metabolism and OSA are incompletely understood. OSA is associated with chronic intermittent hypoxia and sleep loss due to sleep fragmentation, both of which contribute to insulin resistance [9], [17]. Inducement of a pro-inflammatory state, generation of reactive oxygen species, increased sympathetic tone, and alterations in the hypothalamus-pituitary-adrenal axis, are all putative mechanisms linking OSA to changes in glucose metabolism [18], [19]. In addition, beta cells are highly sensitive to hypoxia, and the subsequent shift to glycolytic metabolism favors insulin resistance. In addition, exposure to altitude worsens insulin sensitivity, as indicated by a lower glucose AUC in healthy subjects [20].

Consistent with the above-proposed mechanisms, we found, using a multiplex assay with high sensitivity, that a wide range of functionally related cytokines and chemokines were elevated in patients with OSA. Specifically, subjects with OSA had higher circulating concentrations of IL-2, IL-4, IL-5, IL-6, IL-8, IFN-gamma, and TNF-alpha and tended to have higher concentrations of TNF-beta, clearly indicating an activation of the Th-1 and Th-2 immune response. Increased cytokine levels have previously been observed in association with sleep deprivation, OSA, obesity, and insulin resistance in smaller samples using a limited number of cytokines [21]. The anti-inflammatory cytokine IL-10 was not elevated in subjects with OSA, indicating the lack of a counter-regulatory response. Our findings add novel information on IL-2, IL-4, IL-5, IL-10, IL-13, and IL-15. Since cytokines are secreted in a cascade, determination of one or a few cytokines may provide incomplete and potentially misleading information. In addition, traditional ELISA assays may not be sensitive enough to reliably determine cytokine concentrations in subjects without an overt clinical inflammatory or autoimmune condition. C-reactive protein (CRP) concentrations were abnormal in 66% of subjects. The synthesis of the acute phase mediator CRP by the liver is triggered by IL-6 and other cytokines. CRP is an accepted marker of cardiovascular risk with values ≥3-mg/L indicating increased risk [22].

Subjects with OSA had 60% more visceral fat by CT. Visceral fat is a major source of inflammatory cytokines. Inflammatory cytokines are produced by adipocytes, as well as by a heterogeneous aggregate of immune cells made up mostly of macrophages, but also by T and NK cells embedded among adipocytes. Hypoxia represents a potent stimulus for cytokine production from the adipose tissue via the intracellular pathways of c-Jun and ATF2 [23]. Of note, mean oxygen saturation was within normal limits in subjects with OSA and only 1% lower than in subjects without OSA. These findings suggest that even a small decrease in oxygen desaturation within the normal range of may have a significant impact in obese, sleep-deprived subjects. Based on our multivariate model, the effect size of the number of episodes of OSA on fasting glucose was much more important than that of visceral fat. Our observation has clinical implications for the prevention and treatment of diabetes: in obese, chronically sleep deprived subjects, treating OSA may be more effective than losing abdominal fat.

TABLE 6: Multivariate statistical models of sleep apnea (as quantified by RDI score) predicting fasting glucose concentration.

Dependent variable: Fasting Glucose (mg/dL)	Step 0 Unadjusted	Step 1 Adjusted for visceral fat	Step 2 Adjusted for visceral fat and age	Step 3 Adjusted for visceral fat, age, gender, and sleep duration
Intercept (mg/dL)	82.4 (78.1 – 86.7)	80.2 (74.9 – 85.4)	78.4 (64.1 – 92.6)	77.1 (52.8 – 101.3)
Goodness of fit	**R^2 = 0.106, p = 0.001**	**R^2 = 0.144, p = 0.001**	**R^2 = 0.144, p = 0.005**	**R^2 = 0.162, p = 0.014**
RDI (logarithmic values)	**7.3* (3.0 – 11.6)**	**5.4* (0.3 – 10.5)**	**5.3* (0.2 – 10.5)**	**5.8* (0.3 – 11.3)**
Visceral fat by CT (cm^3)		0.012 (–0.002 – 0.026)	0.012 (–0.002 – 0.026)	0.016 (–0.001 – 0.032)
Age (yrs)			0.047 (–0,301 – 0.395)	0.084 (–0.277 – 0.446)
Gender (female = 0, male = 1)				–2.7 (–8.7 – 3.2)
Actigraphy sleep duration (min/night)				0.004 (–0.044 – 0.052)

Beta coefficients in each cell were calculated after adjustment for the other independent variables in the multivariate model, and reported as mean values with 95% CI
** p<0.05*

There were some hormonal differences between subjects with and without OSA. Morning plasma ACTH and urinary norepinephrine were higher in subjects with OSA, suggesting an activation of the stress system.

Single time-point serum GH levels were significantly lower in subjects with SA, which is compatible with the decreased activity of the GH axis in obese subjects [24], but IGF-1 levels were normal in both groups. These findings should be considered exploratory, given that both the HPA and the GH axes were studied under basal conditions and hormonal measurements conducted on single time-point samples.

At variance with previous reports, sleep duration and glucose parameters were not related in our sample [2], [3], [5], [25], [26]. Most of the existing studies applied protocols of acute sleep deprivation to healthy, non- chronically sleep-deprived lean subjects [27]. We included only obese and chronically sleep deprived subjects and as such it is likely that chronic sleep deprivation may have already produced its negative effects on glucose metabolism.

Several studies have reported on the relationship between OSA and glucose metabolism [2], [3], [5], [25], [26], [28], [29]. The prevalence of OSA in our cohort was higher than the prevalence reported in the Wisconsin Sleep Cohort Study [4]. In the latter study, representing a large, random sample of 30 to 60 year old state agency employees reporting habitual snoring, 9% of women and 24% of men had OSA. Our higher prevalence may be due to the fact that our sample consisted exclusively of obese subjects with short sleep duration. In addition, 60% of our subjects were African American, an ethnic group in which both obesity and OSA are common.

Polysomnography is the gold standard for diagnosing OSA. This method requires an overnight stay in the hospital, is associated with considerable cost and inconvenience and may interfere with sleep. Therefore, in the current study we used for practical purposes portable devices designed for home use. Given the already high and increasing prevalence of OSA, we recommend using these devices more routinely to make large-scale screening practical, while polysomnography should be reserved for more complicated cases in which a formal sleep study may be required. By analogy, while for research purposes insulin resistance is determined by insulin clamp, for clinical purposes determination of fasting glucose and insulin are used. As recently stated by the Centers for Disease Control and Prevention (CDC), universal screening for type 2 diabetes in middle aged African-American, a segment of the population very similar to our sample, is considered very cost-effective [30]; similarly, diagnosis and treatment of OSA is considered cost-effective [31]. It is therefore likely that screening would be quite advantageous in subjects with OSA and obesity. An effort should be made to further develop simple devices that could be used at home; in addition, algorithms using parameters such as snoring, the degree of severity of sleepiness, neck circumference and other measures, should be used for the screening and diagnosis of OSA.

Study limitations include the fact that we did not characterize sleep architecture, that this cross-sectional evaluation was not designed to assess causality, and that the composition of the sample did not allow analyses of gender or ethnic differences. In addition, measurements of OSA were available in 96 of 125 subjects randomized, whereas CRP measurements were available in 87 subjects. As study merits, we would like to note the relatively large and well characterized sample in a real life setting, and the determination of a large variety of cytokines measured simultaneously with a sensitive assay. Finally, this cohort was exclusively composed of obese subjects.

In summary, OSA was more prevalent in our chronically sleep-deprived obese population than previously reported, its presence and severity were closely linked to abnormalities of glucose metabolism and insulin resistance to a greater extent than abdominal fat. OSA should be suspected, diagnosed and treated early in this population. The general public and healthcare providers should be made more aware of the health consequences of OSA, including abnormal glucose metabolism. Ongoing and future studies determining optimal interventions for OSA to improve glycemia and lower cardiometabolic risk are of upmost importance.

REFERENCES

1. Cizza G, Skarulis M, Mignot E (2005) A link between short sleep and obesity: building the evidence for causation. Sleep 10: 1217–20.
2. Punjabi NM, Sorking JD, Katzel LI, Goldberg AP, Schwarts AR, et al. (2002) Sleep-disordered breathing and insulin resistance in middle-aged and overweight men. Am J Respir Crit Care Med 165: 677–82. doi: http://dx.doi.org/10.1164/ajrccm.165.5.2104087.

3. Vgontzas AN, Papanicolaou DA, Bixler EO, Hopper K, Lotsikas A, et al. (2000) Sleep apnea and daytime sleepiness and fatigue: relation to visceral obesity, insulin resistance and hypercytokinemia. J Clin Endocrinol Metab 85: 1151–1158. doi: http://dx.doi.org/10.1210/jc.85.3.1151.
4. Young T, Palta M, Dempsey J, Skatrud J, Weber S, et al. (1993) The occurrence of sleep-disordered breathing among middle-aged adults. N Engl J Med 328: 1230–1235. doi: http://dx.doi.org/10.1056/nejm199304293281704.
5. Tassone F, Lanfranco F, Gianotti L, Pivetti S, Navone F, et al. (2003) Obstructive sleep apnoea syndrome impairs insulin sensitivity independently of anthropometric variables. Clin endocrinol (Oxf) 59: 374–379. doi: http://dx.doi.org/10.1046/j.1365-2265.2003.01859.x.
6. Pamidi S, Wroblewski K, Broussard J, Day A, Hanlon EC, et al. (2012) Obstructive sleep apnea in young lean men: impact on insulin sensitivity and secretion. Diabetes Care. 35: 2384–9. doi: http://dx.doi.org/10.2337/dc12-0841.
7. Spiegel K, Leproult R, Van Cauter E (1999) Impact of sleep debt on metabolic and endocrine function. Lancet 354: 1435–39. doi: http://dx.doi.org/10.1016/s0140-6736(99)01376-8.
8. Spiegel K, Leproult R, L'Hermite-Baleriaux M, Copinschi G, Penev PD, et al. (2004) Leptin levels are dependent on sleep duration: relationships with sympathovagal balance, carbohydrate regulation, cortisol, and thyrotropin. J Clin Endocrinol Metab 89: 5762–5771. doi: http://dx.doi.org/10.1210/jc.2004-1003.
9. Stamatakis KA, Punjabi NM (2010) Effects of sleep fragmentation on glucose metabolism in normal subjects. Chest 137: 95–101. doi: http://dx.doi.org/10.1378/chest.09-0791.
10. Cizza G, Marincola P, Mattingly M, Williams L, Mitler M, et al. (2010) Treatment of obesity with extension of sleep duration: a randomized, prospective, controlled trial. Clin Trials 7: 274–85. doi: http://dx.doi.org/10.1177/1740774510368298.
11. Yao J, Sussman DL, Summers RM (2011) Fully automated adipose tissue measurement on abdominal CT. Proceedings of SPIE 7965: 7965Z.
12. Knutson KL, Zhao X, Mattingly M, Galli G, Cizza G (2012) Predictors of sleep-disordered breathing in obese adults who are chronic short sleepers. Sleep Med 13: 484–9. doi: http://dx.doi.org/10.1016/j.sleep.2011.11.009.
13. Buysse DJ, Reynolds CF, 3rd, Monk TH, Berman SR, Kupfer DJ (1989) The Pittsburgh Sleep Quality Index: a new instrument for psychiatric practice and research. Psychiatry Res 28: 193–213. doi: http://dx.doi.org/10.1016/0165-1781(89)90047-4.
14. Johns MW (1991) A new method for measuring daytime sleepiness: The Epworth Sleepiness Scale. Sleep 14: 540–5. doi: http://dx.doi.org/10.1378/chest.103.1.30.
15. Ayappa I, Norman RG, Seelall V, Rapoport DM (2008) Validation of a self-applied unattended monitor for sleep disordered breathing. J Clin Sleep Med 4: 26–37.
16. Westbrook PR, Levendowski DJ, Cvetinovic M, Zavora T, Velimirovic V, et al. (2005) Description and validation of the apnea risk evaluation system: a novel method to diagnose sleep apnea-hypopnea in the home. Chest 128: 2166–2175. doi: http://dx.doi.org/10.1378/chest.128.4.2166.
17. Tasali E, Mokhlesi B, Van Cauter E (2008) Obstructive sleep apnea and type 2 diabetes: interacting epidemics. Chest. 133: 496–506. doi: http://dx.doi.org/10.1378/chest.07-0828.

18. Louis M, Punjabi NM (2009) Effects of acute intermittent hypoxia on glucose metabolism in awake healthy volunteers. J Appl Physiol. 106: 1538–44. doi: http://dx.doi.org/10.1152/japplphysiol.91523.2008.
19. Peltier AC, Bagai K, Artibee K, Diedrich A, Garland E, et al. (2012) Effect of mild hyperglycemia on autonomic function in obstructive sleep apnea. Clin Auton Res. 22: 1–8. doi: http://dx.doi.org/10.1007/s10286-011-0131-9.
20. Kelly KR, Williamson DL, Fealy CE, Kriz DA, Krishnan RK, et al. (2010) Acute altitude-induced hypoxia suppresses plasma glucose and leptin in healthy humans. Metabolism. 59: 200–5. doi: http://dx.doi.org/10.1016/j.metabol.2009.07.014.
21. Vgontzas AN, Papanicolaou DA, Bixler EO, Kales A, Tyson K, et al. (1997) Elevation of plasma cytokines in disorders of excessive daytime sleepiness: role of sleep disturbance and obesity. J Clin Endocrinol Metab. 82: 1313–6. doi: http://dx.doi.org/10.1210/jc.82.5.1313.
22. Cizza G, Eskandari F, Coyle M, Krishnamurthy P, Wright EC, et al. (2009) Plasma CRP levels in premenopausal women with major depression: a 12-month controlled study. Horm Metab Res. 41: 641–8. doi: http://dx.doi.org/10.1055/s-0029-1220717.
23. O'Rourke RW, White AE, Metcalf MD, Olivas AS, Mitra P, et al. (2011) Hypoxia-induced inflammatory cytokine secretion in human adipose tissue stromovascular cells. Diabetologia. 54: 1480–90. doi: http://dx.doi.org/10.1007/s00125-011-2103-y.
24. Van Cauter E, Latta F, Nedeltcheva A, Spiegel K, Leproult R, et al.. (2004) Reciprocal interactions between the GH axis and sleep. Growth Horm IGF Res. 4 Jun; 14 Suppl A: S10–7.
25. Fredheim JM, Rollheim J, Omland T, Hofsø D, Røislien J, et al. (2011) Type 2 diabetes and pre-diabetes are associated with obstructive sleep apnea in extremely obese subjects: a cross-sectional study. Cardiovasc Diabetol. 10: 84. doi: http://dx.doi.org/10.1186/1475-2840-10-84.
26. Lam JC, Tan KC, Lai AY, Lam DC, Ip MS (2012) Increased serum levels of advanced glycation end-products is associated with severity of sleep disordered breathing but not insulin sensitivity in non-diabetic men with obstructive sleep apnoea. Sleep Med. 1: 15–20. doi: http://dx.doi.org/10.1016/j.sleep.2011.07.015.
27. Van Cauter E (2011) Sleep disturbances and insulin resistance. Diabet Med. 28: 1455–62. doi: http://dx.doi.org/10.1111/j.1464-5491.2011.03459.x.
28. Gruber A, Horwood F, Sithole J, Ali NJ, Idris I (2006) Obstructive sleep apnoea is independently associated with the metabolic syndrome but not insulin resistance state. Cardiovasc Diabetol 5: 22. doi: 10.1186/1475-2840-5-22.
29. Papaioannou I, Patterson M, Twigg GL, Vazir A, Ghatei M, et al. (2011) Lack of association between impaired glucose tolerance and appetite regulating hormones in patients with obstructive sleep apnea. J Clin Sleep Med 7: 486–92B. doi: http://dx.doi.org/10.5664/jcsm.1314.
30. Li R, Zhang P, Barker LE, Chowdhury FM, Zhang X (2010) Cost-effectiveness of interventions to prevent and control diabetes mellitus: a systematic review. Diabetes Care. 33: 1872–94. doi: http://dx.doi.org/10.2337/dc10-0843.
31. Pietzsch JB, Garner A, Cipriano LE, Linehan JH (2011) An integrated health-economic analysis of diagnostic and therapeutic strategies in the treatment of moderate-to-severe obstructive sleep apnea. Sleep. 34: 695–709. doi: http://dx.doi.org/10.5665/sleep.1030.

CHAPTER 11

CLUSTER ANALYSIS OF OBESITY AND ASTHMA PHENOTYPES

E. RAND SUTHERLAND, ELENA GOLEVA, TONYA S. KING, ERIK LEHMAN, ALLEN D. STEVENS, LEISA P. JACKSON, AMANDA R. STREAM, JOHN V. FAHY, and DONALD Y. M. LEUNG FOR THE ASTHMA CLINICAL RESEARCH NETWORK

11.1 INTRODUCTION

Cluster analyses of cross-sectional data from clinical populations have identified phenotypic subsets of patients with asthma, and the assessment of BMI in recent asthma cluster analyses has allowed assessment of the relationship of BMI to clinical features of asthma. Haldar and colleagues reported that obesity was associated with increased symptom expression, reduced eosinophilic airway inflammation, adult age of onset, and female sex, while also being associated with reduced clinical responsiveness to inhaled corticosteroids (ICS) [1]. A separate cluster analysis of patients participating in the NIH Severe Asthma Research Program indicated that elevated body mass index (BMI) was associated with specific clinical features in severe asthma, with the identification of a cluster of patients in

This chapter was originally published under the Creative Commons Attribution License. Lehman E, Stevens AD, Jackson LP, Stream AR, Fahy JV, and Leung DYM. Cluster Analysis of Obesity and Asthma Phenotypes. PLoS ONE *7,5 (2012), doi:10.1371/journal.pone.003663.*

whom elevated BMI was associated with female sex, adult onset asthma, a greater likelihood of complicated asthma treatment regimens, and more frequent health care utilization and need for systemic glucocorticoids (GC) [2]. These two studies have supported the conclusion that asthma phenotype is relatively homogenous in obese patients, with high symptom expression, low atopy and airway eosinophilia, and relative insensitivity to GC, a phenomenon that has been reported by others in both clinical [3]–[5] and in vitro [6] settings.

These reports notwithstanding, other analyses using standard comparative analytical approaches between asthmatics categorized by BMI have suggested that there is phenotypic heterogeneity among obese asthmatics, with some studies suggesting that asthma is more severe in obese asthmatics [7], [8], possibly due to increased airway or systemic inflammation [9], and others suggesting that obesity has a more modest effect, independent of inflammation or altered lung mechanics [10], [11]. Given these disparate observations, and given that over 50% of adult asthmatics are overweight or obese [12], more information is needed to enhance our understanding of asthma in obese patients. In this context, we conducted an analysis of data from two NIH-sponsored clinical trials to evaluate the relationship of obesity to markers of asthma phenotype in adults. A priori, we incorporated measurements of adipokines and systemic inflammation and clinical measures of response to inhaled corticosteroids into a cluster-based analytical approach. We then evaluated differences in in vitro markers of glucocorticoid sensitivity between phenotype clusters identified in the hypothesis-independent analysis.

11.2 METHODS

11.2.1 OBJECTIVE

To define the contribution of obesity and related variables to asthma phenotype.

11.2.2 PARTICIPANTS

Data from adults with persistent asthma participating in the common run-in period of the TALC [13] (NCT00565266) and BASALT trials (NCT00495157) of the NHLBI Asthma Clinical Research Network were utilized to assemble a cohort of rigorously characterized asthmatic subjects. Participants at all centers were assessed for biomarkers of obesity and systemic inflammation. Inclusion/exclusion criteria and design of the common run-in period have been reported previously [13]. Of the 826 participants enrolled in the common run-in period, all participants with complete clinical, physiologic and inflammatory data (n = 250) were eligible for inclusion in these analyses.

11.2.3 DESCRIPTION OF PROCEDURES

During the common run-in period, all participants received hydrofluoroalkane beclomethasone dipropionate (HFA-BDP) at a dose of 80 mcg (2 puffs of 40 mcg) twice daily for a 4-week period and were provided an albuterol metered-dose inhaled for rescue use. Clinical and inflammatory parameters were assessed as reported previously [13]. Peripheral blood mononuclear cells (PBMC) were isolated by Ficoll-Hypaque gradient centrifugation [14] and cultured in medium ± dexamethasone (DEX, 10^{-6} M) for 3 hours. RNA was extracted and expression of GC receptor-alpha (GCRα) and MAP kinase phosphatase-1 (MKP-1) were analyzed by real-time PCR, normalized to corresponding levels of 18 sRNA, and reported as fold-change in expression induced by dexamethasone [15], [16]. 25(OH)D concentrations were assayed by liquid chromatography-tandem mass spectrometry at Mayo Clinical Laboratories (Rochester, Minnesota). Assays for serum concentrations of leptin, adiponectin, interleukin 6 (IL-6), tumor necrosis factor-alpha (TNFα) and C-reactive protein were performed by ELISA or highly-sensitive immunoturbidometric assay (hsCRP).

11.2.4 ETHICS

All participants provided written informed consent. The protocol was reviewed and approved at each institutional IRB listed in the Appendix S1.

11.2.5 STATISTICAL METHODS

Ward's minimum-variance hierarchical clustering method [17] with standardization of incorporated variables was performed in SAS (v. 9.2, SAS Institute Inc., Cary, N.C.). Analyzed variables included sex, race (white versus nonwhite), age at asthma onset, asthma duration, body mass index (BMI), % predicted forced expiratory volume in one second ($FEV_{1\%}$), forced vital capacity (FVC), airway hyperresponsiveness (PC_{20} FEV_1 to methacholine (mg/mL)), Juniper Asthma Control Questionnaire score (ACQ) [18], Asthma Evaluation Questionnaire score (AEQ, a composite of asthma symptoms over the prior two weeks [13]), exhaled nitric oxide (F_ENO, ppb), percent eosinophils in induced sputum, serum IgE (IU/mL), hsCRP, serum IL-6, serum TNFα, serum adiponectin, serum leptin, prior controller use, and change in AEQ and ACQ scores (after 4 and 2 weeks, respectively, of HFA-BDP). Discriminant analysis was then performed to identify significant determinants of cluster membership, and a reclassification procedure determined the accuracy of the discriminant function model for predicting cluster membership. Generalized squared distances were utilized to determine the proximity of clusters.

Differences between clusters were evaluated using analysis of variance or Student's t-test for normally-distributed continuous variables. Chi-square analysis was used for categorical measures. Non-normally distributed data were log-transformed for analysis. Unadjusted analyses correlating continuous variables were performed using simple linear regression, with least-squares regression was used to perform adjusted analyses. Numeric data are presented as mean (standard deviation), except in the case of geometric mean (coefficient of variation) for log-transformed data.

TABLE 1: Characteristics of study population.

Measured at study initiation	
n, subjects	250
Sex (% male)	32
Race (% white)	59
Age (years)	37.6 (12.5)
Age of asthma onset (years)	15.4 (14.7)
Asthma duration (years)	22.2 (12.2)
BMI (kg/m^2)	29.9 (8.3)
FEV_1 (L)	2.8 (0.8)
FVC (L)	3.9 (1.1)
FEV1/FVC (%)	71.8 (8.7)
FEV_1 (predicted)	82.2 (13.8)
PC_{20} (mg/mL)$^+$	1.2 (1.2)
Asthma evaluation questionnaire score	0.7 (0.8)
Measured after 2 weweks HFA-BDP	
Asthma control questionnaire score	1.0 (0.8)
IgE (IU/mL)$^+$	105.4 (1.6)
hsCRP (mg/L)$^+$	1.8 (1.4)
Interleukin-6 (pg/mL)$^+$	1.4 (0.9)
TNFα (pg/mL)$^+$	1.7 (0.8)
Adiponectin (mcg/mL)$^+$	7.0 (0.7)
Leptin (ng/mL)$^+$	10.8 (1.3)
Measured after 4 weeks HFA-BDP	
F_ENO (ppb)$^+$	19.9 (0.6)
Sputum eosinophils (%)$^+$	0.8 (1.0)
Asthma evaluation questionnaire score	0.6 (0.7)
Asthma control questionnaire score	0.9 (0.8)

Numeric data presented as mean (standard deviation), except $^+$geometric mean (coefficient of variation), log-transformed for analysis.

11.3 RESULTS

11.3.1 PARTICIPANT CHARACTERISTICS

Data from 250 participants were analyzed (Table 1). The population was 32% male, 59% white and had a mean (SD) age of 37.6 (12.5) years. The study population had a mean BMI of 29.9 (8.3) kg/m^2, with a mean FEV_1 of 82.2 (13.8) % predicted and airway hyperresponsiveness as reflected by a methacholine PC_{20} FEV_1 of 1.2 (1.2) mg/mL. Serum IgE was 105.4 (1.6) IU/mL, F_ENO was 19.9 (0.6) ppb, and sputum eosinophils were 0.8 (1.0)% (geometric mean and coefficient of variation).

11.3.2 DETERMINANTS OF CLUSTER MEMBERSHIP

Discriminant analysis revealed that 16 variables (Table 2) were significant determinants of cluster membership, with reclassification indicating that the discriminant function model achieved 89% accuracy for predicting cluster membership. BMI was the most significant determinant of cluster membership ($F = 57.1$, $p<0.0001$), followed by asthma symptoms ($F = 44.8$, $p<0.0001$). Less significant were degree of asthma control (ACQ, $F = 12.5$, $p<0.0001$), race ($F = 9.4$, $p<0.0001$), degree of improvement in asthma symptoms after 4 weeks of treatment with HFA-BDP ($F = 9.1$, $p<0.0001$), age of onset/disease duration, lung function, airway hyperresponsiveness (PC_{20}), leptin, adiponectin, biomarkers of systemic (hsCRP, TNFα), airway inflammation (F_ENO) and atopy (IgE). Generalized squared distances between the clusters ranged from 7.8 to 16.0, with pair-wise differences as follows: cluster 1 vs. 2, 9.2; cluster 1 vs. 3, 15.3; cluster 1 vs. 4, 7.8; cluster 2 vs. 3, 16.0; cluster 2 vs. 4, 13.1; and cluster 3 vs. 4, 13.3.

TABLE 2: Results of discriminant analysis demonstrating relative contribution of variables in determining cluster membership.

Variable	Partial R-square	F	p
BMI	0.4105	57.1	<0.0001
AEQ (symptoms)	0.3542	44.8	<0.0001
ACQ (control)	0.1339	12.5	<0.0001
Race	0.1039	9.4	<0.0001
Change in AEQ after 4 weeks for HFA-BDP	0.1021	9.1	<0.0001
Age of asthma onset	0.0991	8.8	<0.0001
F_ENO	0.0845	7.4	<0.0001
Asthma controller type	0.0724	6.2	0.0005
$FEV_{1\%}$ predicted	0.0696	5.9	0.0007
Leptin	0.0651	5.5	0.0012
Asthma duration	0.0630	5.2	0.0017
Adiponectin	0.0601	5.0	0.0022
TNFα	0.0587	4.9	0.0027
PC_{20}	0.0474	3.9	0.0100
IgE	0.0385	3.1	0.0282
FVC	0.0358	2.9	0.0372

11.3.3 ASTHMA CLUSTERS

Analysis revealed four unique clusters of asthma patients, with characteristics as reported in Table 3. These four clusters differed from each other significantly with regard to BMI, with mean BMI in clusters 1 and 2 falling within the overweight range (BMI = 25.8 (5.0) and 26.9 (4.4)). In contrast, BMI in clusters 3 and 4 was indicative of class I and class II obesity [19] (34.7 (8.0) and 38.5 (9.2), respectively), $p<0.01$ for comparison between the four clusters. As shown in Table 3, FEV_1 was highest and IgE, hsCRP and leptin were all lower in the non-obese clusters when compared with the two obese clusters. All clusters were marked by low sputum eosinophils and did not differ significantly from each other (Table 3). Concentrations of hsCRP were highest in the two obese clusters, with hsCRP concentration of 4.2 (1.2) and 4.5 (1.1) in clusters 3 and 4 and 1.3 (1.3) and 0.8 (1.1) mg/L in clusters 1 and 2.

11.3.4 PHENOTYPIC HETEROGENEITY IN OBESE ASTHMATICS

As reported in Table 3, obese clusters 3 and 4 were similar with regard to lung function, sex distribution, racial composition, age and concentrations of the adipokines leptin and adiponectin and hsCRP, a marker of systemic inflammation. There was a trend toward a significant BMI difference between the two obese clusters that did not achieve statistical significance, with cluster 3 demonstrating an average BMI of 34.7 (8.0) kg/m^2, versus 38.5 (9.2) kg/m^2 in cluster 4 ($p = 0.06$). Age of asthma onset differed between the two clusters with members of cluster 3 having asthma onset during childhood at 10.0 (10.8) years of age, and members of cluster 4 having disease onset during adolescence, at 16.1 (13.9) years of age. The two obese clusters differed with regard to degree of symptom expression and asthma control despite 4 weeks' treatment with HFA-BDP: cluster 3 demonstrated persistently high symptom expression, with an AEQ score of 1.3 (0.9) versus 0.7 (0.8) ($p<0.01$), and also demonstrated persistently worse asthma control, with an ACQ score of 1.8 (1.0) versus 0.9 (0.9) ($p<0.01$). Cluster 3 also demonstrated the highest concentration of F_ENO at 24.8 (0.7) vs. 14.9 (0.7) ppb ($p<0.01$) and the greatest degree of airway hyperresponsiveness of the four clusters, with a PC_{20} FEV_1 of 0.7 mg/mL methacholine. In both clusters, IgE and hsCRP were elevated when compared with non-obese clusters but were not significantly different from each other ($p = 0.32$ and 0.82, respectively). Thus, while obese individuals shared similar degrees of lung function impairment, adipokines, atopy and systemic inflammation (as indicated by hsCRP), a more severe group could be identified that had asthma of childhood onset, greater airway hyperresponsiveness, greater airway inflammation (as reflected by F_ENO), and persistence of symptoms and suboptimal asthma control despite treatment with ICS.

TABLE 3: Characteristics of asthma disease clusters.

	Non-obese female asthmatics	Non-obese male asthmatics	Obese uncontrolled asthma	Obese well-controlled asthma	P
Cluster number	1	2	3	4	--
n	114	52	30	54	--
Sex (% male)	18	83	17	24	<0.01
Race (% white)	77	67	37	26	<0.01
Age at onset (years)	19.1 (16.1)	9.8 (11.8)	10.0 (10.8)*	16.1 (13.9)*	<0.01
Asthma duration (years)	18.3 (11.3)	26.2 (11.5)	25.9 (12.0)	24.6 (12.9)	<0.01
BMI (kg/m^2)	25.8 (5.0)	26.9 (4.4)	34.7 (8.0)	38.5 (9.2)	<0.01
FVC (L)	3.8 (0.7)	4.9 (1.3)	3.2 (0.9)	3.3 (0.9)	<0.01
FEV_1 (% predicted)	87.7 (12.1)	82.3 (16.4)	73.5 (9.0)	75.5 (11.1)	<0.01
FEV1/FVC (%)	74.1 (8.7)	68.5 (8.7)	71.5 (8.0)	69.7 (8.0)	<0.01
PC_{20} (mg/mL)$^+$	1.2 (1.2)	1.6 (1.3)	0.7 (1.2)*	1.5 (0.9)*	0.02
ACQ score	0.8 (0.7)	0.8 (0.6)	1.8 (1.0)*	0.9 (0.9)*	<0.01
AEQ score	0.5 (0.6)	0.4 (0.5)	1.3 (0.9)*	0.7 (0.8)*	<0.01
F_ENO (ppb)$^+$	20.8 (0.6)	21.6 (0.6)	24.8 (0.7)*	14.9 (0.7)*	<0.01
Eosinophils (%)$^+$	0.8 (0.9)	0.9 (1.0)	0.8 (1.1)	0.7 (0.9)	0.44
IgE (IU/mL)$^+$	78.1 (1.7)	99.8 (1.3)	201.9 (1.5)	146.1 (1.4)	<0.01
hsCRP (mg/L)$^+$	1.3 (1.3)	0.8 (1.1)	4.2 (1.2)	4.5 (1.1)	<0.01
Interleukin-6 (pg/mL)$^+$	1.2 (1.0)	0.9 (0.6)	1.9 (0.7)	2.1 (0.7)	<0.01
TNFα (pg/mL)$^+$	2.0 (1.0)	1.4 (0.4)	1.4 (0.6)	1.5 (0.7)	0.03
Adiponectin (mcg/mL)$^+$	10.2 (0.6)	4.8 (0.6)	6.3 (0.7)	4.9 (0.7)	<0.01
Leptin (ng/mL)$^+$	9.3 (1.0)	3.4 (1.3)	23.1 (0.9)	29.3 (0.8)	<0.01
Use of medium/high-dose ICS (%)	26	21	37	43	0.06

Table p values from Pearson chi-square test (Exact or CMH test) or analysis of variance comparing all 4 clusters.

**indicated $p<0.05$ for comparison of clusters 3 and 4*

Numeric data presented as Mean (standard deviation) except $^+$Geometric Mean (Coefficient of Variation), log-transformed for analysis.

ACQ: asthma control questionnaire score after 4 weeks of HFA-BDP, AEQ: asthma evaluation questionnaire score after 4 weeks of HFA-BDP.

11.3.5 CHARACTERISTICS OF NON-OBESE ASTHMATICS

Non-obese clusters 1 and 2 differed from each other with regard to baseline lung function, with $FEV_{1\%}$ predicted of 87.7% (12.1) in cluster 1 and 82.3% (16.4) in cluster 2 ($p = 0.02$). A similar trend was seen with FEV_1/FVC ratio, which was 74.1 (8.7)% in cluster 1 and 68.5 (8.7)% in cluster 2 ($p<0.01$). These two clusters also differed with regard to the percent of subjects who were male, at 18 vs. 83% ($p<0.01$) and age at asthma onset, at 19.1 (16.1) vs. 9.8 (11.8) years ($p<0.01$). Asthma symptom expression (AEQ scores of 0.5 (0.6) and 0.4 (0.5), $p = 0.66$) and degree of asthma control (ACQ scores of 0.8 (0.7) and 0.8 (0.6), $p = 0.81$) were similar between the two clusters, and these clusters were also similar with regard to biomarkers of inflammation (F_ENO, IgE and hsCRP), indicating that the observed differences between clusters in lung function, sex, and age at disease onset were not linked with a distinct inflammatory phenotype (Table 3).

11.3.6 CLUSTER MEMBERSHIP, BMI AND IN VITRO GC SENSITIVITY

Markers of in vitro GC response were assessed in 49 participants in a single center translational mechanistic substudy. In members of obese clusters 3 and 4 ($n = 12$), PBMC GCRα expression (pg/ng 18 s RNA, log-transformed) was significantly less than in members of the non-obese clusters 1 and 2, at 6.6 (0.3) versus 6.9 (0.3), $p = 0.004$, corresponding with an approximately 25% reduction in the absolute values of GCRα expression in obese asthmatics (742.8 (184.5) vs. 984.7 (276.1) pg/ng 18 s RNA, $p = 0.007$).

When we analyzed the correlation between log-transformed GCRα expression in all 49 participants, we observed an inverse correlation ($r = -0.23$) that was not statistically significant ($p = 0.1$). Next, due to prior reports suggesting a relationship between vitamin D and biomarkers of steroid responsiveness [20], [21], we measured 25(OH)D concentrations in these participants. Members of clusters 3 and 4 demonstrated reduced

25(OH)D when compared with cluster 1 and 2 members, at 21.2 (7.6) vs. 29.2 (9.9) ng/mL ($p = 0.01$). We then analyzed the relationship between GCRαexpression and BMI in subjects who had 25(OH)D concentrations ≤30 ng/mL [20]. In this subset, an inverse correlation between BMI and log-transformed GCRαexpression was observed, with $r = -0.52$ ($p = 0.02$). This exploratory analysis suggested that the negative effect of BMI on GCRαexpression is augmented by 25(OH)D concentrations. Of note, 25(OH)D was not significantly correlated with GCRαexpression.

Finally, to determine if reduced GCRα expression might be one factor leading to reduced in vitro responsiveness to GCs reported in obese asthmatics [6], the correlation between GCRα expression (log-transformed) and MKP-1 expression both before and after exposure to dexamethasone was examined. Expression of GCRαwas significantly and positively correlated with baseline (pre-DEX, log-transformed) expression of MKP-1, with an unadjusted $r = 0.47$ ($p = 0.008$, Figure 1) and an $r = 0.47$ ($p =$

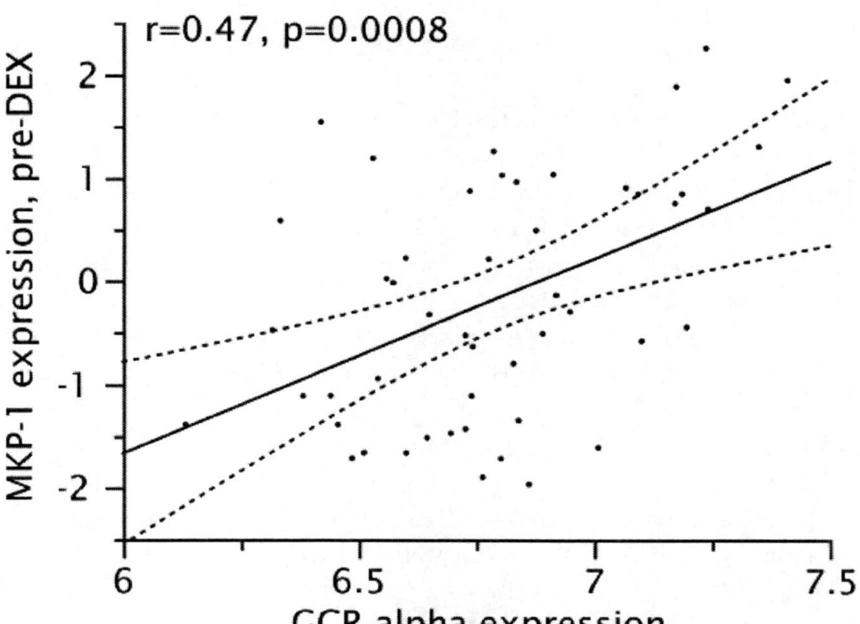

FIGURE 1: Correlation between expression of GCRα and baseline expression of MKP-1 in PBMC (both log-transformed).

0.004) when adjusted for 25(OH)D concentrations. A significant positive correlation between GCRα and fold-induction of MKP-1 expression by DEX was also observed, with an adjusted $r = 0.38$ ($p = 0.03$). Additionally, concentrations of hsCRP, which were increased in obese cluster members, were found to be inversely correlated with GCRα expression, with an $r = -0.39$ ($p = 0.005$, Figure 2). Due to small sample size in clusters 3 and 4, we were unable to demonstrate a correlation between the differential clinical response to GC and in vitro markers of GC response in clusters 3 and 4.

11.4 DISCUSSION

The application of an hypothesis-free cluster analytical approach to a well-characterized cohort of adults with mild-to-moderate persistent asthma demonstrates that obesity is a determinant of clinical phenotype in asthma, playing a more significant role than other commonly-assessed clinical, physiologic or inflammatory variables. Of the four distinct clusters of asthma revealed, two had BMI in the obese range and two did not. There was heterogeneity of airway inflammation, symptoms and control in the obese clusters, suggesting that asthma phenotype is not uniform in obese individuals. In the two non-obese clusters, sex emerged as an important determinant of cluster membership; one cluster had a predominance of males the other a predominance of females, with comparatively earlier age of onset and lower lung function (as reflected by $FEV_{1\%}$ predicted) in the male-predominant cluster. Additionally, we have demonstrated that in vitro GC insensitivity in obese asthmatics (as represented by a reduced ability of dexamethasone to induce the expression of MKP-1, an anti-inflammatory marker of GC-induced transactivation [22]) appears to be mediated by reduced expression of GCRα, the dominant isoform of the receptor and a ligand-dependent transcription factor necessary for glucocorticoid-induced transactivation [23]. Exploratory analysis also suggests an important role for 25(OH)D concentrations in mediating this relationship.

Our findings also suggest that the mechanisms which underlie clinical response to GC in obese asthmatics are complex and likely involve an interaction between alterations in GC-mediated anti-inflammatory processes and both systemic and airway inflammation. This conclusion is based on

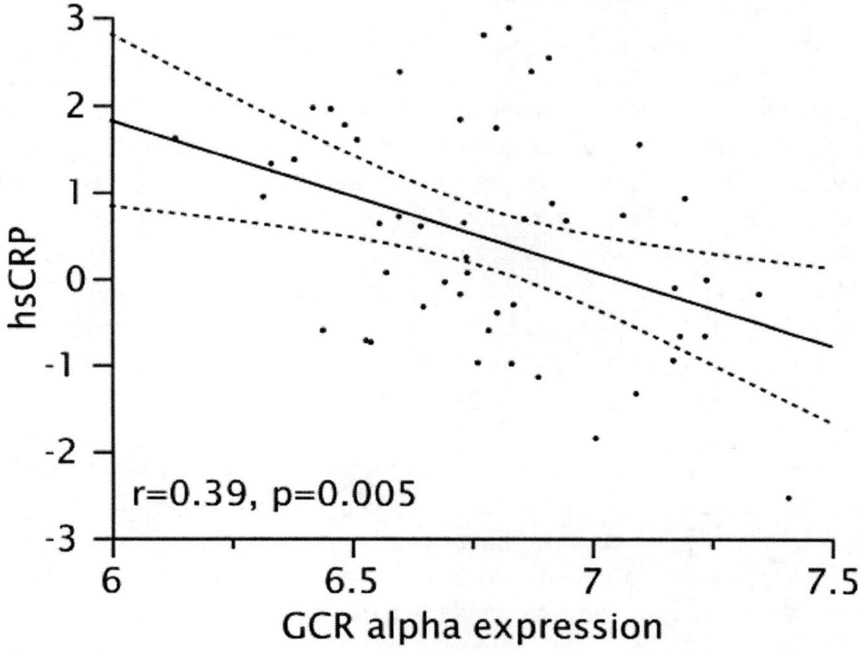

FIGURE 2: Correlation between expression of GCRα in PBMC and serum hsCRP concentrations of (both log-transformed).

our observation that while evidence of in vitro GC insensitivity was observed across both obese clusters, persistently poor asthma control and increased symptoms were observed in the cluster of asthmatics with the earliest onset of asthma, a greater degree of airway hyperresponsiveness and increased concentration of nitric oxide in exhaled breath. The GC insensitivity observed in obese asthmatics was also directly associated with the degree of systemic inflammation, as indicated by the inverse association between hsCRP and GCRα expression, and also is enhanced in the presence of reduced serum 25(OH) vitamin D concentrations. It is also interesting to note that our findings appear to minimize the role of comparative differences in sputum eosinophils as a reason for GC insensitivity in obese asthmatics. Independent of BMI, sputum eosinophils averaged less than 1% in the study population, suggesting that the GC insensitivity observed in obese patients with asthma is likely attributable to the defects in molecular GC response or increased inflammation that we have demonstrated, rather than to a pauci-eosinophilic airway inflammatory phenotype specific to obese asthmatics, as has been suggested in other reports [1].

Potential limitations of our must be considered: first, our analytical approach is hypothesis-independent. While this provides the opportunity to identify new associations that one might not be able (on the basis of current knowledge) to prespecify, it runs the risk of returning results that are counterintuitive or which differ from current hypothetical constructs of disease. Second, as with any meta-analytical technique, the results are entirely dependent on the data available for entry into the analysis. Thus, while we have attempted to include all clinically-relevant data, the derivation of our data from a clinical trial dataset limits the availability of certain data (e.g. socioeconomic or environmental status) and may introduce issues of generalizability given the highly-selected nature of clinical trial participants. Next, as with any cross-sectional data, we are unable to comment on causation, per se, and thus can only conclude that there are specific aspects of the obesity-asthma relationship that are clinically relevant. In fact, a number of questions regarding causal aspects of the relationship between obesity and asthma remain unanswered. Although many epidemiologic studies suggest that antecedent obesity increases subsequent asthma risk, asthma could also increase the risk of becoming overweight or obese. Factors that may play a role in this regard include chronic glucocorticoid use leading to weight gain, as well as respiratory impairment leading to sedentariness, reduced participation in physical, educational or occupational activities, as well as overall reductions in quality of life, all of which may lead to or be associated with increases in body mass.

Our analytical approach and validation of clinical phenotypes with studies of the molecular mechanisms of GC insensitivity in asthma strengthen the assertion that patients with asthma, both adult and pediatric [3], [5], [24]–[27], who are overweight or obese bear a disproportionate burden of illness when compared with non-obese asthmatics. Notwithstanding, the mechanisms of GC insensitivity are complex [28], and the mechanisms by which obesity reduces molecular response to GC require further study. In this light, recent studies have shown that monokines secreted by adipose tissue activate blood monocytes and recruit activated macrophages to adipose tissue, significantly amplifying pro-inflammatory cytokine generation [29]–[32]. This phenomenon can be associated with classical activation [32] which has been documented in both blood monocytes and alveolar macrophages in glucocorticoid-insensitive asthma [33], [34], and may be relevant in obese patients with asthma as well. Additionally, these data provide additional support to the importance of recent observations [6], [21], [35]–[38], that low serum vitamin D concentrations are associated with impaired glucocorticoid response in asthma.

Clinicians frequently encounter obese asthmatics who do not respond optimally to therapy, but no specific guidance currently exists in national and international guidelines as to the optimal therapeutic approach to the obese asthmatic [39], [40]. Many obese asthmatics receive complicated asthma treatment regimens to which they do not respond [2] and which may subject them to increased risk of treatment-related adverse effects. Given this, and given the prevalence of both obesity and asthma, additional information on which to base therapeutic decision making is critical. This study used unbiased analytical approaches to further validate reports that asthma phenotype differs between obese and non-obese asthmatics, while also demonstrating that asthma phenotype is not homogenous in all obese individuals, particularly with regard to the degree of control achieved with ICS treatment. Thus, clinical GC response may not be uniformly attenuated in obese asthmatics, and more work is needed to identify the pathways by which GC signaling mechanisms, systemic inflammation and airway inflammation interact to lead to clinical insensitivity to GC in some, but not all, obese asthmatics.

REFERENCES

1. Haldar P, Pavord ID, Shaw DE, Berry MA, Thomas M, et al. (2008) Cluster Analysis and Clinical Asthma Phenotypes. Am J Respir Crit Care Med 178: 218–224. doi: 10.1164/rccm.200711-1754OC.
2. Moore WC, Meyers DA, Wenzel SE, Teague WG, Li H, et al. (2009) Identification of Asthma Phenotypes Using Cluster Analysis in the Severe Asthma Research Program. Am J Respir Crit Care Med 181: 315–323. doi: 10.1164/rccm.200906-0896OC.
3. Peters-Golden M, Swern A, Bird SS, Hustad CM, Grant E, et al. (2006) Influence of body mass index on the response to asthma controller agents. Eur Respir J 27: 495–503. doi: 10.1183/09031936.06.00077205.
4. Sutherland ER, Lehman EB, Teodorescu M, Wechsler ME (2009) Body mass index and phenotype in subjects with mild-to-moderate persistent asthma. J Allergy Clin Immunol 123: 1328–1334 e1321: doi: 10.1016/j.jaci.2009.04.005.

5. Forno E, Lescher R, Strunk R, Weiss S, Fuhlbrigge A, et al. (2011) Decreased response to inhaled steroids in overweight and obese asthmatic children. J Allergy Clin Immunol 127: 741–749. doi: 10.1016/j.jaci.2010.12.010.
6. Sutherland ER, Goleva E, Strand M, Beuther DA, Leung DY (2008) Body mass and glucocorticoid response in asthma. Am J Respir Crit Care Med 178: 682–687. doi: 10.1164/rccm.200801-076oc.
7. Mosen DM, Schatz M, Magid DJ, Camargo CA Jr (2008) The relationship between obesity and asthma severity and control in adults. J Allergy Clin Immunol 122: 507–511.e506. doi: 10.1016/j.jaci.2008.06.024.
8. Taylor B, Mannino D, Brown C, Crocker D, Twum-Baah N, et al. (2008) Body mass index and asthma severity in the National Asthma Survey. Thorax 63: 14–20. doi: 10.1136/thx.2007.082784.
9. Dixon AE, Holguin F, Sood A, Salome CM, Pratley RE, et al. (2010) An Official American Thoracic Society Workshop Report: Obesity and Asthma. Proc Am Thorac Soc 7: 325–335. doi: 10.1513/pats.200903-013st.
10. Farah CS, Kermode JA, Downie SR, Brown NJ, Hardaker KM, et al. (2011) Obesity Is a Determinant of Asthma Control, Independent of Inflammation and Lung Mechanics. Chest 140: 659–666. doi: 10.1378/chest.11-0027.
11. Sutherland TJ, Cowan JO, Young S, Goulding A, Grant AM, et al. (2008) The association between obesity and asthma: interactions between systemic and airway inflammation. Am J Respir Crit Care Med 178: 469–475. doi: 10.1164/rccm.200802-301OC.
12. Beuther DA, Sutherland ER (2007) Overweight, Obesity, and Incident Asthma: A Meta-analysis of Prospective Epidemiologic Studies. Am J Resp Crit Care Med 175: 661–666. doi: 10.1164/rccm.200611-1717OC.
13. Peters SP, Kunselman SJ, Icitovic N, Moore WC, Pascual R, et al. (2010) Tiotropium bromide step-up therapy for adults with uncontrolled asthma. N Engl J Med 363: 1715–1726. doi: 10.1056/NEJMoa1008770.
14. Li LB, Goleva E, Hall CF, Ou LS, Leung DY (2004) Superantigen-induced corticosteroid resistance of human T cells occurs through activation of the mitogen-activated protein kinase kinase/extracellular signal-regulated kinase (MEK-ERK) pathway. J Allergy Clin Immunol 114: 1059–1069. doi: 10.1016/j.jaci.2004.08.005.
15. Nomura I, Goleva E, Howell MD, Hamid QA, Ong PY, et al. (2003) Cytokine milieu of atopic dermatitis, as compared to psoriasis, skin prevents induction of innate immune response genes. J Immunol 171: 3262–3269.
16. DeRijk RH, Schaaf M, Stam FJ, de Jong IE, Swaab DF, et al. (2003) Very low levels of the glucocorticoid receptor beta isoform in the human hippocampus as shown by Taqman RT-PCR and immunocytochemistry. Brain Res Mol Brain Res 116: 17–26. doi: 10.1016/S0169-328X(03)00209-2.
17. Ward JH Jr (1963) Hierarchical grouping to optimize an objective function. Journal of the American statistical association 58: 236–244. doi: 10.2307/2282967.
18. Juniper EF, O'Byrne PM, Guyatt GH, Ferrie PJ, King DR (1999) Development and validation of a questionnaire to measure asthma control. Eur Respir J 14: 902–907. doi: 10.1034/j.1399-3003.1999.14d29.x.
19. (2000) Obesity: preventing and managing the global epidemic. Report of a WHO consultation. World Health Organization technical report series 894: i-xii, 1–253: doi: 10.1017/S0021932003245508.

20. Sutherland ER, Goleva E, Jackson LP, Stevens AD, Leung DY (2010) Vitamin D levels, lung function, and steroid response in adult asthma. Am J Respir Crit Care Med 181: 699–704. doi: 10.1164/rccm.200911-1710OC.
21. Xystrakis E, Kusumakar S, Boswell S, Peek E, Urry Z, et al. (2006) Reversing the defective induction of IL-10-secreting regulatory T cells in glucocorticoid-resistant asthma patients. J Clin Invest 116: 146–155. doi: 10.1172/JCI21759.
22. Kassel O, Sancono A, Kratzschmar J, Kreft B, Stassen M, et al. (2001) Glucocorticoids inhibit MAP kinase via increased expression and decreased degradation of MKP-1. Embo J 20: 7108–7116. doi: 10.1093/emboj/20.24.7108.
23. Goleva E (2005) Increased Glucocorticoid Receptor beta Alters Steroid Response in Glucocorticoid-insensitive Asthma. Am J Respir Crit Care Med 173: 607–616. doi: 10.1164/rccm.200507-1046OC.
24. Camargo CA, Boulet L-P, Sutherland ER, Busse WW, Yancey SW, et al. (2010) Body Mass Index and Response to Asthma Therapy: Fluticasone Propionate/Salmeterol versus Montelukast. Journal of Asthma 47: 76–82. doi: 10.3109/02770900903338494.
25. Dixon AE, Shade DM, Cohen RI, Skloot GS, Holbrook JT, et al. (2006) Effect of obesity on clinical presentation and response to treatment in asthma. Journal of Asthma 43: 553–558. doi: 10.1080/02770900600859123.
26. Kattan M, Kumar R, Bloomberg GR, Mitchell HE, Calatroni A, et al. (2010) Asthma control, adiposity, and adipokines among inner-city adolescents. J Allergy Clin Immunol 125: 584–592. doi: 10.1016/j.jaci.2010.01.053.
27. Michelson PH, Williams LW, Benjamin DK, Barnato AE (2009) Obesity, inflammation, and asthma severity in childhood: data from the National Health and Nutrition Examination Survey 2001–2004. Ann Allergy Asthma Immunol 103: 381–385. doi: 10.1016/S1081-1206(10)60356-0.
28. Barnes PJ, Adcock IM (2009) Glucocorticoid resistance in inflammatory diseases. Lancet 373: 1905–1917. doi: 10.1016/S0140-6736(09)60326-3.
29. Kanda H, Tateya S, Tamori Y, Kotani K, Hiasa K, et al. (2006) MCP-1 contributes to macrophage infiltration into adipose tissue, insulin resistance, and hepatic steatosis in obesity. J Clin Invest 116: 1494–1505. doi: 10.1172/JCI26498.
30. Dahlman I, Kaaman M, Olsson T, Tan GD, Bickerton AS, et al. (2005) A unique role of monocyte chemoattractant protein 1 among chemokines in adipose tissue of obese subjects. J Clin Endocrinol Metab 90: 5834–5840. doi: 10.1210/jc.2005-0369.
31. Gordon S (2003) Alternative activation of macrophages. Nat Rev Immunol 3: 23–35. doi: 10.1038/nri978.
32. Lumeng CN, Bodzin JL, Saltiel AR (2007) Obesity induces a phenotypic switch in adipose tissue macrophage polarization. J Clin Invest 117: 175–184. doi: 10.1172/JCI29881.
33. Goleva E, Hauk PJ, Hall CF, Liu AH, Riches DW, et al. (2008) Corticosteroid-resistant asthma is associated with classical antimicrobial activation of airway macrophages. J Allergy Clin Immunol 122: 550–559 e553: doi: 10.1016/j.jaci.2008.07.007.
34. Hakonarson H, Bjornsdottir US, Halapi E, Bradfield J, Zink F, et al. (2005) Profiling of genes expressed in peripheral blood mononuclear cells predicts glucocorticoid sensitivity in asthma patients. Proc Natl Acad Sci U S A 102: 14789–14794. doi: 10.1073/pnas.0409904102.

35. Brehm JM, Celedon JC, Soto-Quiros ME, Avila L, Hunninghake GM, et al. (2009) Serum vitamin D levels and markers of severity of childhood asthma in Costa Rica. Am J Respir Crit Care Med 179: 765–771. doi: 10.1164/rccm.200808-1361OC.
36. Brehm JM, Schuemann B, Fuhlbrigge AL, Hollis BW, Strunk RC, et al. (2010) Serum vitamin D levels and severe asthma exacerbations in the Childhood Asthma Management Program study. J Allergy Clin Immunol 126: 52–58. doi: 10.1016/j.jaci.2010.03.043.
37. Majak P, Olszowiec-Chlebna M, Smejda K, Stelmach I (2011) Vitamin D supplementation in children may prevent asthma exacerbation triggered by acute respiratory infection. J Allergy Clin Immunol 127: 1294–1296. doi: 10.1016/j.jaci.2010.12.016.
38. Searing DA, Zhang Y, Murphy JR, Hauk PJ, Goleva E, et al. (2010) Decreased serum vitamin D levels in children with asthma are associated with increased corticosteroid use. J Allergy Clin Immunol 125: 995–1000. doi: 10.1016/j.jaci.2010.03.008.
39. Expert Panel Report 3: Guidelines for the Diagnosis and Management of Asthma (EPR-3 2007). NIH Publication Number 07– (4051) Bethesda, MD: U.S. Department of Health and Human Services; National Institutes of Health; National Heart Lung and Blood Institute; National Asthma Education and Prevention Program, 2007.
40. management Global strategy for asthma2011)GlobalInitiativeforAsthma(GINA) Url: prevention (updatedhttp://www.ginasthma.org; 2011

There is online supporting information that is not included in this version of the article. To see these additional files, please use the citation in the beginning of the chapter to view the original article.

CHAPTER 12

DIET, PHYSICAL EXERCISE, AND COGNITIVE BEHAVIORAL TRAINING AS A COMBINED WORKPLACE BASED INTERVENTION TO REDUCE BODY WEIGHT AND INCREASE PHYSICAL CAPACITY IN HEALTH CARE WORKERS: A RANDOMIZED CONTROLLED TRIAL

JEANETTE R. CHRISTENSEN, ANNE FABER, DORTE EKNER, KRISTIAN OVERGAARD, ANDREAS HOLTERMANN, and KAREN SØGAARD

12.1 BACKGROUND

Overweight and obesity are well documented to be associated with major chronic illnesses, including hypertension, diabetes, arthritis, heart diseases, cancer and all-cause mortality [1-3]. Moreover, excessive body weight has also been shown to increase the risk for musculoskeletal pain [4], sick leave [5] and early retirement from the workforce before they are entitled to state pension [6], causing high socioeconomic costs [7]. Effective inter-

This chapter was originally published under the Creative Commons Attribution License. Christensen JR, Faber A, Ekner D, Overgaard K, Holtermann A, and Søgaard K. Diet, Physical Exercise and Cognitive Behavioral Training as a Combined Workplace Based Intervention to Reduce Body Weight and Increase Physical Capacity in Health Care Workers: A Randomized Controlled Trial. BMC Public Health ***11****,671 (2011), doi:10.1186/1471-2458-11-67.*

ventions for weight reduction and addressing obesity are therefore a high priority.

It is well documented that being overweight or obese is inversely associated with educational level and occupational class in developed countries [8], particularly among women [9]. Because education and gender often works as stratification into certain labor market sectors, workplaces may be optimal arenas for reaching high-risk populations for overweight and obesity. Health care workers represent a high risk population with high physical demands, involving patient handling and other manual work tasks with high peak force, walking and standing as well as awkward postures [10]. Health care work is predominantly performed by female employees with high prevalence of overweight and low physical capacities and a high prevalence of musculoskeletal pain [11]. Studies suggests, it may be the combination of high body weight, low physical capacity and high physical work demands that causes the high prevalence of musculoskeletal pain [12-15]. Effective well-documented initiatives for reducing weight, improving physical capacity and reducing musculoskeletal pain among health care workers are therefore needed.

Strength training has been shown to improve physical capacity and reduce musculoskeletal pain [16]. Meanwhile, different strategies to reduce overweight have been suggested, as well as several consensus statements regarding weight loss maintenance for individualized interventions, for taxes, tariffs and trade laws policies, and the built environment [17,18]. Diet alone has shown limited effectiveness for long term weight loss maintenance [19]. Programs combining diet and physical exercise are therefore recommended to avoid reductions in energy metabolism with dietary restrictions [20]. Grave and colleagues suggest that weight regain is due to failure to keep up physical activity, as maintenance of physical activity is fundamental for long-term weight loss [21]. The key to maintaining physical activity is new cognitive procedures and strategies that will help weight-loser's to build a mind-set of long-term weight control. In summary, more multidisciplinary interventions are recommended [21] and should include a combination of the three elements—dietary change, physical exercise and cognitive behavioral training [22]. However, only few studies have combined these initiatives [23] and to our knowledge, no previous studies have investigated the combined effects of these initiatives on weight loss at a high-risk group like health care workers in a workplace setting.

Therefore, the main aim of this study was to investigate the effects of a workplace intervention combining diet, physical exercise and cognitive behavioral training on body weight, general health variables and physical capacity in health care workers. The secondary aim was to study if these health promotions could affect musculoskeletal pain among health care workers. This paper presents results from the first three months of a one year intervention.

12.2 METHODS

12.2.1 STUDY DESIGN

The study is part of the FINALE program, which has the long-term aim to reduce physical deterioration indicated by musculoskeletal disorders, work ability and sickness absence among workers with high physical work demands. Details of the background, design and conceptual model of FINALE are previously reported [24]. The present study, FINALE-health is a cluster randomized single-blinded controlled trial conducted from May 2009 to the end of June 2010. The 14 months included 12 months intervention with tests performed at baseline, after three months, and after one year. In this paper, the effects of the first three months of intervention are reported. All participants worked as personnel in care units in the western part of Denmark. The project was ethically approved by The Central Denmark Region Committees on Biomedical Research Ethics (M-20090050), and qualified for registration in the International Standard Randomized Controlled Trial Number Registry (NCT01015716).

12.2.2 WORKPLACE RECRUITMENT

Initially, three Danish municipalities in Central Jutland (DK) were contacted. Randers municipality agreed to participate immediately, and the project was initiated there. Randers Municipality consisted of nine care areas that were considered for the project. For practical implementation of the intervention, only care areas meeting inclusion criteria of at least 50 health care workers with a minimum employment of 15 hours/week were considered. Furthermore, it was requested that the care area was not involved in other health related projects. Four care areas had too few health care workers, three were already involved in health projects, and one suddenly acquired new management and could not find resources to enroll in the project. This left one care area that was eligible to participate.

12.2.3 RECRUITMENT PROCEDURE AND STUDY POPULATION

It was a management demand that all employees working at least 15 hours/week should be invited to participate in the project. The recruitment of participants was therefore based on the complete payroll of employees. Three introductory one-hour meetings were held in April and May 2009, and a total of 159 (out of 202 invited) employees attended one of these meetings. The employees filled out a screening questionnaire handed out at the meetings, with questions about health, and if they wanted to participate in the study. Employees, who did not attend the meetings, were given written information and screening questionnaires from their closest manager. Questionnaires and possible consent were returned in a sealed envelope. The primary target group for the intervention included those fulfilling the following inclusion criteria; being female and overweight, defined as BMI > 25 or having body fat % > 33 (age 18-40 years) or > 34 (age > 40 years) [25] as well as working primarily as health care workers, or with elderly care as primary work task.

All who consented to participate in the study were subsequently invited for a physical test the following week and through their closest manager handed a questionnaire, to be returned at the test session. Help with understanding the questionnaire was offered by the test leader of the physical tests, which took place during working hours at the worksite. Subsequently, the consenters were enrolled and randomly allocated to either intervention or reference group. For an overview of the procedure, see Figure 1.

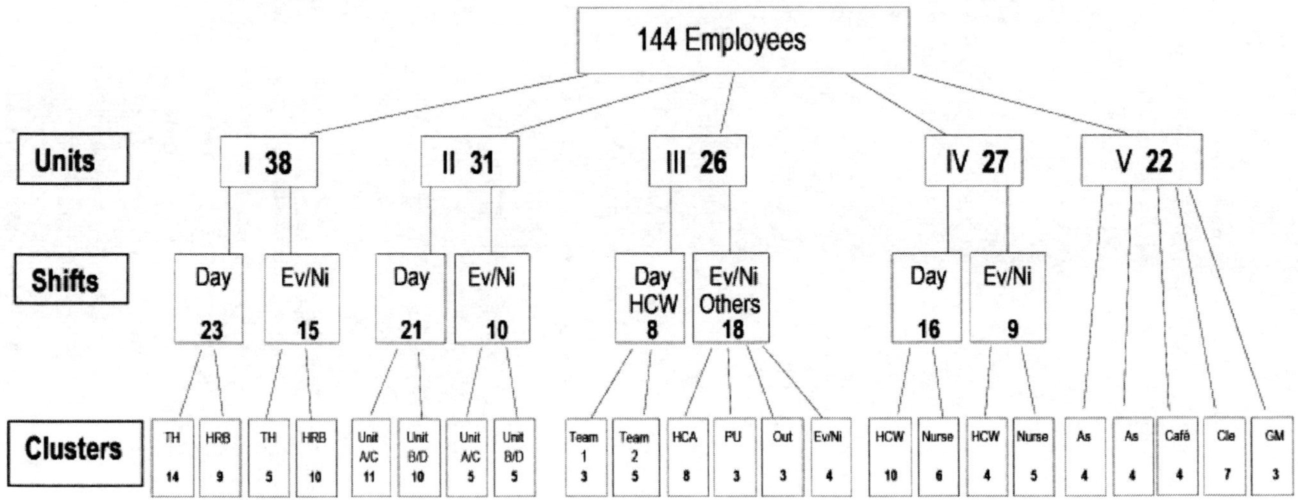

FIGURE 1: Flow of the cluster randomization. Cluster flow of consenting employees stratified in levels of work units (Units), day and evening/night shifts (Shifts) and clusters for randomization based on daily contact at work between participants (Clusters). Day = Day shifts, Ev/Ni = Evening/Night shifts, HCW = Home Care Worker, AS = Administration Staff, Cle = Cleaners, GM = Grounds Men, TH = Home Care Workers in a Terraced House, HRB = Home, Care Workers in a high-rise block, HCA = Health Care Assistants, PU = Psychiatric Unit.

12.2.4 CLUSTER-RANDOMIZATION PROCEDURE

Groups were created based on information from the screening questionnaire and the management of working teams, day and evening/night shifts and close working relations. This approach was chosen to avoid contamination between the intervention and the reference group, and so that the participants could benefit from the social support of colleagues in their unit. The aim was to increase compliance and to facilitate the necessary practical arrangement at the work place. It was therefore decided to integrate the intervention into work time. A cluster formation of the groups was performed to assure equal allocation in the intervention and reference groups balanced on sex, age, job seniority or job type with cluster size varying from 3 to 15. The randomization was done by an external research group, which had no knowledge of the work place or the participants. Clusters were randomly allocated to intervention and control by the drawing of sealed envelopes from a bag. An overview of the resulting allocation is given in Figure 1.

12.2.5 INTERVENTION

The intervention lasted 12 months and consisted of two parts. The first part (0-3 months) focused on weight loss and included advice on dietary change based on the Danish Dietary recommendations, calorie counting, weight measurements, weight loss targets, strengthening exercises and initiating leisure time fitness exercise. The remaining part that focused on weight loss maintenance (3-12 months) is not described in this paper.

12.2.6 INSTRUCTORS AND INSTRUCTION

Instruction was given as a weekly one hour session during work time. The intervention group consisted of 70 participants divided into seven training teams - each with its own instructor. The aim was to create a close-knit team spirit, which hopefully would help prevent dropouts. The project manager (JRC) and two employed instructors with sports degrees taught the seven teams. The instructors served as substitutes for each other during holidays and sick leave. Prior to the start the instructors were acquainted with the project, its aim, hypotheses, etc. They were also encouraged to read a literature list consisting of the Danish Dietary recommendations, "Overvægtens psykologi" (The Psychology of Obesity), by Tove Hvid [26], "At tale om forandring" (Talk About Change) by the The Danish Council on Smoking and Health [27] as well as a micro-compendium describing the cognitive behavioral training specifically tailored for this intervention. The three instructors also met for a whole day before each phase, going through the phase, the materials and outlining the content of each session. At the start of the intervention, JRC supervised all training for the first month, and subsequently offered support when required. Two-hour weekly meetings were held with instructors and JRC with fixed agendas, including follow-up on the previous week's session, next week's session, team compliance and good and bad experiences.

12.2.7 DIETARY INTERVENTION

A subsample of the study population filled out dietary records which were used to obtain information on dietary preferences. This information was adjusted according to the Danish Dietary recommendations, and used to create different exemplary courses with specific calorie amounts. These courses were proposed for every mealtime in amounts adjusted to suit an individual calorie prescription. To obtain an estimate of daily energy requirement, each individual's resting metabolism was calculated, based on gender, age and weight and multiplied by a Physical Activity Level factor (PAL) of 1.8 [28]. Then 1200 calories were subtracted from the estimated daily energy requirements giving an individual calorie prescription. These values were chosen to achieve a weight reduction rate of 1 kg per week [29]. If weight loss after two weeks was less than expected, the participants were given meal plans which further lowered their planned daily calorie intake by 300 kcal a day. Prescribed calorie amount was lowered in steps of 300 kcal a day throughout the intervention as participants decreased their weight. The dietary advises and the weight check occupied approximately 30 min of the weekly session.

12.2.8 PHYSICAL EXERCISE TRAINING

Ten to 15 minutes physical exercise training was included in the weekly session at the workplace. Focus during sessions was on strength training to increase muscle mass in the lower extremities in order to increase resting metabolism and maintain physical capacity. These exercises consisted of both one and two legged squats, with and without dumb bells and core balls, and lunges walking forward and to each side. Other exercises focused more on general strength, and included exercises for abdominal and back extension, shoulders and arms. Participants brought home a strength training program, picturing these exercises, and were encouraged to perform them twice a week at home. In addition to the brief training sessions, participants were encouraged to initiate aerobic leisure time exercises such as biking, walking, running, swimming or attending different sports in the local area for two hours weekly. The dose of the instructed physical exercises in the sessions progressed in intensity throughout the weeks of the intervention, by increasing weights and repetitions. To motivate participants and individualize feedback from the instructors log books to monitor leisure time exercises was given to the participants and were shown to the instructor at each session.

12.2.9 COGNITIVE BEHAVIORAL TRAINING

From a cognitive behavior program, designed by Linton aiming to prevent chronic musculoskeletal pain [30], a specific cognitive behavioral training (CBT) tool were modified and tailored to support a change to a more physically active lifestyle and by addressing the distress and challenges involved with weight loss. Whereas general counseling are not obliged to follow specific methods, traditionally cognitive behavior therapy aims at reflecting on dysfunctional attitudes and coping behaviors, discussing functional alternatives, and training the implementation of these in everyday life [30]. This included helping the participants to make realistic weight loss targets, find personal strategies to ease hunger, continue healthy behaviors, cope with social contexts and situations involving alcohol, food etc. These elements were discussed in the groups based on a specifically tailored guideline, containing 15 exercises such as pro-and-con schemes and positive thinking strategies with homework between each session. The CBT was offered as a 15 min part of the weekly sessions.

12.2.10 REFERENCE GROUP

The reference group was offered a monthly two-hour oral lecture during working hours. The three presentations were based on the Danish National Board of Health and the Ministry of Food, Agriculture and Fisheries public websites and concerned the Danish Dietary recommendations.

12.3 DATA COLLECTION AND STUDY MATERIALS

12.3.1 OBJECTIVE MEASURES

All participants were tested at baseline and after three months. Each test session lasted an hour and consisted of anthropometrical, health-related and physical capacity measures specified as the following. Height was measured to the nearest mm without shoes. Body weight was measured wearing light clothes, but without socks and shoes. One kilogram was subtracted from the weight measure to compensate for clothing. Body Fat was measured using a bio impedance device (TANITA SC-330), which was set to 'standard' while body frame and the participant's age, height and gender were entered. Waist circumference was measured over the umbilicus standing up and with clothes on, using an ergonomic circumference measuring tape (Seco 203 Girth measuring tape) and clothes thickness was noted. Blood pressure was measured in seated position after 10 minutes of rest with an electronic blood pressure monitoring device (Artsana CS 410). Three measurements were done one minute apart and an average calculated [31]. Aerobic fitness was measured using a Monark E327 bicycle ergometer and a pulse oximeter (Nellcor OxiMax N-65) fitted on the ring finger. Participants cycled for five minutes at 70 watts (60 rpm,

1 kp). During the first five minutes, the test subject was asked to answer the question: "How would you rate your fitness? Respond with one of the following classes:" Extremely good/very good/average/poor/very poor. Hereafter load was increased by 35 watts (1/2 kp) every other minute until the test subject was forced to stop because of exhaustion. With 30 seconds to the next work-load increase, participants were asked to assess the level of perceived exertion using the Borg Scale (rate of perceived exertion on a scale from 6-20) and heart rate was measured. The total number of seconds elapsed and the subject's maximum heart rate were noted. An algorithm was used to estimate maximal oxygen uptake (VO_2-max) [32]. VO_2-max values were expressed either as absolute values in L O_2/min or relative to body weight in ml O_2/kg/min (aerobic fitness).

Isometric maximal voluntary strength was obtained with a reproducible standardized setup [33], measuring maximal voluntary handgrip, shoulder elevation, and back flexion and extension force [34]. The participants performed a minimum of three attempts with steady increasing force to reach maximum within 3-5 seconds. The test was repeated until a maximal of five contractions if the last attempt showed a more than 5% increase. The participant rested at least 30 seconds between each attempt. The maximal attempt was recorded for further analysis. Standardized verbal command and encouragement was given to maximize the effort. Handgrip in both hands was measured using a grip strength measurer (La Fayette) [35]. Shoulder elevation was measured with a Bofors dynamometer with the subject seated erect in a chair with legs hanging freely, arms hanging along the side and head facing forward. The distance from pressure point to sternoclavicular joint was measured as the moment arm [36]. Back flexion and extension were measured with the subject standing, facing/backing onto beam and support plate at the spina iliaca anterior superior. The Bofors dynamometer was fixed to pull horizontal with a belt positioned at the vertical level of m. deltoid insertion on the humerus. The distance from the belt to a line through the crista iliaca and lumbalcolumna (L4L5 level) was measured for the moment calculation [37].

Prior to the test session, participants were screened in accordance with the exclusion criteria for the test. The exclusion criteria for one or more of the tests were elevated blood pressure, defined as systolic values higher than 110 mmHg + age in years, or diastolic values higher than 100 mmHg regardless of age [31], angina pectoris, heart or lung prescription medication, current or pervious illnesses and trauma, herniated disc, tennis elbow, golf elbow, Carpal Tunnel Syndrome, significant level of musculoskeletal pain at the time of the test and pregnancy. The test manager was blinded regarding the participants' intervention status, and whenever possible the same test manager tested the subject both before and after the three-month intervention.

12.3.2 QUESTIONNAIRE

A questionnaire was completed twice, approximately one week before each test round. The questionnaire was developed for use in all workplaces participating in the FINALE program and consisted of 140 questions mainly of standardized and validated scales [24]. In the present paper, responses to questions on musculoskeletal disorders are reported. Musculoskeletal disorders were measured with the Nordic questionnaires of musculoskeletal disorders [38], supplemented with questions about localized pain intensity [39].

12.3.3 STATISTICAL ANALYSES

A power calculation was carried out for the main outcomes - weight change, comparing two groups of equal size. Power was set to 0.8 with a significant level of 0.05. At least 30 participants in each group were needed to detect a difference in weight loss of at least 3 kg. With an estimated 30% drop out, 43 participants were needed in each group. PASW statistics 18 was used for the statistical analysis. Differences between intervention and reference group at baseline were tested with Pearson's x^2 for distribution in sex, education (health care workers), current smoking status and the dichotomized parameter for musculoskeletal symptoms in neck, shoulders, upper- and lower back. All other parameters were tested with a Student's t-test. When comparing intervention group and reference group over time, ANCOVA analysis were performed in accordance to the intention-to-treat principle, i.e. all randomized participants are included in the analyses with missing values substituted with carried forward or backwards measured variables. Clusters, age and the investigated value at baseline were included as covariates. All results are given as mean (SD). $p < 0.05$ are considered statistically significant.

10.4 RESULTS

10.4.1 EMPLOYEE FLOW

A flow-chart of the project is presented in Figure 2. From the employee list, 202 persons (8 men and 194 women), working at least 15 hours/week were invited to participate in the study. Among these, 144 fulfilled the inclusion criteria and consented to participate, and were randomly allocated to either the intervention or the reference group. Among these, 139 were women, 105 worked with health care as main task, and 98 met the full criteria to enter target group (i.e. women, overweight based on BMI or fat percentage, health care workers or having similar education with daily patient care). Among the 98 female overweight health care workers, 91 were still taking part in the study after three months (five left the company and two were on long-term sick leave).

10.4.2 BASELINE CHARACTERISTICS OF WORKPLACE POPULATION

The participants in the study were on average 45.5 (9.5) years of age, 77.4 (16.8) kg body weight, 36.8 (8.2)% in fat percentage, 28.1 (5.8) in BMI and 94.6 (15.0) cm in waist circumference. A BMI ≥ 25 was found for 64.5% of the employees, and a critically high waist circumference (> 88 cm) was recorded for 61.1%. Average blood pressure was 130/82 mmHg, and 31.6% had elevated blood pressure (> 139/89 mmHg) [31]. There were no anthropometrical differences between the intervention and the reference group. In Table 1, details are given on intervention and reference group within the workplace population.

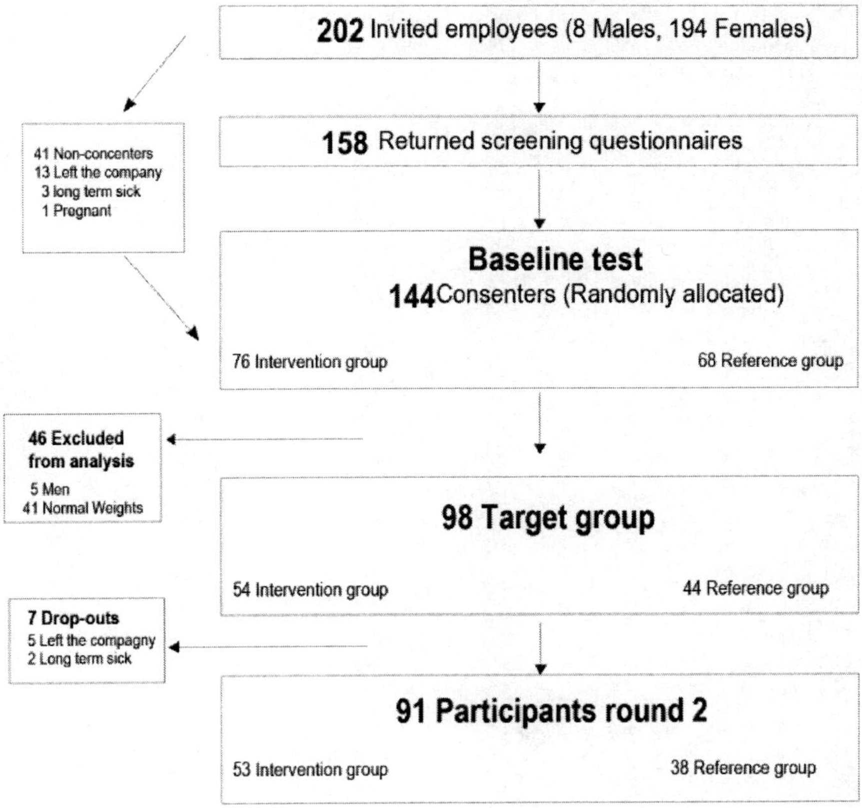

FIGURE 2: Flow of the participants.

TABLE 1: Anthropometric, lifestyle and work related characteristics at baseline of the whole and the target population.

		Whole population (n = 144)			Target population (n = 98)		
		Intervention group (n = 76)	Reference group (n = 68)	P-values	Intervention group (n = 54)	Reference group (n = 44)	P-values
Sex (females)	N %	75 98.7	64 94.1	0.189	54 100	44 100	1.000
Education (healthcare worker)	N %	58 80.6	49 74.2	0.302	41 77.4	35 79.5	0.497
Current smoking	N %	21 32.8	18 32.7	0.430	18 35.3	9 26.5	0.244
Age (years)	Mean SD	44.8 9.5	46.4 9.5	0.314	45.7 8.7	46.0 8.6	0.893
Job Seniority (months)	Mean SD	176.0 105.2	158.7 122.4	0.418	188.8 105.1	152.0 120.9	0.146
Working hours (hours/week)	Mean SD	32.3 3.5	32.0 4.1	0.708	32.1 3.4	32.3 3.4	0.744
Height (cm)	Mean SD	166.0 5.9	165.5 6.9	0.649	166.2 5.8	165.1 6.7	0.410
Weight (kg)	Mean SD	78.3 17.3	76.3 16.3	0.499	84.3 16.0	83.0 14.4	0.660
Body mass index (kg/m^2)	Mean SD	28.4 6.0	27.8 5.6	0.558	30.5 5.4	30.4 4.9	0.898
Fat percentage (%)	Mean SD	37.5 7.9	36.0 8.6	0.274	40.9 5.8	40.5 5.7	0.744
Waist circumference (cm)	Mean SD	94.8 15.0	94.3 15.2	0.856	99.7 13.7	101.6 12.4	0.492
Systolic blood pressure (mmHg)	Mean SD	132.1 18.6	127.0 13.4	0.077	134.1 19.3	129.3 11.9	0.162
Diastolic blood pressure (mmHg)	Mean SD	83.7 10.7	80.1 9.1	0.042*	85.1 10.8	81.7 8.3	0.108

Because of some missing data, the number of responders on the different measures varied from 53-76 of the whole population and 34-54 of the target group.
Where N is displayed, percentages are based on the number of responses.

TABLE 2: Physical capacity and musculoskeletal pain at different body regions at baseline of the target population.

		Intervention group (n = 54)	Reference group (n = 44)	P-values
Handgrip Dom side (N)	Mean (SD)	298.9 (52.9)	308.2 (56.0)	0.420
Right shoul. elevation (Nm)	Mean (SD)	73.6 (22.9)	61.4 (24.2)	0.085
Left shoul. elevation (Nm)	Mean (SD)	62.0 (22.1)	54.7 (24.4)	0.283
Back flexion (Nm)	Mean (SD)	127.2 (31.7)	133.1 (49.9)	0.613
Back extension (Nm)	Mean (SD)	117.3 (39.9)	118.4 (42.5)	0.927
VO_2 Max (L/min)	Mean (SD)	2.07 (0.36)	2.13 (0.34)	0.517
Physical fitness (ml/min/kg)	Mean (SD)	25.80 (4.62)	26.72 (5.12)	0.474
Neck pain				
Last 12 months (N = yes)	N (%)	42 (82.4)	25 (73.5)	0.282
Last 7 days (N = yes)	N (%)	23 (45.1)	12 (35.3)	0.500
Intensity last 7 days (1-10)	Mean (SD)	2.6 (2.6)	2.1 (2.4)	0.493
Shoulder pain (right)				
Last 12 months (N = yes)	N (%)	29 (56.9)	18 (52.9)	0.699
Last 7 days (N = yes)	N (%)	18 (36.0)	8 (23.5)	0.242
Intensity last 7 days (1-10)	Mean (SD)	2.1 (2.7)	1.0 (1.6)	0.062
Upper back pain				
Last 12 months (n = yes)	N (%)	30 (58.2)	18 (54.5)	0.372
Last 7 days (n = yes)	N (%)	15 (29.4)	9 (26.5)	0.811
Intensity last 7 days (1-10)	Mean (SD)	1.9 (2.3)	1.5 (2.5)	0.562
Lower back pain				
Last 12 months (N = yes)	N (%)	41 (80.4)	27 (79.4)	0.139
Last 7 days (N = yes)	N (%)	24 (47.1)	15 (44.1)	0.827
Intensity last 7 days (1-10)	Mean (SD)	2.6 (2.4)	2.9 (3.1)	0.651

Due to missing data, the number of responders on the different measures varies from 22-54. Where N is displayed, percentages are based on the number of responses.

10.4.3 BASELINE CHARACTERISTICS IN TARGET POPULATION

At baseline there were no significant differences between the intervention and the reference group in anthropometric measures in the target group (Table 1). In addition, physical capacity measured as muscle strength and maximal oxygen uptake was similar in the intervention and the reference groups (Table 2). Mean hand grip for both groups was 303 (54) N, shoulder elevation was 66 (24) Nm and 58 (24) Nm for right and left shoulder, respectively and trunk flexion and extension were 127 (39) Nm and 122 (40) Nm, respectively. VO_2 max was 2.1 (0.4) l/min, and aerobic fitness was 26.2 (4.8) ml/min/kg. Corresponding data are given for intervention and reference group separately (Table 2). Musculoskeletal pain at baseline showed no difference between the intervention and the reference group in any body region. The 12 months prevalence in both groups was 75-80% for the neck and low back, while for the upper back and shoulders it was around 55%. The seven days prevalence for the neck and lower back was about 45%, with mean pain intensity of 2.5 on a scale from 0-10. The 7 days prevalence for the lower back was about 20%, with mean intensity about 2.

10.4.4 CHANGES AFTER 3 MONTHS IN TARGET POPULATION

Table 3 presents average changes in the target group from baseline to 3 months of all measures in the intervention and the reference group. A highly significant Intervention group* Test round interaction was found for weight loss, BMI, fat percentage, waist circumference and diastolic blood pressure. In the intervention group, body weight decreased from 84.2 to 80.6 kg, corresponding to a decrease in BMI from 30.5 to 29.1. Fat percentage fell from 40.9 to 39.3% and waist circumference decreased from 99.3 to 95.1 cm. Blood pressure was lowered from 134.1/85.2 to 126.6/79.8 mmHg. For the reference group, no significant changes were found except for an increased BMI from 30.4 to 30.7. Regarding physical capacity, no significant Intervention group* Test round interaction was found for muscle strength. VO_2 max was unchanged in both groups, while an Intervention group* Test round interaction ($p < 0.011$) was found for aerobic fitness with the intervention group increasing from 25.9 to 28.0 ml/min/kg. Regarding musculoskeletal pain, no significant Intervention group* Test round interactions were found.

TABLE 3: Mean change from baseline to 3 months test in anthropometric characteristics of the target population.

	Intervention group (n = 54)		Reference group (n = 44)		Time vs. group interaction
	Δ mean	P	Δ mean	P	P
Weight (kg)	-3.59 (3.80)	0.000	+0.68 (2.37)	0.064	0.000
Body mass index (kg/m²)	-1.31 (1.39)	0.000	+0.27 (0.85)	0.039	0.000
Fat percentage (%)	-1.56 (2.78)	0.000	+0.33 (1.25)	0.093	0.000
Waist circumference (cm)	-4.24 (6.10)	0.000	-0.91 (4.18)	0.165	0.001
Systolic blood pressure (mmHg)	-7.52 (12.97)	0.000	-2.11 (9.25)	0.148	0.067
Diastolic blood pressure (mmHg)	-5.43 (7.79)	0.000	-0.68 (7.17)	0.543	0.016
Hand grip Dom side (N)	+10.28 (31.80)	0.022	-6.22 (33.97)	0.248	0.102
Right shoul. Elevation (Nm)	-0.03 (23.78)	0.994	+5.57 (19.41)	0.164	0.087
Left shoul. Elevation (Nm)	+1.49 (15.73)	0.548	+5.66 (18.53)	0.140	0.218
Back flexion (Nm)	+9.02 (23.94)	0.016	-3.99 (33.95)	0.555	0.068
Back extension (Nm)	+1.26 (31.56)	0.796	+18.04 (34.46)	0.013	0.045
VO_2 (L/min)	+0.14 (0.22)	0.003	+0.01 (0.21)	0.834	0.185
Physical fitness (ml/min/kg)	+3.33 (3.48)	0.000	-0.11 (2.87)	0.889	0.011
Intensity of musculoskeletal pain last 7 days					
Neck	-0.67 (2.15)	0.028	-0.24 (2.24)	0.538	0.452
Shoulder (right)	-0.00 (1.59)	1.000	-0.03 (1.54)	0.913	0.427
Upper back	-0.25 (1.55)	0.249	-0.11 (1.39)	0.634	0.476
Lower back	+0.06 (2.08)	0.837	+0.15 (1.99)	0.664	0.552

10.5 DISCUSSION

The main result of this workplace randomized controlled trial consisting of diet, physical exercise and cognitive behavioral training was a mean weight loss of 3.6 kg in the intervention group. In addition, a substantial effect was found for systolic and diastolic blood pressure with decreases of 7.5 and 5.4 mmHg, respectively. A remarkably large adherence was obtained with only seven out of 98 participants dropping out during the three-month intervention. The results will be discussed in more detail below.

Among the 105 female health care workers, 93% was overweight, showing that efficient weight loss programs are highly relevant as health promotion for this sector. To our knowledge, this is the first randomized controlled workplace intervention among health care workers with the specific aim to reduce body weight. One previous Danish workplace health promotion study among health care workers, consisting of 20 weeks with weight training, fitness training and advice on healthy living did not show any positive effects on body weight [40]. In a non-randomized study by Rigsby and colleagues from 2009 among 454 female employees at a hospital and nursing home, eight weeks weight loss intervention in groups reduced mean body weight by 3.8 kg [41]. Other workplace studies not specifically targeting health care workers but aiming at weight loss with intervention periods from 10 to 16 weeks have shown weight losses from 1.3 - 4.5 kg [42-45]. In comparison to these workplace studies targeting similar populations or using comparable intervention programs, the present study shows an equal or even larger effect. Also the decrease in blood pressure was in line with or even larger than reported in previous studies on weight loss and blood pressure [46].

The intervention consisting of diet, physical exercise and cognitive behavioral training during working hours one hour/week was shown to be very effective, generating a significant weight loss, decreased blood pressure and increased aerobic fitness after three months. These findings support the recommendations of combining these three initiatives for successful weight loss [23]. However, the long-term effects of this combined intervention remain to be investigated.

The intervention was not able to increase muscle strength, indicating that no changes in muscle mass occurred. Increasing muscle mass was considered a means to further ease weight loss by raising resting metabolism. Therefore, 10 - 15 minutes per week of physical exercise seems insufficient if the aim is to increase muscle strength while simultaneously encouraging weight loss. However, it was sufficient to maintain muscle strength alongside the weight loss. Similarly, no increase in VO_2 max was found. However due to the weight loss, the aerobic fitness being relative to the body weight was increased. The maintained physical capacity in combination with the reduction in body fat % indicates that the weight loss achieved during the intervention is primarily due to loss of fat tissue. The increased aerobic fitness may represent a functional benefit, decreasing the relative physical workload of the health care workers, and therefore their risk of cardiovascular disease [47].

Only seven participants dropped out during the three months intervention. The adherence rate was therefore higher than in most other weight loss studies at the workplace [48,49]. The successful adherence may be due to a number of initial precautions taken. First, workplaces adopting this intervention study were obliged by contract to provide time for the intervention during working hours. Second, each of the seven intervention groups was, as far as possible, guided by a single instructor to personalise the interventions. Third, a close collaboration between managers ensured that obstacles for the intervention were quickly solved. In summary, the workplace approach is likely to explain the high adherence and therefore the positive results of the study. Other studies have pointed out that workplace-initiated weight loss programs promote a team spirit among the employees [50,51]. The participants tend to form into particular groups at workplaces, often based on gender, educational backgrounds and interests, which makes group counseling easier. The participants see each other on a daily basis during the intervention period and tend to share meals and have opportunities to meet immediately after work for exercise [41]. In the present study, employees without weight problems were also invited to take part in the intervention. Not excluding them from the intervention may have contributed to a positive team spirit regarding the initiative.

The present study was conducted as a cluster randomized single-blinded controlled trial. It was carried out at a workplace that enabled us to target a high-risk group and obtain a very high adherence. The results in this paper were tested using intention-to-treat analyses (ITT), where missing observations are carried forwards or backwards. In spite of this conservative approach, we were able to reveal significant effects on weight loss and related outcomes such as fat percentage, waist circumference and blood pressure.

For a weight reduction program, a three months perspective is a short time frame. This study showed strong results after three months, but the main aim of the project is to maintain the weight loss for a longer period of time. Maintenance of the improved bodyweight, blood pressure and aerobic fitness is well known to reduce the risk of chronic diseases such as cardiovascular diseases and Type 2 diabetes, which in turn may reduce the risk for sick leave [52]. There was no observed effect on musculoskeletal pain after three months of the intervention. However, because weight loss will lower the mechanical load on joints and potentially improve work postures, it may have a positive effect on musculoskeletal pain in the long run.

A limitation in the study is the lack of quantitative registration of physical training doses in leisure time. The logbook was primarily used to facilitate the individual coaching and serve as a motivating factor. Another limitation is that in the integrated multiple intervention concept of this study the importance of each of the components cannot be evaluated. A four-armed design where each of the components as well as the combined concept is tested against a control group would have been ideal, but also unrealistic with the current resources and the workplaces available. A qualitative process analysis with focus group interview is another approach that would have been possible, but unfortunately not performed. Finally, the target group only consists of females and the results cannot be extrapolated to males. Concerning statistics, several ANCOVA models were carried out for testing effects of the intervention on multiple outcomes. The risk for a chance finding may therefore be resent. However, reducing the level of significance would substantially increase the risk for a type II error. This aspect ought to be included in the interpretation of the study results.

10.6 CONCLUSIONS

This workplace-initiated intervention enabled us to target a high-risk group. The combination of diet, physical exercise and cognitive behavioral training resulted in significant weight loss, decreased blood pressure and increased aerobic fitness after three months. The positive results are encouraging regarding the use of workplace initiated weight loss interventions. The long-term effects of the intervention remain to be investigated.

REFERENCES

1. Koh-Banerjee P, Wang Y, Hu FB, Spiegelman D, Willett WC, Rimm EB: Changes in body weight and body fat distribution as risk factors for clinical diabetes in US men. Am J Epidemiol 2004, 159:1150-1159.
2. van Dam RM, Willett WC, Manson JE, Hu FB: The relationship between overweight in adolescence and premature death in women. Ann Intern Med 2006, 145:91-97.
3. Yusuf S, Hawken S, Ounpuu S, Bautista L, Franzosi MG, Commerford P, et al.: Obesity and the risk of myocardial infarction in 27,000 participants from 52 countries: a case-control study. Lancet 2005, 366:1640-1649.
4. Han TS, Schouten JS, Lean ME, Seidell JC: The prevalence of low back pain and associations with body fatness, fat distribution and height. Int J Obes Relat Metab Disord 1997, 21:600-607.
5. Tunceli K, Li K, Williams LK: Long-term effects of obesity on employment and work limitations among U.S. Adults, 1986 to 1999. Obesity (Silver Spring) 2006, 14:1637-1646.
6. Houston DK, Cai J, Stevens J: Overweight and obesity in young and middle age and early retirement: the ARIC study. Obesity (Silver Spring) 2009, 17:143-149.
7. Konnopka A, Bodemann M, Konig HH: Health burden and costs of obesity and overweight in Germany. Eur J Health Econ 2010.
8. Kautiainen S, Koivisto AM, Koivusilta L, Lintonen T, Virtanen SM, Rimpela A: Sociodemographic factors and a secular trend of adolescent overweight in Finland. Int J Pediatr Obes 2009, 4:360-370.
9. Marques-Vidal P, Bovet P, Paccaud F, Chiolero A: Changes of overweight and obesity in the adult Swiss population according to educational level, from 1992 to 2007. BMC Public Health 2010, 10:87.
10. Torgen M, Nygard CH, Kilbom A: Physical work load, physical capacity and strain among elderly female aides in home-care service. Eur J Appl Physiol Occup Physiol 1995, 71:444-452.
11. Pohjonen T: Age-related physical fitness and the predictive values of fitness tests for work ability in home care work. J Occup Environ Med 2001, 43:723-730.
12. Kivimaki M, Makinen A, Elovainio M, Vahtera J, Virtanen M, Firth-Cozens J: Sickness absence and the organization of nursing care among hospital nurses. Scand J Work Environ Health 2004, 30:468-476.
13. Caruso CC, Waters TR: A review of work schedule issues and musculoskeletal disorders with an emphasis on the healthcare sector. Ind Health 2008, 46:523-534.

14. Torgen M, Punnett L, Alfredsson L, Kilbom A: Physical capacity in relation to present and past physical load at work: a study of 484 men and women aged 41 to 58 years. Am J Ind Med 1999, 36:388-400.
15. Nygard CH, Luopajarvi T, Suurnakki T, Ilmarinen J: Muscle strength and muscle endurance of middle-aged women and men associated to type, duration and intensity of muscular load at work. Int Arch Occup Environ Health 1988, 60:291-297.
16. Andersen LL, Christensen KB, Holtermann A, Poulsen OM, Sjogaard G, Pedersen MT, et al.: Effect of physical exercise interventions on musculoskeletal pain in all body regions among office workers: a one-year randomized controlled trial. Man Ther 2010, 15:100-104.
17. Atlantis E, Lange K, Wittert GA: Chronic disease trends due to excess body weight in Australia. Obes Rev 2009, 10:543-553.
18. Proper KI, Hildebrandt VH, van der Beek AJ, Twisk JW, van MW: Effect of individual counseling on physical activity fitness and health: a randomized controlled trial in a workplace setting. Am J Prev Med 2003, 24:218-226.
19. Wu T, Gao X, Chen M, van Dam RM: Long-term effectiveness of diet-plus-exercise interventions vs. diet-only interventions for weight loss: a meta-analysis. Obes Rev 2009, 10:313-323.
20. Shaw K, Gennat H, O'Rourke P, Del MC: Exercise for overweight or obesity. Cochrane Database Syst Rev 2006, :CD003817.
21. Dalle GR, Calugi S, Centis E, El GM, Marchesini G: Cognitive-behavioral strategies to increase the adherence to exercise in the management of obesity. J Obes 2011, 2011:348293.
22. Atlantis E, Chow CM, Kirby A, Fiatarone Singh MA: Worksite intervention effects on physical health: a randomized controlled trial. Health Promot Int 2006, 21:191-200.
23. Shaw K, O'Rourke P, Del MC, Kenardy J: Psychological interventions for overweight or obesity. Cochrane Database Syst Rev 2005, :CD003818.
24. Holtermann A, Jorgensen MB, Gram B, Christensen JR, Faber A, Overgaard K, et al.: Worksite interventions for preventing physical deterioration among employees in job-groups with high physical work demands: background, design and conceptual model of FINALE. BMC Public Health 2010, 10:120.
25. Gallagher D, Heymsfield SB, Heo M, Jebb SA, Murgatroyd PR, Sakamoto Y: Healthy percentage body fat ranges: an approach for developing guidelines based on body mass index. Am J Clin Nutr 2000, 72:694-701.
26. Hvid T: Overvægtens psykologi. Copenhagen, Modtryk; 2004.
27. The Danish Council on Smoking and Health: At tale om forandring. Copenhagen; 2000.
28. Nordic Council of Ministers: Nordic Nutrition Recommendation 2004 Integrating nutrition and physical activity. 4th edition. Copenhagen, Norden; 2004.
29. Franz MJ, VanWormer JJ, Crain AL, Boucher JL, Histon T, Caplan W, et al.: Weight-loss outcomes: a systematic review and meta-analysis of weight-loss clinical trials with a minimum 1-year follow-up. J Am Diet Assoc 2007, 107:1755-1767.
30. Linton SJ, Andersson T: Can chronic disability be prevented? A randomized trial of a cognitive-behavior intervention and two forms of information for patients with spinal pain. Spine (Phila Pa 1976) 2000, 25:2825-2831.

31. Appleyard M: The Copenhagen City Heart Study, Østerbroundersøgelsen. A book of tables with data from the first examination (1976-78) and a five year follow-up (1981-83). Scand J Soc Med 1989, (Supplementum 41):1-160.
32. Andersen LB: A maximal cycle exercise protocol to predict maximal oxygen uptake. Scand J Med Sci Sports 1995, 5:143-146.
33. Essendrop M, Maul I, Laubli T, Riihimaki H, Schibye B: Measures of low back function: a review of reproducibility studies. Clin Biomech (Bristol, Avon) 2002, 17:235-249.
34. Schibye B, Hansen AF, Sogaard K, Christensen H: Aerobic power and muscle strength among young and elderly workers with and without physically demanding work tasks. Appl Ergon 2001, 32:425-431.
35. Fairfax AH, Balnave R, Adams RD: Variability of grip strength during isometric contraction. Ergonomics 1995, 38:1819-1830.
36. Backman E, Johansson V, Hager B, Sjoblom P, Henriksson KG: Isometric muscle strength and muscular endurance in normal persons aged between 17 and 70 years. Scand J Rehabil Med 1995, 27:109-117.
37. Yates JW, Kamon E, Rodgers SH, Champney PC: Static lifting strength and maximal isometric voluntary contractions of back, arm and shoulder muscles. Ergonomics 1980, 23:37-47.
38. Kuorinka I, Jonsson B, Kilbom A, Vinterberg H, Biering-Sorensen F, Andersson G, et al.: Standardised Nordic questionnaires for the analysis of musculoskeletal symptoms. Appl Ergon 1987, 18:233-237.
39. Videman T, Nurminen T, Tola S, Kuorinka I, Vanharanta H, Troup JD: Low-back pain in nurses and some loading factors of work. Spine (Phila Pa 1976) 1984, 9:400-404.
40. Lüders K, Andersen B, Berggren F: Det Batter. Institute of Sport Sciense & Clinical Biomechanics, University of Suthern Denmark; 1996.
41. Rigsby A, Gropper DM, Gropper SS: Success of women in a worksite weight loss program: Does being part of a group help? Eat Behav 2009, 10:128-130.
42. Abrams DB, Follick MJ: Behavioral weight-loss intervention at the worksite: feasibility and maintenance. J Consult Clin Psychol 1983, 51:226-233.
43. Wier LT, Ayers GW, Jackson AS, Rossum AC, Poston WS, Foreyt JP: Determining the amount of physical activity needed for long-term weight control. Int J Obes Relat Metab Disord 2001, 25:613-621.
44. Crouch M, Sallis JF, Farquhar JW, Haskell WL, Ellsworth NM, King AB, et al.: Personal and mediated health counseling for sustained dietary reduction of hypercholesterolemia. Prev Med 1986, 15:282-291.
45. Briley ME, Montgomery DH, Blewett J: Worksite nutrition education can lower total cholesterol levels and promote weight loss among police department employees. J Am Diet Assoc 1992, 92:1382-1384.
46. Stevens VJ, Obarzanek E, Cook NR, Lee IM, Appel LJ, Smith WD, et al.: Long-term weight loss and changes in blood pressure: results of the Trials of Hypertension Prevention, phase II. Ann Intern Med 2001, 134:1-11.
47. Holtermann A, Mortensen OS, Burr H, Sogaard K, Gyntelberg F, Suadicani P: Physical demands at work, physical fitness, and 30-year ischaemic heart disease and all-cause mortality in the Copenhagen Male Study. Scand J Work Environ Health 2010, 36:357-365.

48. Malone M, Alger-Mayer SA, Anderson DA: The lifestyle challenge program: a multidisciplinary approach to weight management. Ann Pharmacother 2005, 39:2015-2020.
49. Benedict MA, Arterburn D: Worksite-based weight loss programs: a systematic review of recent literature. Am J Health Promot 2008, 22:408-416.
50. Brownell KD, Cohen RY, Stunkard AJ, Felix MR, Cooley NB: Weight loss competitions at the work site: impact on weight, morale and cost-effectiveness. Am J Public Health 1984, 74:1283-1285.
51. Peregrin T: Weighing in on corporate wellness programs and their impact on obesity. J Am Diet Assoc 2005, 105:1192-1194.
52. Diabetes Prevention Program Research Group: Reduction in the incidence of type 2 diabetes with lifestyle intervention or metformin. N Engl J Med 2002, 346(6):393-403.

CHAPTER 13

REDUCTION IN ADIPOSITY, β-CELL FUNCTION, INSULIN SENSITIVITY, AND CARDIOVASCULAR RISK FACTORS: A PROSPECTIVE STUDY AMONG JAPANESE WITH OBESITY

MAKI GOTO, AKEMI MORITA, ATSUSHI GOTO, KIJO DEURA, SATOSHI SASAKI, NAOMI AIBA, TAKURO SHIMBO, YASUO TERAUCHI, MOTOHIKO MIYACHI, MITSUHIKO NODA, and SHAW WATANABE, FOR THE SCOP STUDY GROUP

13.1 INTRODUCTION

Since the identification of obesity as the a strong risk factor for various diseases, such as cardiovascular disease (CVD), stroke, and type 2 diabetes, lifestyle modification and weight loss have become major strategies for disease prevention. The development of CVD may be mediated through obesity, decreased insulin sensitivity, dyslipidemia, or high blood pressure [1]-[3]. Previous studies have investigated the associations between obesity and CVD risk factors [2], [4]-[7], but few studies have examined

---

This chapter was originally published under the Creative Commons Attribution License. Goto M, Morita A, Goto A, Deura K, Sasaki S, Aiba N, Shimbo T, Terauchi Y, Miyachi M, Noda M, and Watanabe S. Reduction in Adiposity, β-Cell Function, Insulin Sensitivity, and Cardiovascular Risk Factors: A Prospective Study among Japanese with Obesity. PLoS ONE ***8**,3 (2013), doi:10.1371/journal.pone.0057964.*

the associations between changes in adiposity measures and changes in CVD risk factors [8], [9]. Furthermore, simple adiposity assessments (e.g., body mass index [BMI], waist circumference, or waist-to-hip ratio) might underestimate the contribution of adiposity to the risk of CVD [10]. Therefore, the use of the visceral fat area (VFAT) and the subcutaneous fat area (SFAT) determined using computed tomography might detect important relations between changes in adiposity and changes in CVD risk factors [9].

In light of effective diabetes prevention, strategies for preserving β-cell function are of great importance. It has now been recognized that a compensatory period (i.e., a compensatory increase in insulin secretion secondary to insulin resistance with little change in the glucose levels) exists before the diagnosis of diabetes, and the insulin secretion decreases after the diagnosis of diabetes [11]. Insulin resistance is considered to be responsible for the increase in insulin levels during the compensatory period. Therefore, it is of great interest to investigate whether reduction in adiposity is associated with improvement in insulin secretion as well as insulin resistance. However, the relationship between the changes in adiposity and insulin resistance or β-cell function has not been well-understood.

Therefore, we investigated the associations between changes in adiposity, including SFAT and VFAT evaluated using computed tomography, and changes in insulin secretion and sensitivity as well as CVD risk factors in 196 Japanese participants with obesity over a 1-year period.

13.2 MATERIALS AND METHODS

13.2.1 ETHICS STATEMENT

This study was reviewed and approved by the Ethical Committee of the National Institute of Health and Nutrition and Saku Central Hospital. Participants received a precise explanation of the study and provided their written informed consent.

13.2.2 SUBJECTS

This study is a secondary analysis of a randomized controlled trial, the Saku Control Obesity Program (SCOP), examining the effect of behavioral treatment and exercise at the Saku Central Hospital Human Dock Center. The details and design of the study have been previously described elsewhere [12 reatment at the Saku Health Dock Center. People who had undergone health checkups at the center were registered in the database, and 976 members between the ages of 40 and 64 years who did not have type 1 diabetes or severe diseases, such as stroke, cardiovascular disease, advanced cancer or significant renal or hepatic dysfunction, and had a body mass index (BMI) in the upper five percentile of all examinees (28.3 or above) were invited. A total of 237 people participated in the study and were randomly assigned to two groups: group A, who participated in a lifestyle intervention program during year 1; and group B, who participated in the same intervention program during year 2. The intervention group received individual-based counseling on diet and physical activity, and by 1 year, the intervention group had significantly lost more weight than the control group (−5.0 kg vs. 0.1 kg among men, $P < 0.01$; −2.9 kg vs. −0.2 kg among women, $P < 0.01$) [15].

In this study, we excluded 29 patients who had already been diagnosed as having diabetes and were receiving treatment at baseline or at 1 year (27 participants and 2 participants, respectively), 3 participants not in fasting states at the time of blood sampling, and 9 participants who did not complete the study. Finally, 196 participants were included in the analysis.

13.2.3 ANTHROPOMETRIC MEASUREMENTS

The height (cm) and weight (kg) of the subjects were measured using an automatic scale (BF-220; Tanita, Tokyo, Japan), and the BMI was calculated as the weight (kg) divided by the squared height (m^2). The waist circumference was measured twice in a standing position at the umbilicus level using a fiber glass measuring tape, and the average was used for the analysis. Blood pressure was measured in a sitting position using a validated automated blood pressure monitor (HEM-907; Omron, Kyoto, Japan) [16].

The VFAT and SFAT were assessed based on a CT scan at the level of the umbilicus while the subject was in a supine position (Fat scan; N2 system Corp., Japan) [6]. Physical activity levels were obtained from a questionnaire that aimed to identify activity levels during the recent month as follows: light activity, approximately 1 hour of walking or 3 hours of standing per day; medium activity, approximately 2 hours of walking or 6 to 7 hours of standing per day; moderately-to-heavy activity, approximately 1 hour of intense activity plus 9 hours of walking or standing per day; heavy activity, approximately 2 hours of intense activity plus 9 hours of walking or standing per day.

13.2.4 LABORATORY PROCEDURES

Following an overnight fast, blood samples were collected at the time of each health checkup at the Saku Health Dock Center. Blood samples were collected in tubes containing EDTA and heparin for the measurement of fasting plasma glucose (FPG), insulin, and HbA1c and in serum gel separator tubes for the measurement of total cholesterol, high-density lipoprotein cholesterol (HDL), and triglyceride (TG) levels. Routine laboratory blood analyses were performed at the Saku Central Hospital. HbA1c levels were measured using a high-performance liquid chromatography method (TOSOH HLC-723 G8, Tosoh Corporation, Tokyo, Japan) with intra- and inter-assay coefficients of variation (CVs) $\leq$1.4%. The plasma glucose levels were analyzed using an enzymatic method (ECO glucose buffer; A&T Corporation, Kanagawa, Japan), with intra- and inter-assay CVs $\leq$0.8%. The plasma insulin levels were analyzed using an electrochemiluminescence immunoassay (Modular E170; Roche Diagnostics, Mannheim, Germany) with intra- and inter-assay CVs $\leq$3.6%. The serum total cholesterol, HDL, and TG concentrations were determined using enzymatic methods (Detaminar L TC II, Kyowa Medex, Tokyo, Japan; Cholestest N HDL, Sekisui Medical Co Ltd, Tokyo, Japan; and Mizuho TG-FR Type II, Mizuho Medi, Saga, Japan, respectively) and an autoanalyzer BM-2250 (Nihon Denshi, Tokyo, Japan) with intra- and inter-assay CVs of ≤2.3%. The HbA1c values were determined as Japan Diabetes Society (JDS) values and then converted to National Glycohemoglobin Standardization Program (NGSP) values using the following conversion formula: HbA1c (NGSP) = 1.02×HbA1c (JDS)+0.25% [17]. The low-density lipoprotein cholesterol levels (LDL) were calculated using the Friedewald equation: LDL = total cholesterol-(HDL + [TG/5]).

To evaluate insulin sensitivity, we used the homeostasis model assessment for insulin resistance (HOMA-IR)[18] and the insulin sensitivity index (ISI) with reduced time points [19]; to evaluate β cell function, we used the homeostasis model assessment β cell function (HOMA-β) [20] and the insulinogenic index[21], [22] based on a 75 g oral glucose tolerance test (OGTT). The HOMA-IR was calculated as follows: fasting insulin (I_0) (μIU/ml) × fasting glucose (G_0) (mg/dL)/405 [18]. We calculated the ISI using reduced time points because of the absence of 90-minute glucose-load values from the OGTTs, with the measurement of the insulin and glucose levels at 0, 60 and 120 minutes as follows: ISI = 10,000/[square root of ($G_0 \times I_0$ × mean OGTT glucose concentration × mean OGTT insulin concentration)] [23]. This index has been reported to be well correlated with the original composite index; we did not use G30 and I30 in our calculations because this time point was not recommended when using reduced time points to calculate the ISI [23]. The HOMA-β was calculated using the formula: 360 × I_0 (μIU/mL)/[G_0 (mg/dL) −63]. The insulinogenic index was calculated as follows: $(I_{30}-I_0)/(G_{30}-G_0)$ [24].

13.2.5 DATA ANALYSIS

The characteristics of the study population are presented as the mean for continuous variables. We calculated the means (± SDs) and the proportions of the covariates. A visual inspection of the histograms did not reveal any violations of the assumption of normality; we conducted the analysis without the use of log transformation. To compare the characteristics of the participants at baseline and at 1 year, we used a paired t test (Table 1). Then, we investigated the associations of CVD risk factors and insulin secretion and sensitivity using adiposity measures (Tables 2, 3, 4). We used multiple linear regression models to estimate the point estimates, the

95% confidence intervals (95% CIs), and the P-values with adjustments for potential confounding factors including age, sex, baseline adiposity measures, baseline insulin related indexes, intervention group assignment, and physical activity level. In addition, we conducted the following sensitivity analyses: (i) stratification according to sex, (ii) stratification according to WHO diagnostic criteria for impaired glucose tolerance (IGT) and diabetes, and (iii) exclusion of participants with medications for hyperlipidemia. We also examined the associations with stratification according to the intervention assignment, but the direction and strength of the associations remained consistent across the subgroups. Thus, we focused primarily on the associations for the full sample (i.e., the product terms were not included in the models).

TABLE 1: Baseline characteristics of participants.

	Baseline	1 year	P value*
N	196	196	
Male/Female (n)	96/100		
Age (years)	53.8 ± 6.4		
BMI (kg/m²)	30.5 ± 3.1	29.6 ± 3.5	<0.001
Subcutaneous fat area (cm²)	294 ± 102	268 ± 94	<0.001
Visceral fat area (cm²)	139 ± 48	123 ± 47	<0.001
Waist circumference (cm)	102 ± 8	100 ± 9	<0.001
HbA1c (%)	6.0 ± 0.8	5.8 ± 0.5	<0.001
Fasting plasma glucose (mg/dL)	106 ± 13	107 ± 14	0.21
Fasting insulin (μIU/mL)	11.3 ± 8.0	9.4 ± 10.0	0.01
HOMA-IR	3.0 ± 2.2	2.6 ± 3.3	0.14
HOMA-β	100 ± 72	77 ± 62	<0.001
Insulin Senstitivity Index	4.8 ± 3.4	6.5 ± 4.2	<0.001
Insulinogenic index	0.84 ± 0.90	0.91 ± 1.8	0.57
LDL (mg/dL)	126 ± 34	128 ± 30	0.37
HDL (mg/dL)	53 ± 12	52 ± 13	0.21
Tryglyceride (mg/dL)	162 ± 106	142 ± 72	<0.001
Systolic blood pressure (mmHg)	132 ± 19	132 ± 20	<0.001
Diastolic blood pressure (mmHg)	85 ± 14	83 ± 14	0.07

*Data are (n) or means ± SD. *P value for paired t-test.*
Abbreviations: BMI, body mass index; HOMA-IR, homeostasis model assessment ratio; HOMA-β, homeostasis model assessment β cell function.

TABLE 2: Associations between changes in adiposity measures and glucose indices from baseline to 1 year.

	Δ HbA1c (%)		Δ FPG (mg/dL)	
	Coef.	P value	Coef.	P value
Explanatory variables	(95% CL)		(95% CL)	
Δ BMI (kg/m²)	0.09	<0.001	1.90	0.001
	(0.05, 0.12)		(0.79, 3.02)	
Δ Subcutaneous fat area (cm²)	0.003	<0.001	0.07	0.003
	(0.002, 0.005)		(0.03, 0.12)	
Δ Visceral fat area (cm²)	0.005	<0.001	0.08	0.01
	(0.003, 0.007)		(0.02, 0.14)	
Δ Waist circumference (cm)	0.03	<0.001	0.48	0.01
	(0.01, 0.04)		(0.11, 0.86)	

Abbreviations: BMI, body mass index; FPG, fasting plasma glucose; Coef., coefficient; CL, confidence limit.
A multiple linear regression model was used to adjust for potential confounding factors including age, sex, physical activity levels, intervention assignment, the baseline adiposity measure of interest, and the baseline value of the outcome variable.

Two-sided P values <0.05 were considered to be statistically significant. Analyses were performed using Stata software (version 12; Stata Corp, College Station, TX).

13.3 RESULTS

Among a total of 196 participants aged 40 to 64 years, the mean age was 53.8 years. At baseline, all the participants had obesity with relatively high average glucose levels accompanied by insulin resistance and hyperinsulinemia (Table 1). Over a 1-year period, reductions in all adiposity measures, HbA1c, insulin secretion, TG, and systolic blood pressure were observed, possibly because of the trial intervention (Table 1).

After adjustments for age, sex, physical activity, intervention assignment, baseline adiposity measures, and the baseline value of the outcome variable, reductions in all adiposity measures, including BMI, SFAT, VFAT, and waist circumference, were associated with reductions in the

TABLE 3: Associations between changes in adiposity measures and insulin related indexes from baseline to 1 year.

Outcome variables	Δ Insulin (μIU/mL)		Δ HOMA-IR		Δ ISI		Δ HOMA-β		Δ Insulinogenic index	
	Coef	P value	Coef.	P value	Coef.	P value	Coef.	P value	Coef.	P value
Explanatory variables	(95% CL)		(95% CL)		(95% CL)		(95% CL)		(95% CL)	
Δ BMI (kg/m²)	1.09	0.02	0.32	0.045	−1.05	<0.001	7.43	0.007	0.14	0.12
	(0.16, 2.01)		(0.01, 0.64)		(−1.32, −0.78)		(2.02, 12.8)		(−0.04, 0.31)	
Δ Subcutaneous fat area (cm²)	0.02	0.29	0.01	0.39	−0.03	<0.001	0.12	0.31	0.003	0.39
	(−0.02. 0.06)		(−0.01, 0.02)		(−0.04, −0.02)		(−0.11, 0.36)		(−0.004, 0.01)	
Δ Visceral fat area (cm²)	0.06	0.01	0.02	0.048	−0.05	<0.001	0.50	0.001	−0.0005	0.92
	(0.01. 0.11)		(0.0001, 0.03)		(−0.06, −0.03)		(0.21, 0.79)		(−0.01, 0.009)	
Δ Waist circumference (cm)	0.25	0.10	0.07	0.18	−0.29	<0.001	1.80	0.053	0.04	0.15
	(−0.05, 0.56)		(−0.03, 0.18)		(−0.39, −0.20)		(−0.02, 3.62)		(−0.02, 0.10)	

Abbreviations: BMI, body mass index; HOMA-IR, homeostatic model assessment for insulin resistance; ISI, insulin sensitivity index; HOMA-β, homeostasis model assessment for β-cell function; Coef., coefficient; CL, confidence limit.
A multiple linear regression model was used to adjust for potential confounding factors including age, sex, physical activity levels, intervention assignment, the baseline adiposity measure of interest, and the baseline value of insulin related indices.

TABLE 4: Associations between changes in adiposity measures and lipid levels and blood pressure from baseline to 1 year.

Outcome variables	Δ LDL (mg/dL)		Δ HDL (mg/dL)		Δ Triglyceride (mg/dL)		Δ Systolic blood pressure (mmHg)		Δ Diastolic blood pressure (mmHg)	
	Coef	P value	Coef.	P value	Coef.	P value	Coef.	P value	Coef.	P value
Explanatory variables	(95% CL)		(95% CL)		(95% CL)		(95% CL)		(95% CL)	
Δ BMI (kg/m²)	0.47	0.67	–0.63	0.06	9.37	<0.001	2.03	0.01	1.48	0.01
	(–1.71, 2.66)		(–1.28, 0.03)		(4.75, 14.0)		(0.47, 3.59)		(0.35, 2.62)	
Δ Subcutaneous fat area (cm²)	0.04	0.39	–0.01	0.49	0.19	0.06	0.03	0.32	0.03	0.19
	(–0.05. 0.13)		(–0.04, 0.02)		(–0.01, 0.39)		(–0.03, 0.10)		(–0.02, 0.08)	
Δ Visceral fat area (cm²)	–0.03	0.56	–0.05	0.01	0.48	<0.001	0.12	0.005	0.07	0.04
	(–0.15, 0.08)		(–0.08, –0.01)		(0.23, 0.72)		(0.04, 0.20)		(0.004, 0.13)	
Δ Waist circumference (cm)	0.33	0.36	–0.17	0.11	2.61	0.001	0.66	0.01	0.45	0.02
	(–0.38, 1.05)		(–0.39, 0.04)		(1.07, 4.15)		(0.15, 1.18)		(0.08, 0.82)	

Abbreviations: BMI, body mass index; LDL, low density cholesterol; HDL, high density cholesterol; Coef., coefficient; CL, confidence limit. A multiple linear regression model was used to adjust for potential confounding factors including age, sex, physical activity levels, intervention assignment, the baseline adiposity measure of interest, and the baseline value of lipid levels.

HbA1c and FPG levels (Table 2). The relations between the changes in adiposity and glucose levels were consistent with previous findings. In this study, we were able to further examine the associations of changes in adiposity with the changes in insulin secretion and resistance. As expected, reductions in BMI and VFAT were associated with an improvement in insulin sensitivity as measured using the HOMA-IR and ISI (Table 3). Furthermore, reductions in all adiposity measures were associated with an elevation in the ISI. Decreases in BMI and visceral fat area were related to reduced insulin secretion as measured using the HOMA-β. In contrast, changes in the insulinogenic index were not related to changes in any adiposity measure (Table 3).

Changes in any of the adiposity measures were not associated with the change in the LDL level, but a change in VFAT was inversely associated with a change in HDL while changes in the BMI, VFAT, and waist circumference were positively associated with a change in the TG level (Table 4). In addition, changes in the BMI, VFAT, and waist circumference were positively associated with changes in the systolic and diastolic blood pressure (Table 4).

A sensitivity analysis stratified according to sex did not substantially change the results; and furthermore, the exclusion of the participants with hyperlipidemia medications (n = 38) did not materially alter the results (data not shown). According to the WHO diagnostic criteria [25], there were 86 participants with normal glucose tolerance (NGT), 11 participants with impaired fasting glycemia (IFG), 76 participants with impaired glucose tolerance (IGT), and 23 participants with diabetes. The adiposity-HbA1c association was slightly stronger among the participants with IFG, IGT, and diabetes (n = 110), compared with those with NGT. After excluding participants with diabetes, the associations between the changes in HOMA-β and the changes in adiposity measures (e.g., VFAT) became stronger (coefficient, 0.62; 95%CI 0.31, 0.92).

13.4 DISCUSSION

In this prospective study, changes in all the examined adiposity measures were positively associated with changes in glycemia in 196 Japanese participants with obesity. Furthermore, we found that reductions in BMI, visceral fat area, and waist circumference were associated with a reduction in HOMA-β, while no association was observed for the insulinogenic index. Reductions in BMI and VFAT were also associated with an improvement in insulin sensitivity. In addition, changes in adiposity were related to changes in TG and blood pressure. These findings suggest that controlling adiposity among obese individuals may effectively improve CVD risk factors and insulin sensitivity.

These results were consistent with a preceding study among obese individuals with type 2 diabetes, in which weight loss was associated with an improvement in glycemia, blood pressure, TG, and HDL [8], [9]. In the current study, we were able to assess VFAT and SFAT changes using computed tomography. We found that a reduction in visceral adiposity as well as the BMI was associated with an improvement in the CVD risk factors. Consistent with the previous study [8], the adiposity change was not associated with the LDL change in the current study. In another study reviewing weight loss effects and lipid outcomes [26], weight loss was reported to be associated with the LDL reduction. This dissociation may be because, in a previous review [26], studies with a large weight reduction (22 to 55 kg) as a result of surgical intervention were included. In the current study, the mean weight reduction within 1 year was 2.4 kg (SD 4.3), so the amount of the weight reduction may have been insufficient to detect any changes.

Among adiposity measures, changes in BMI and VFAT were positively associated with changes in insulin and HOMA-IR and were inversely associated with changes in ISI. Indeed, the change in ISI was inversely associated with changes in all the adiposity measures. These findings indicate that a reduction in adiposity may lead to an improvement in insulin sensitivity. This finding is consistent with a preceding study showing that baseline adiposity measures were inversely associated with future insulin sensitivity indices [6]. Although changes in SFAT and the waist circumference were also related to some of the insulin related indices, our findings may suggest that BMI and VFAT may be better markers of adiposity in this obese population. This finding is consistent with the results of preceding studies among Japanese-Americans, which have shown that the baseline VFAT, but not the SFAT, was associated with future insulin resistance [6].

Reductions in BMI, VFAT, and waist circumference were associated with a decrease in HOMA-β. Importantly, a previous study has shown that HOMA β-cell function, another measure of β-cell function, is elevated 3–4 years before the diagnosis of diabetes, and then decreases until the time of diagnosis, indicating that a period of compensation for insulin resistance exists [27]. In our study, a reduction in adiposity was related to a reduction in insulin resistance, which was accompanied by a reduction in HOMA-β. Furthermore, the associations between the HOMA-β change and the adiposity changes became stronger after the exclusion of participants with diabetes (coefficient for ΔVFAT-ΔHOMA-β, 0.50 to 0.62). This finding may suggest that a compensatory period actually exists among obese individuals who did not develop diabetes—and the adiposity reduction may reduce the needs for compensatory hyperinsulinemia.

Preceding studies have also reported that a decrease in the early-phase insulin response to glucose is a major feature of glucose tolerance among Japanese [22], [28], [29]. However, the change in the insulinogenic index was not related to changes in any adiposity measures in our study. This finding may suggest that the insulinogenic index may not measure compensatory hyperinsulinemia observed during the compensatory period, but might instead evaluate residual β-cell function. Thus, the null association between the insulinogenic index change and the adiposity change suggests that a reduction in adiposity may be insufficient to improve residual β-cell function.

Some limitations of the present study need to be addressed. First, participants in this study were Japanese individuals with obesity, and the sample size was limited; thus generalizability may be a problem. Second, although smoking has been reported to be related to CVD and weight reduction [2], smoking data was not available, and the analysis could not be adjusted for smoking. Third, we did not have intermediate measurements. Finally, because the follow up period was relatively short, a longer period observation period is needed to confirm the results. The major strengths of this study were the high compliance of our study participants, which enabled us to assess CVD risk factors, and the observation of adiposity changes using computed tomography over a 1-year period with few participant dropouts.

13.5 CONCLUSIONS

Our findings suggest that the reduction of obesity, especially the BMI and visceral fat area, may be associated with an improvement in CVD risk factors. Furthermore, we found that reductions in BMI and visceral adiposity were associated with a reduced HOMA-β and HOMA-IR. These findings support the notion that controlling adiposity among obese individuals may effectively improve CVD risk factors and insulin resistance.

REFERENCES

1. Donahue RP, Abbott RD, Bloom E, Reed DM, Yano K (1987) Central obesity and coronary heart disease in men. Lancet 1: 821–824. doi: 10.1016/S0140-6736(87)91605-9.
2. Fujimoto WY, Leonetti DL, Bergstrom RW, Shuman WP, Wahl PW (1990) Cigarette smoking, adiposity, non-insulin-dependent diabetes, and coronary heart disease in Japanese-American men. Am J Med 89: 761–771. doi: 10.1016/0002-9343(90)90219-4.
3. Look ARG, Wing RR (2010) Long-term effects of a lifestyle intervention on weight and cardiovascular risk factors in individuals with type 2 diabetes mellitus: four-year results of the Look AHEAD trial. Arch Intern Med 170: 1566–1575. doi: 10.1001/archinternmed.2010.334.
4. Carr DB, Utzschneider KM, Boyko EJ, Asberry PJ, Hull RL, et al. (2005) A reduced-fat diet and aerobic exercise in Japanese Americans with impaired glucose tolerance decreases intra-abdominal fat and improves insulin sensitivity but not beta-cell function. Diabetes 54: 340–347. doi: 10.2337/diabetes.54.2.340.
5. Pouliot MC, Despres JP, Nadeau A, Moorjani S, Prud'Homme D, et al. (1992) Visceral obesity in men. Associations with glucose tolerance, plasma insulin, and lipoprotein levels. Diabetes 41: 826–834. doi: 10.2337/diabetes.41.7.826.
6. Hayashi T, Boyko EJ, McNeely MJ, Leonetti DL, Kahn SE, et al. (2008) Visceral adiposity, not abdominal subcutaneous fat area, is associated with an increase in future insulin resistance in Japanese Americans. Diabetes 57: 1269–1275. doi: 10.2337/db07-1378.
7. Albu JB, Murphy L, Frager DH, Johnson JA, Pi-Sunyer FX (1997) Visceral fat and race-dependent health risks in obese nondiabetic premenopausal women. Diabetes 46: 456–462. doi: 10.2337/diabetes.46.3.456.
8. Wing RR, Lang W, Wadden TA, Safford M, Knowler WC, et al. (2011) Benefits of modest weight loss in improving cardiovascular risk factors in overweight and obese individuals with type 2 diabetes. Diabetes Care 34: 1481–1486. doi: 10.2337/dc10-2415.

9. Matsushita Y, Nakagawa T, Yamamoto S, Takahashi Y, Yokoyama T, et al. (2012) Effect of longitudinal changes in visceral fat area and other anthropometric indices to the changes in metabolic risk factors in Japanese men: the Hitachi Health Study. Diabetes Care 35: 1139–1143. doi: 10.2337/dc11-1320.
10. Goncalves FB, Koek M, Verhagen HJ, Niessen WJ, Poldermans D (2011) Body-mass index, abdominal adiposity, and cardiovascular risk. Lancet 378: 227; author reply 228. doi: 10.1016/S0140-6736(11)61121-5.
11. Tabák AG, Jokela M, Akbaraly TN, Brunner EJ, Kivimäki M, et al. Trajectories of glycaemia, insulin sensitivity, and insulin secretion before diagnosis of type 2 diabetes: an analysis from the Whitehall II study. The Lancet 373: 2215–2221.
12. Watanabe S, Morita A, Aiba N, Miyachi M, Sasaki S, et al. (2007) Study Design of the Saku Control Obesity Program (SCOP). Anti-Aging Medicine 4: 70–73. doi: 10.3793/jaam.4.70.
13. Morita A, Ohmori Y, Suzuki N, Ide N, Morioka M, et al. (2008) Anthropometric and Clinical Findings in Obese Japanese: The Saku Control Obesity Program (SCOP). Anti-Aging Medicine 5: 13–16. doi: 10.3793/jaam.5.13.
14. Tanaka T, Morita A, Kato M, Hirai T, Mizoue T, et al. (2011) Congener-specific polychlorinated biphenyls and the prevalence of diabetes in the Saku Control Obesity Program. Endocrine journal doi: 10.1507/endocrj.K10E-361.
15. Nakade M, Aiba N, Suda N, Morita A, Miyachi M, et al. (2012) Behavioral change during weight loss program and one-year follow-up: Saku Control Obesity Program (SCOP) in Japan. Asia Pac J Clin Nutr 21: 22–34.
16. White WB, Anwar YA (2001) Evaluation of the overall efficacy of the Omron office digital blood pressure HEM-907 monitor in adults. Blood Press Monit 6: 107–110. doi: 10.1097/00126097-200104000-00007.
17. Kashiwagi A, Kasuga M, Araki E, Oka Y, Hanafusa T, et al. (2012) International clinical harmonization of glycated hemoglobin in Japan: From Japan Diabetes Society to National Glycohemoglobin Standardization Program values. Journal of Diabetes Investigation 3: 39–40. doi: 10.1111/j.2040-1124.2012.00207.x.
18. Matthews DR, Hosker JP, Rudenski AS, Naylor BA, Treacher DF, et al. (1985) Homeostasis model assessment: insulin resistance and beta-cell function from fasting plasma glucose and insulin concentrations in man. Diabetologia 28: 412–419. doi: 10.1007/BF00280883.
19. DeFronzo RA, Matsuda M (2010) Reduced time points to calculate the composite index. Diabetes Care 33: e93. doi: 10.2337/dc10-0646.
20. Wallace TM, Levy JC, Matthews DR (2004) Use and abuse of HOMA modeling. Diabetes Care 27: 1487–1495. doi: 10.2337/diacare.27.6.1487.
21. Kosaka K, Hagura R, Kuzuya T (1977) Insulin responses in equivocal and definite diabetes, with special reference to subjects who had mild glucose intolerance but later developed definite diabetes. Diabetes 26: 944–952.
22. Yoneda H, Ikegami H, Yamamoto Y, Yamato E, Cha T, et al. (1992) Analysis of early-phase insulin responses in nonobese subjects with mild glucose intolerance. Diabetes Care 15: 1517–1521. doi: 10.2337/diacare.15.11.1517.
23. DeFronzo RA, Matsuda M (2010) Reduced time points to calculate the composite index. Diabetes Care 33: e93. doi: 10.2337/dc10-0646.

24. Wareham NJ, Phillips DI, Byrne CD, Hales CN (1995) The 30 minute insulin incremental response in an oral glucose tolerance test as a measure of insulin secretion. Diabet Med 12: 931. doi: 10.1111/j.1464-5491.1995.tb00399.x.
25. Alberti KG, Zimmet PZ (1998) Definition, diagnosis and classification of diabetes mellitus and its complications. Part 1: diagnosis and classification of diabetes mellitus provisional report of a WHO consultation. Diabet Med 15: 539–553. doi: 10.1002/(SICI)1096-9136(199807)15:7<539::AID-DIA668>3.0.CO;2-S.
26. Poobalan A, Aucott L, Smith WC, Avenell A, Jung R, et al. (2004) Effects of weight loss in overweight/obese individuals and long-term lipid outcomes-a systematic review. Obes Rev 5: 43–50. doi: 10.1111/j.1467-789X.2004.00127.x.
27. Tabak AG, Jokela M, Akbaraly TN, Brunner EJ, Kivimaki M, et al. (2009) Trajectories of glycaemia, insulin sensitivity, and insulin secretion before diagnosis of type 2 diabetes: an analysis from the Whitehall II study. Lancet 373: 2215–2221. doi: 10.1016/S0140-6736(09)60619-X.
28. Kosaka K, Kuzuya T, Hagura R, Yoshinaga H (1996) Insulin response to oral glucose load is consistently decreased in established non-insulin-dependent diabetes mellitus: the usefulness of decreased early insulin response as a predictor of non-insulin-dependent diabetes mellitus. Diabet Med 13: S109–119.
29. Matsumoto K, Miyake S, Yano M, Ueki Y, Yamaguchi Y, et al. (1997) Glucose tolerance, insulin secretion, and insulin sensitivity in nonobese and obese Japanese subjects. Diabetes Care 20: 1562–1568. doi: 10.2337/diacare.20.10.1562.

CHAPTER 14

BARIATRIC SURGERY: THE CHALLENGES WITH CANDIDATE SELECTION, INDIVIDUALIZING TREATMENT, AND CLINICAL OUTCOMES

K.J. NEFF, T. OLBERS, and C.W. LE ROUX

14.1 BACKGROUND

The rates of obesity are increasing with at least 300 million people worldwide now classified as obese [1]. Obesity is associated with reduced life expectancy, increased morbidity and mortality, and greater healthcare costs [2,3]. Bariatric surgery is more effective than non-surgical treatments of obesity with a reduction in overall mortality of 30% demonstrated in surgical recipients [4-7]. Greater reductions are seen in cancer and diabetes mortality [6,7].

Recommendations for referring candidates for bariatric surgery are available but they seldom give guidance to help a specific patient. We will examine the evidence for the magnitude and duration of the positive effects and negative side effects of bariatric surgery. Finally, we will offer a synopsis of the data on post-operative outcomes, and on what to expect in the months and years following surgery.

14.2 REVIEW

14.2.1 INDIVIDUALIZING TREATMENT: AVAILABLE OPTIONS IN BARIATRIC SURGERY

Several bariatric procedures are available. The most commonly performed procedures are Roux-en-Y gastric bypass (RYGB), adjustable gastric banding (AGB), and sleeve gastrectomy (SG) [8]. Biliopancreatic diversion, with or without duodenal switch (BPD and BPD-DS), is less commonly performed but is often considered in extremely obese individuals [9]. All procedures can be performed laparoscopically with a lower rate of complications such as wound infection and incisional hernias [10].

In RYGB, the stomach is divided into an upper gastric pouch, which is 15 to 30 mL in volume and a lower gastric remnant. The gastric pouch is anastomosed to the jejunum after it has been divided some 30 to 75 cm distal to the ligament of Treitz; this distal part is brought up as a 'Roux-limb'. The excluded biliary limb, including the gastric remnant, is connected to the bowel some 75 to 150 cm distal to the gastrojejunostomy (see Figure 1).

In AGB, a band with an inner inflatable silastic balloon is placed around the proximal stomach just below the gastroesophageal junction. The band can be tightened through a subcutaneous access port by the injection or withdrawal of a saline solution [11] (see Figure 2).

In SG, the stomach is transected vertically over a 34 or 36F bougie creating a gastric tube and leaving a pouch of 100 to 200 mL (see Figure 3). Although many regard SG as a restrictive procedure, it is increasingly recognized as a metabolic procedure [12].

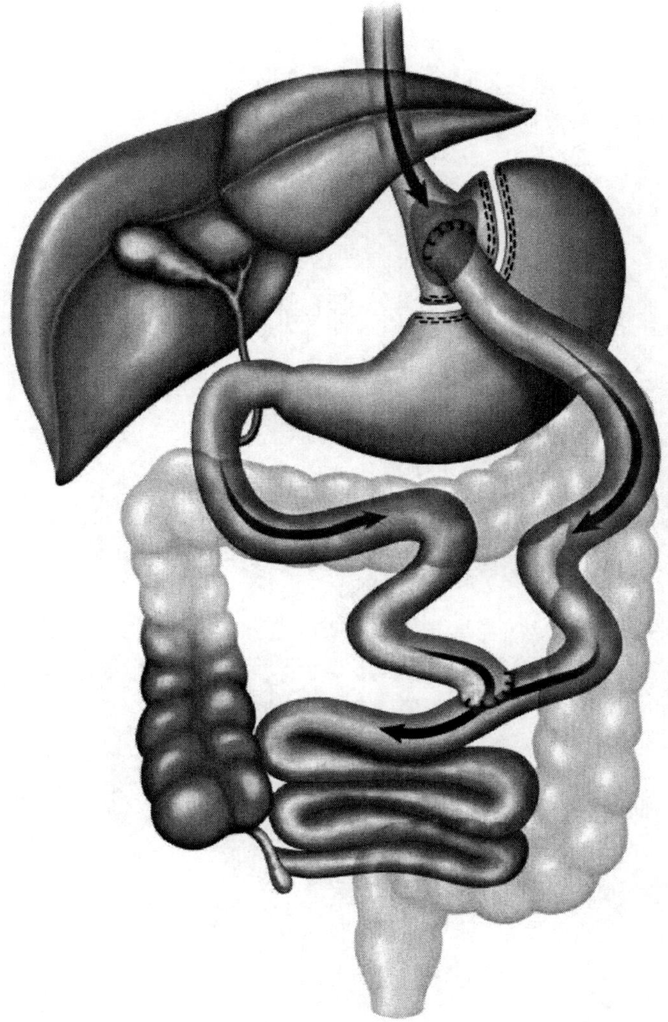

FIGURE 1: RYGB: Roux-en-Y gastric bypass. An upper gastric pouch, of 15 to 30 mL in volume, and a lower gastric remnant is formed from the stomach. The jejunum is divided some 30 to 75 cm distal to the ligament of Treitz, and anastomosed to the gastric pouch. The distal jejunum is brought up as a 'Roux-limb'. The excluded biliary limb, including the gastric remnant, is anastomosed to the bowel some 75 to 150 cm distal to the gastrojejunostomy. The included figures are the property of Johnson and Johnson and Ethicon Endo-Surgery (Europe). They are reproduced here with their kind permission.

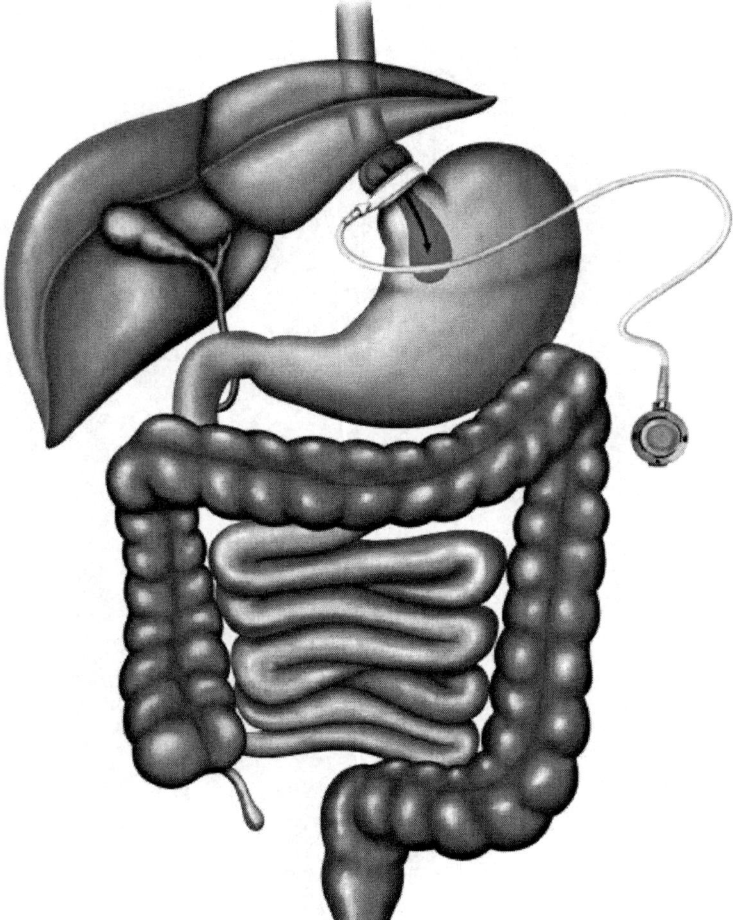

FIGURE 2: AGB: Adjustable gastric band. A band with an inner inflatable silastic balloon is placed around the proximal stomach just below the gastroesophageal junction. The band is adjusted through a subcutaneous access port by the injection or withdrawal of solution. The included figures are the property of Johnson and Johnson and Ethicon Endo-Surgery (Europe). They are reproduced here with their kind permission.

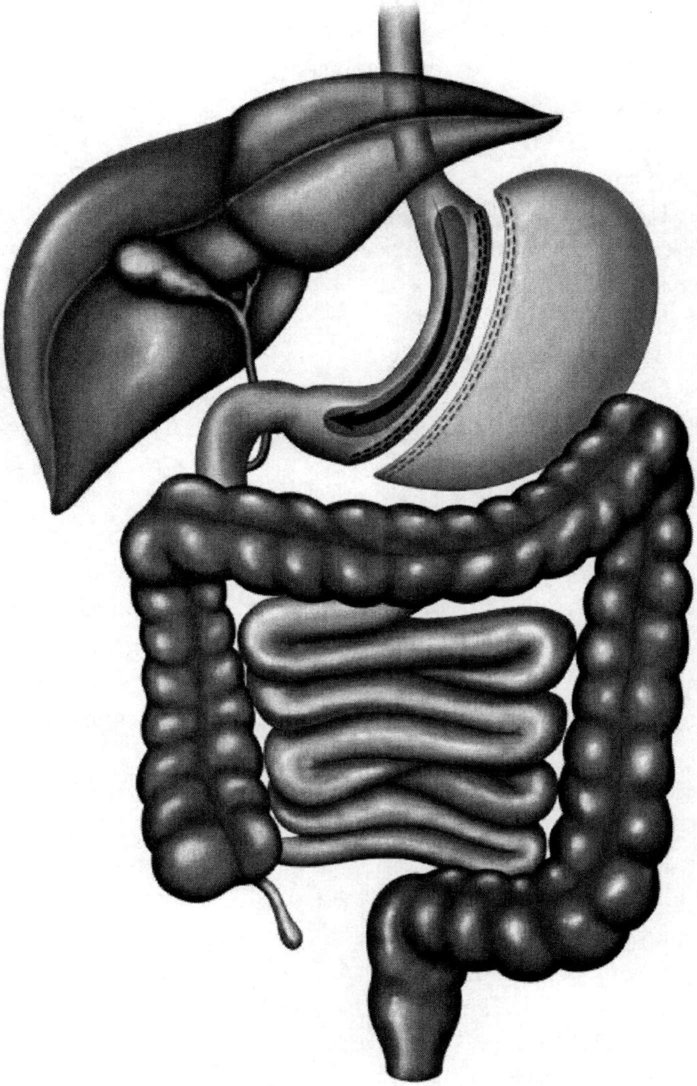

FIGURE 3: SG: Sleeve gastrectomy. The stomach is transected vertically creating a gastric tube and leaving a pouch of 100 to 200 mL. The included figures are the property of Johnson and Johnson and Ethicon Endo-Surgery (Europe). They are reproduced here with their kind permission.

BPD involves a partial gastrectomy that results in a 400 mL gastric pouch [13]. The small bowel is divided 250 cm proximal to the ileocecal valve, and the alimentary limb is connected to the gastric pouch to create a Roux-en-Y gastroenterostomy. An anastomosis is performed between the excluded biliopancreatic limb and the alimentary limb 50 cm proximal to the ileocecal valve (see Figure 4). In BPD-DS, a vertical SG is constructed and the division of the duodenum is performed immediately beyond the pylorus. The alimentary limb is connected to the duodenum, whereas the iliopancreatic limb is anastomosed to the ileum 75 cm proximal to the ileocecal valve [14].

Endoscopically placed synthetic duodenojejunal bypass liners such as the EndoBarrier® have been recently developed and are associated with a mean weight loss of 10% to 20% [15,16]. These devices establish duodenal exclusion and result in greater weight loss than diet and exercise alone up to 12 weeks post-insertion [17]. They may also improve glycemic control in those with type 2 diabetes mellitus (T2DM) [18].

However, long-term data remain to be reported and the device is often poorly tolerated [18]. Complications include sleeve migration and obstruction, which can occur with a frequency of 15% to 20% [15,16,18]. It can also be difficult to insert the device with placement failure in up to 13% [18]. While the concept of endoscopic techniques such as Endobarrier® remains attractive, the permanence of the weight loss and the clinical role of the device itself remain to be determined.

Other techniques for the treatment of obesity include the intra-gastric balloon, which can be effective for short-term weight loss [16]. However, these newer techniques remain in the experimental realm and data on long-term clinical efficacy are not available. The EndoBarrier® may not be any better or worse than gastric balloons or very low calorie diets at reducing operative risk in patients with extreme obesity. The device may be developed for use in those with diabetes and obesity who decline laparoscopic bariatric surgery. If other non-surgical treatments such as exogenous satiety gut hormones, or weight loss maintenance diets, can show that the weight loss after removal of the EndoBarrier® can be maintained, then a comparison with established bariatric procedures may be feasible.

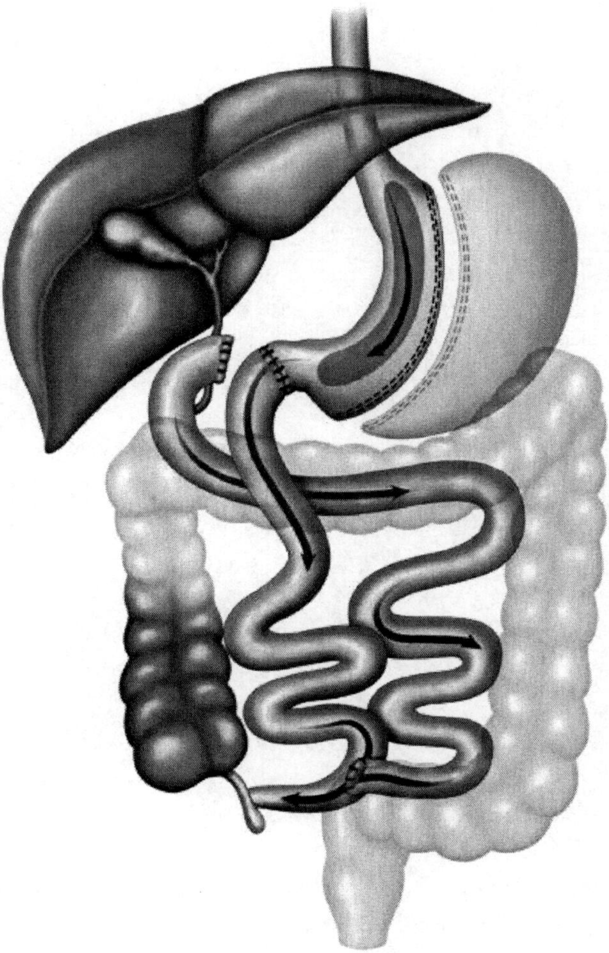

FIGURE 4: BPD: Biliopancreatic diversion. A 400 mL gastric pouch is formed from the stomach. The small bowel is divided 250 cm proximal to the ileocecal valve and is connected to the gastric pouch to create a Roux-en-Y gastroenterostomy. An anastomosis is performed between the excluded biliopancreatic limb and the alimentary limb 50 cm proximal to the ileocecal valve. In BPD-DS, a vertical sleeve gastrectomy is constructed and the division of the duodenum is performed immediately beyond the pylorus. The alimentary limb is connected to the duodenum, whereas the iliopancreatic limb is anastomosed to the ileum 75 cm proximal to the ileocecal valve. The included figures are the property of Johnson and Johnson and Ethicon Endo-Surgery (Europe). They are reproduced here with their kind permission.

14.2.2 CANDIDATE SELECTION AND PRE-OPERATIVE ASSESSMENT

Patient selection criteria for bariatric surgery include body mass index (BMI), the presence of co-morbidities and a history of prior weight loss attempts. National Institute of Clinical Excellence (NICE) and National Institutes of Health (NIH) guidelines state that bariatric surgery should be offered to patients with a BMI of 35 to 40 kg/m^2 who have obesity related conditions such as diabetes mellitus or obstructive sleep apnea, or in those with a BMI of 40 kg/m^2 or greater regardless of weight related co-morbidities [19,20]. Bariatric surgery for individuals with a BMI less than 35 kg/m^2 with obesity related co-morbidities is under investigation but is not currently recommended [21].

If a candidate meets the criteria for surgery, then a multi-disciplinary team assessment is made as to the suitability of the candidate. This is a complex process involving psychological, surgical, dietetic and medical review. The individual must be physically and psychologically fit to proceed to surgery. Expectations must be managed and a determination must be made as to the individuals' ability to comply with post-operative care. The decision to operate will take into account the benefits the candidate is likely to gain, and the risks peri-operatively and post-operatively.

This is an individualized assessment, and the role of the psychologist and/or psychiatrist should be central. Some reports suggest an increased risk of suicide after bariatric surgery, although the etiology remains unclear [6]. Major failures of bariatric surgery are due to poor psychological adaptation, especially if the patient's expectations were not adequately managed. All candidates should be given the correct and realistic information on what the procedure can achieve. If this is addressed, then the risk of surgical failure can often be mitigated [22,23]. This personalized assessment is a vital part of the pre-operative assessment.

For each patient the benefits of the procedure should outweigh the operative risk. In general, obese patients have an increased prevalence of cardiopulmonary disease that may be undiagnosed pre-operatively [24]. An individualized pre-operative assessment should be completed by a multidisciplinary team [25]. Pre-operative investigations should focus on screening for cardiac arrhythmia, prolonged QT syndrome, and cardiomyopathy

[25]. Almost 70% of individuals awaiting bariatric surgery can be diagnosed with obstructive sleep apnea, with over 40% meeting the criteria for severe disease [26,27]. However, this is not associated with a greater rate of peri-operative complications [28]. Male gender, age older than 50 years, congestive heart failure, peripheral vascular disease and renal impairment are associated with greater mortality [29].

14.2.3 PREDICTING OUTCOMES

Once the candidate has been selected, then the appropriate procedure must be chosen. Unfortunately, there is no evidence based medical approach for procedure selection, and this remains one of the most frustrating shortfalls in bariatric practice for clinicians and patients. Clinicians take a pragmatic approach to the choice of procedure, and the decision is determined by the individuals' clinical phenotype, the aims of therapy, and peri-operative risk.

Clinicians and patients can often be disappointed when surgical outcomes are not as impressive as may have been hoped and look for objective evidence that can allow them to predict outcomes. The most damaging outcome of surgical procedures that do not perform as expected is to blame the recipient for not performing well enough with regard to diet and exercise, when in fact, the failure is almost always rooted in biology. Weight loss prediction is one of the common aims of these predictive models. Pre-operative weight loss can predict post-operative weight loss, putatively as a marker of 'intrinsic motivation' [30,31]. These data are contentious and not without bias as many of them are retrospective uncontrolled studies [32]. The available prospective data are of short duration [31,32]. A systematic review shows that 50% of the published results find that pre-operative weight loss has an association with weight change post-operatively, and the remaining 50% refute these findings [32]. In the context of this evidence, pre-operative weight loss cannot be relied on to predict surgical outcomes at this time.

Genetic disorders such as melanocortin-4 receptor (MC4R) deficiency may have an inherent physiological role in these mixed results, as animals with MC4R deficiency have a resistance to weight loss after bariatric surgery [33]. There is interest in these genotypes, as identifying them may aid the prediction of outcomes. However, identified phenotypes such as MC4R are not common in the obese population, with heterogeneous mutations identified in less than 3% of European and North American obese cohorts [34]. Culprit genes that have been associated with obesity, with approximately 20 implicated to date, are still only found in 5% of obese people [35].

Investigation of genetic factors that may predict individual responses to bariatric surgery is ongoing and controversial [35-37]. While certain genotypes are associated with improved outcomes after bariatric surgery, they are not procedure specific and, therefore, while potentially aiding prediction of weight loss post-operatively, will not aid procedure selection [35-37]. It is also well recognized that the genetic influence on obesity may be much more complex than we currently understand, with the inevitable influence of environment making the situation less clear. For now, study of identified genotypes, with a correlation between genotype and treatment outcomes, may answer questions on the clinical utility and predictive ability of genotyping in bariatric surgery [33].

To date, any potential genetic markers or biomarkers of weight loss following bariatric surgery have been limited by clinical utility, and sensitivity and specificity [38,39]. Some data identifying potential markers of weight loss are inadequately controlled and unmatched [38]. The positive findings are in the context of complex interactions, without clinically usable tests that could be applied in daily practice [39].

While there is some potential in this field, usable techniques are still many years away [40].

The factors most consistently negatively associated with post-operative weight loss include higher BMI levels and personality disorders [32]. Given the impact of psychological markers on outcomes, techniques such the artificial neural network, which can incorporate psychological and biological measurements, have been tested to predict surgical outcomes [41]. Such techniques rely on established data that have been shown to effect outcomes, but may incorrectly predict response in as many as 30% of bariatric surgery recipients [41]. These models are multi-factorial, prone to bias and socio-cultural differences [41]. They are also time-consuming and expensive [41]. As the techniques are refined, we may develop a useful model that could be employed in routine practice, although we have not arrived at that point as of yet.

While weight loss remains difficult to predict, there are increasing amounts of data on prediction of diabetes remission. Markers of insulin secretion, such as C-peptide may aid pre-operative prediction of diabetes remission [42]. These results report an increased rate of diabetes remission with higher C-peptide levels [42,43]. The highest cut-off can predict diabetes remission with a specificity of approximately 90% [42]. Shorter duration of diabetes, lower glycosylated hemoglobin (HbA1c) levels and insulin independence are also associated with a higher post-operative remission rate [43,44]. These data illustrate a role for C-peptide to be used in conjunction with clinical data to predict diabetes remission. If a validated, sensitive and specific model were developed then it may aid procedure selection. However, the models currently studied can provide great specificity, but only at the cost of sensitivity [45].

The use of incretin and bile acid profiles has been investigated for use in predicting weight loss and metabolic outcomes following bariatric surgery [46,47]. The findings suggest that the restoration of peptide YY (PYY) and glucagon-like-peptide- 1 (GLP-1) secretion following RYGB contribute to satiety and weight loss [46,48]. Bile acids also have a role in this process, and the mechanisms underlying this are currently being elucidated [47]. Increased bile acid delivery to the terminal ileum can improve satiety and enhance weight loss [47]. However, these changes occur after surgery, and there is no current evidence that would allow them to be used to select candidates pre-procedure.

Similarly, while the restoration of the PYY and GLP-1 response is associated with satiety and weight loss in RYGB, as opposed to AGB, there are no strong data on differences within this group that allow us to predict the degree of weight loss following RYGB based on the incretin or bile acid response [48,49]. There are data demonstrating a progressive rise in PYY and GLP-1 following RYGB that is associated with increased satiety but without noted differences within the group [49]. The relationship between absolute incretin or bile acid levels, or trends, and weight loss remains to be determined. At this time, the restoration of incretin secretion and increased serum levels of bile acid are associated with enhanced satiety and weight loss, but they cannot be used to predict weight loss [46-49].

14.2.4 PROCEDURE SELECTION

For now, procedure selection is best informed by the candidates' objectives and by how they want to live their lives after surgery. As a primary aim of surgery, the efficacy of weight loss associated with each procedure must be considered. RYGB results in greater weight loss than AGB, although good quality post-operative care can improve the weight loss following AGB, with results comparable to RYGB [50-52]. AGB is associated with a lower rate of immediate post-operative complications but also a higher rate of re-operation for insufficient weight loss [50-52]. The associated mortality rate is higher with RYGB than with AGB but still less than 0.3% [50,51].

Weight loss is comparable between RYGB and SG in the short term [53,54]. Some studies suggest that more patients will regain weight in the medium-term after SG [55]. BPD/BPD-DS results in greater weight loss, but with higher complication rates, than RYGB [56,57]. Therefore, the greatest weight loss would likely be achieved with BPD/BPD-DS. However, this is not generally agreed. BPD/BPD-DS may not be suitable for high-risk operative candidates and some randomized controlled trials have shown no additional benefit of the extra weight loss above RYGB [58].

There are variances in outcome between national health systems, with AGB considered a superior bariatric procedure in systems where there is an excellent post-operative care pathway [52]. This implies that AGB can have comparable results providing that the post-operative care is planned and provided by experienced clinicians.

With regard to diabetes remission or treatment, RYGB offers a greater rate of remission than AGB [50,51]. SG has a remission rate comparable to RYGB in the short-term, but a higher rate of relapse in the medium-term [59]. BPD and BPD-DS may offer a higher rate of diabetes remission than RYGB or AGB [60-62]. While AGB is the least effective in inducing diabetes remission, it can offer substantial improvements in diabetes control, which are greater than those offered by medical therapy in obese cohorts [63,64].

Other conditions can influence a decision on bariatric surgery. Respiratory disease may improve more significantly with greater weight loss [65]. Therefore, those with obstructive sleep apnea (OSA) or asthma could theoretically be considered for more consistently efficacious procedures such as BPD/BPD-DS or RYGB. Conversely, SG and AGB are associated with deteriorations in gastro-esophageal reflux disease (GERD) and, therefore, should be avoided in this cohort [55,66]. In GERD, RYGB is increasingly considered as the treatment of choice as it can remediate the GERD due to the reduction in the stomach pouch and prevention of esophageal reflux [67].

In summary, candidate selection and preparation is key to achieving good surgical outcomes. Each procedure should be considered for each individual, and the data to date do not support the application of a generic selection based on body weight, diabetes or other co-morbidities. The choice of procedure is a complex process with the patient and their interests at its core. The surgeon's experience to deal with the inevitable complications of each procedure and to manage long-term follow-up care remain dominant considerations.

In those with diabetes, BPD/BPD-DS offers the highest rate of remission, but also the highest complication rates. RYGB and SG are comparably efficacious in treating diabetes in the short-term, but questions remain regarding the medium to long-term. It should be noted that the volume of data for RYGB is greater than that for SG and BPD/BPD-DS. For those with GERD, RYGB should be the treatment of choice. SG and AGB should be avoided.

AGB can also lead to weight loss and diabetes remission and can offer greater control than medical therapy, even if remission is not achieved. It should be noted that the choice of AGB should take into account the availability of good quality post-operative care. AGB may be suitable for those who wish to lose weight and improve diabetes control, but not remission, and are at higher surgical risk.

14.2.5 CLINICAL OUTCOMES

The outcomes following bariatric surgery vary between procedures, and predicting individual outcomes following bariatric surgery is difficult, for the reasons outlined in the previous sub-sections. We will review each outcome individually and compare between modalities below.

A. AIRWAY: OBSTRUCTIVE SLEEP APNEA (OSA) AND ASTHMA

Bariatric surgery is associated with impressive remission rates for OSA (68). However, bariatric surgery can improve the severity of OSA more frequently than resulting in full remission, and the improvement can still leave the individual in a moderate or severe category [68]. The symptoms of asthma can improve after bariatric surgery but the mechanism of this effect is unknown, although reduction of subcutaneous tissue with improvement of the restrictive effect on the chest wall may be involved [69].

B. BODY WEIGHT

Bariatric surgery effectively induces weight loss, but the degree varies between procedures [8-10]. RYGB results in greater weight loss than AGB in most studies [51]. The quality of the post-operative care affects weight loss after AGB, with good quality post-operative care resulting in comparable weight loss to RYGB [52]. Weight loss is comparable between RYGB and SG at 36 months post-operatively but long-term data are pending [53]. Weight regain can be frequent following SG [55]. BPD results in greater weight loss, but higher complication rates, than RYGB, with comparable metabolic and quality of life outcomes [56,58].

Weight loss usually reaches a maximum twelve months post-operatively, and some weight regain is common thereafter. The mean ten-year weight reduction is 25% for RYGB and 13% for AGB [4].

C. CARDIOVASCULAR AND CARDIAC DISEASE

Obesity is a risk factor for cardiovascular disease [70]. The available data over a median of almost twenty years show that bariatric surgery is associated with reduced cardiovascular mortality and morbidity [71]. In RYGB a reduction of cardiovascular morbidity of more than 50% is seen when compared to BMI and age matched controls [6,71]. The mechanism is unclear but improvements in glucose metabolism, blood lipid profiles and hypertension probably contribute [71,72]. The reduction in hypertension and dyslipidemia does remit somewhat post-operatively but both remain reduced from baseline at ten years [6,7].

Cardiomyopathy in obesity is associated with left ventricular hypertrophy and diastolic dysfunction with a longer exposure to obesity associated with worse cardiac function and larger ventricular mass [73]. Left atrial dilatation and systolic dysfunction can also develop [74]. This is likely due to a combination of increased cardiac output and increased circulatory volume [74]. Bariatric surgery has been shown to result in improved cardiac function and 'reverse remodeling' of the left ventricle up to three years post-operatively [75].

D. DIABETES

There is a strong association between obesity and diabetes with approximately half of those diagnosed with T2DM classified as obese [76]. Bariatric surgery can induce remission of diabetes by inducing weight loss [61]. There are also enteroendocrine effects following RYGB and BPD, achieving greater remission rates for diabetes when compared to patients who have had similar weight loss after AGB [61]. Diabetes remission is greatest for patients undergoing BPD-DS, followed by RYGB and then AGB [61]. SG has a comparable remission rate to RYGB [59,77]. The remission of diabetes following bariatric surgery can be transient, with 72% free of diabetes two years after bariatric surgery but only 36% remaining free of diabetes at ten years [4].

The most reliable long-term prospective data comes from the Swedish Obese Study in which the majority of participants underwent vertical banded gastroplasty with the remaining undergoing RYGB or AGB [4]. Subgroup analyses report that the RYGB group (N = 34) had a greater reduction in serum glucose at ten years than the rest of the cohort (N = 608) [4]. However, rates of diabetes according to subgroup and other prospective data for RYGB specifically are not available. Retrospective data at nine years following RYGB show a reduced rate of medical treatment of diabetes by more than 65% in parallel with a reduction in mortality of more than 70% [78]. The improvement in mortality was primarily due to a decrease in the number of cardiovascular deaths.

Shorter duration of diabetes, lower HbA1c levels and insulin independence are associated with a higher post-operative remission rate [44].

The presence of diabetes could influence the choice of bariatric procedure with RYGB, BPD and SG considered to result in remission of diabetes in a significant proportion of candidates. In those who do not achieve remission, bariatric surgery, including AGB, results in better glycemic control and a reduced medication burden compared to medical treatment [63,64]. Emerging data also suggest that bariatric surgery may facilitate remission of microvascular complications, such as microalbuminuria [79].

E. ECONOMIC

Obese individuals are more than twice as likely to take sick leave and almost three times as likely to avail of disability benefits [4]. Medical costs are significantly higher for obese individuals, mainly due to the cost of diabetic, hypertensive and lipid therapy, but with additional costs secondary to analgesia, respiratory and psychiatric treatments [80,81]. When classified by BMI, patients in the highest ranges spend more on healthcare [81].

While the presence of obesity may be secondary to lower socio-economic status rather than causative, bariatric surgery has been shown to result in increased productivity and reduced sick leave [82,83]. It is more costly than non-surgical management of obesity in the short-term but a return of investment can be achieved within four years [84].

Medication prescription is reduced by bariatric surgery with resultant reductions in healthcare costs that can persist for up to 20 years [84,85]. Cost effectiveness may also be achieved through reduced healthcare system utility due to the reduction in obesity related co-morbidities [85]. However, the modeling used in this type of cost assessment is open to criticism and there is a dearth of controlled prospective data.

F. FUNCTIONAL

Basic activities of daily living such as walking and personal hygiene can be affected by severe obesity, and this loss of autonomy can be extremely distressing for the affected individuals [86]. Joint pain, including lower back pain, is common in obese populations and can impinge on individual functional status [87]. Bariatric surgery results in improved function status, reduced levels of back pain and greater levels of independence [87].

G. GONADAL FUNCTION AND FERTILITY

In men, obesity can result in erectile dysfunction, reduced serum testosterone levels and reduced sperm quality [88,89]. Bariatric surgery is associated with increased serum testosterone levels but may paradoxically result in a deterioration in sperm quality [90,91]. There are no controlled prospective data to evaluate the effect of bariatric surgery on male fertility.

In women, obesity is associated with high rates of ovulatory dysfunction, increased risk of spontaneous abortion and increased materno-fetal risk in pregnancy [92]. There is evidence that weight reduction via bariatric surgery can improve ovulatory cycles and reduce hyperandrogenism in women [93]. It also probably reduces materno-fetal risk, although the current evidence is mainly limited to observational data [94,95]. To date, there are no randomized controlled data or long-term prospective data available and, therefore, no strong recommendation can be made on advising reproductively active women considering bariatric surgery.

H. PERCEIVED HEALTH STATUS

People who are classified as obese often report poor health perceptions and altered mood [96]. Psychiatric co-morbidities including anxiety and depression are also common [97]. Bariatric surgery improves quality of life and perceived health status, with changes seen in the first year and benefit retained up to ten years [96]. Depression, aggression and low self-concept can all be improved by bariatric surgery [97]. The improvements in perceived health status and quality of life may be correlated with weight loss, with superior results following RYGB compared to AGB [98]. However, factors other than weight loss may be responsible for these psychological benefits as the improvements have been reported in the immediate post-surgical phase [99].

I. IMAGE

Body image dysphoria is found in high frequency in obese cohorts but this sometimes improves post-operatively [86,100]. The improvement in body image satisfaction is associated with improved quality of life scores, and the improvements continue for at least two years following surgery [101,102]. Weight regain is associated with deterioration in self-concept and body image and can be associated with depressive symptoms [102]. In general, changes in body image are very unpredictable.

Eating disorders are common in obese populations [101]. Some evidence suggests that bariatric surgery can be associated with remission of eating disorders, particularly binge eating disorder [103]. The persistence of these disorders is associated with poor outcomes, and eating behavior needs to be regularly reviewed post-operatively [103].

J. JUNCTION OF GASTRO-ESOPHAGUS

The presence of obesity and GERD has been linked with pre-malignant metaplasia of the gastro-esophageal junction, and frank adenocarcinoma of the esophagus [104]. RYGB can reduce the symptoms of GERD and is associated with regression of pre- malignant metaplasia [67,105]. There is concern that AGB may worsen symptoms in a significant proportion of recipients [66]. SG has also been associated with worsening GERD, and patients with pre-existing disease may not be suitable candidates [55].

Surgical treatment of GERD can be ineffective in obese populations, and RYGB can be considered before fundoplication in this group given the improved outcomes [67]. Therefore, the presence of GERD supports use of RYGB as a first line procedure.

K. KIDNEY FUNCTION

While the measurement of glomerular filtration rate in obese cohorts is not well validated, obesity is noted to result in higher rates of chronic kidney disease (CKD) independent of the effect of co-morbid diabetes mellitus, hypertension or dyslipidemia [106,107]. Renal parameters such as serum creatinine and urinary protein excretion can improve after bariatric surgery, but at present it is unknown if the potential benefits outweigh the risks in those with CKD, given the greater peri-operative risk associated with renal impairment [29,108,109].

L. LIVER

Liver disease such as hepatosteatosis, non-alcoholic steatohepatitis (NASH), hepatic fibrosis, and cirrhosis are all associated with obesity [110]. Bariatric surgery improves the histological appearance of the liver and can lead to regression of established liver disease [111]. However, these data are often uncontrolled and some authors have reported worsening in fibrosis rates after bariatric surgery [111]. The presence of fibrotic liver disease needs to be considered in the decision to proceed with surgery and in follow-up plans post-operatively.

M. MEDICATION

Bariatric surgery results in a significant cost reduction in glycemic, lipid and antihypertensive therapy that can take effect within two weeks of surgery [84,85]. There are additional therapies needed following bariatric surgery, with increased prescription of GERD therapy with some procedures [80]. The need for increased GERD treatment and ongoing mineral and vitamin supplementation can partially offset the cost reductions in diabetic and cardiovascular medication [80,85].

O. OTHER

There is emerging evidence that weight loss using bariatric surgery may reduce the incidence of cancer [112]. It seems that the protective effect is strongest for women, and the reduction of risk may be as high as 60% [6,112,113]. The mechanisms underlying this apparent risk reduction are unclear, but may involve mediation of inflammatory pathways and attenuation of obesity associated hyperinsulinism [112].

14.2.6 MORBIDITY AND MORTALITY AFTER BARIATRIC SURGERY

Surgical complications can be defined as early or late, depending on if they occur within the first thirty post-operative days or afterwards. There is a wide range in the reported complication rates. The benchmark for bariatric centers of excellence is the Longitudinal Assessment of Bariatric Surgery consortium [114]. Mortality rates after bariatric surgery are low with a mortality rate after RYGB of 0.3% [114]. Pulmonary and venous thrombo-embolism are early complications and occur in less than 0.5% of bariatric surgery recipients [115]. Other complications can be specific to the modality and include the following.

14.2.6.1 ANASTOMOTIC LEAK AND BOWEL PERFORATION

Anastomotic leak is a feared early complication. Higher BMI, male gender, re-operation, older age and surgeon's experience are all associated with higher rates of anastomotic leakage [115,116]. Leakage can occur at any of the anastomotic junctions in RYGB, SG or BPD/BPD-DS and can result in severe peritonitis, sepsis, and multi-organ failure. Enteric leaks require emergent operative treatment in the context of hemodynamic instability or peritonitis.

Anastomotic leakage appears most commonly at the gastrojejunostomy in RYGB and the incidence associated with mortality is 0.1% [116,117].

The incidence of leakage is up to 3.6% in SG and most commonly occurs as a defect in the staple line [118]. In BPD-DS, leakage from the staple line is more common than anastomotic leakage and the total enteric leakage rate is 5% [119].

In AGB, there is no anastomosis and gastro-esophageal perforation is an uncommon early complication that can result in peritonitis and abdominal sepsis with an incidence of less than 0.5% [120].

14.2.6.2 HEMORRHAGE

Hemorrhage is an early complication that occurs in up to 4% of patients [121]. Using finer anastomotic closure techniques can reduce bleeding rates [122]. The presence of diabetes mellitus has been associated with a higher risk of post-operative hemorrhage [123]. In SG, hemorrhage has an incidence of up to 5.6%, but there is a large range in reported data that is likely explained by surgical experience, the complexity of the case intra-operatively, and the use of buttress material [124,125].

14.2.6.3 BOWEL OBSTRUCTION

Internal hernias can cause bowel obstruction, and can occur early or late post-operatively. The reported frequency ranges from 0.4% to 5.5% in RYGB [126,127]. Long-term data over seven years record a hernia rate of 38% in BPD/BPD-DS [128]. A laparoscopic approach may result in higher rates, but new surgical techniques where the mesentery windows are surgically closed may reduce the rate to as low as 1% [129].

14.2.6.4 ANASTOMOTIC STRICTURE

Anastomotic stricture is a late complication that can occur at any of the anastomotic sites. It is commonly described at the gastrojejunostomy in RYGB and is associated with dysphagia and vomiting [130]. The mean incidence of gastrojejunal stricture is approximately 10%, but rates as high as 20% are reported [130]. The laparoscopic approach and use of circular staplers to make the gastrojejunal anastomosis may result in higher rates of stricture [131].

14.2.6.5 OTHER COMPLICATIONS

Incisional hernias can occur but are less common with the increased use of laparoscopic techniques [10]. Marginal ulcers are usually late complications of bariatric surgery and occur in 2% of patients within the first post-operative year, and then in 0.5% for up to five years [132]. Proton pump inhibition is the preferred treatment but ulcers can be refractory and may require revisional surgery [133].

14.2.6.6 COMPLICATIONS SPECIFIC TO AGB

Band migration is becoming less common since the introduction of the 'pars flaccida' technique and individually sized bands, with rates as low as 1.4% [134]. Band migration can result in acute postoperative stoma obstruction, although this can occur in the absence of migration due to impacted food boluses [135].

Infections of the adjustment port can be an early or late complication. A late adjustment port infection can present years post-operatively, with abdominal pain or port site erythema, caused by band erosion with ascending infection, in up to 1% of cases [136]. This can result in intra-abdominal sepsis requiring removal of the band and high dose intravenous antibiotics. Band erosion is associated with surgical experience, with higher rates in those with less experience [137].

There is a recognition that AGB can have high failure rates in long-term follow-up, although this can likely be remediated by good quality post-operative care [138,139]. The emergence of SG as a procedure with greater weight loss and metabolic effects than AGB, with complication rates comparable or possibly slightly lower than RYGB has led to the consideration of SG before AGB in some cases [139]. However, SG's major

Achilles heel is the lack of long-term data with some authors concerned that the 10-year re-operation rate after SG will be similar to that of AGB.

As long-term data accumulate, SG may come to replace AGB in many cases, although for now AGB is likely to remain more popular given the established experience in its use and the lower complication rate in comparison to the other major bariatric modalities [139].

14.2.7 NUTRITIONAL AND GASTROINTESTINAL COMPLICATIONS AFTER BARIATRIC SURGERY

Deficiencies of iron, vitamin B12, folate, and fat-soluble vitamins can occur after bariatric surgery and are best described in RYGB, BPD and BPD-DS [140]. Vitamin D deficiency can persist despite prescribed replacement in BPD and may tend towards secondary hyperparathyroidism [140]. The risk of nutritional deficiencies depends on postoperative weight loss, the surgical procedure performed and patient compliance with follow up [140,141].

Vomiting is frequent after bariatric surgery but must always be considered to be pathological until proven otherwise after RYGB. An examination and appropriate radiological studies to screen for stricture, stoma stenosis or herniation must be completed. If no pathological cause is found then treatment should be conservative with replacement of fluid and electrolytes [141]. Often, vomiting can be the result of overeating or rapid eating. The patient should be re-educated on eating habits and kept under review.

Diarrhea is reported in up to 40% following bariatric surgery [142]. More than 30% of bariatric surgical recipients report worsening bowel function in the post-operative period and some develop fecal incontinence [143]. The etiology of this is unclear and treatment is based on appropriate dietary modification and anti-diarrheal pharmacotherapy.

There is a variable incidence of the dumping syndrome after bariatric surgery, particularly in RYGB [144]. Dumping syndrome remains a 'waste-basket diagnosis', with the clinical presentation generally considered to include early abdominal pain, diarrhea, nausea, bloating, fatigue, facial flushing, palpitations, hypotension and syncope after high glycemic index meals. These symptoms usually occur within an hour of eating. Similar symptoms that occur two or three hours after a meal include perspiration, palpitations, hunger, tremor, agitation, and syncope [144]. These have been blamed on hypoglycemia and GLP-1, although a definitive etiology remains to be established [145,146].

The treatment of early dumping syndrome is usually straightforward dietary modification, with small regular meals containing protein and carbohydrate with a very low glycemic index. Treatment of the symptoms that occur within two or three hours of a meal also rely on the same dietary modifications, with the added aim of 2 or 3 kg of weight gain which often abolishes the symptoms secondary to the small amount of increased insulin resistance. Pharmacotherapy with acarbose or somatostatin analogues may be needed [147], with transient enteral feeding required in severe cases [144].

There is some overlap in the hypoglycemic syndromes associated with bariatric surgery, with a number of mechanisms likely contributing to each. Obesity-related beta-cell hypertrophy that does not fully regress after weight loss, with improved GLP-1 dynamics and improved peripheral sensitivity, all probably contribute to each syndrome [148]. There can be an exaggerated incretin response in those with hypoglycemic syndromes [145,146]. However, the extent to which the incretin effect is involved can vary by syndrome and even by case [148]. If a post-operative patient presents with dumping syndrome or hypoglycemia that is unresponsive to dietary modification or 3 kg weight gain, or with atypical features such as fasting symptoms, then a full investigation of their insulin dynamics is needed.

14.2.8 OTHER COMPLICATIONS AFTER BARIATRIC SURGERY

Other post-operative complications include alopecia, cholelithiasis and hypoglycemia. Postoperative hair loss has been reported in up to 4.5% of bariatric surgical candidates [149]. This is usually mild and non-progressive. Cholelithiasis can occur in up to 2% of individuals in the months after surgery [150]. Ursodeoxycholic acid has been recommended for prevention [140].

14.3 FUTURE DIRECTIONS

As obesity continues to become more prevalent, bariatric surgery will become necessary for greater numbers of people. The current guidelines are aimed at a grade of obesity considered moderate to severe, but evidence is accumulating for the use of bariatric surgery in those with BMI levels of less than 35 kg/m^2 [151]. This is particularly the case in those with diabetes [151].

The ongoing randomized controlled trials comparing bariatric surgery and intensive medical glycemic therapy may yield results that will lead to bariatric surgery being used for metabolic benefits in those with diabetes, including those with BMIs of less than 35 kg/m2 [63,64]. This is the continuation of the concept of metabolic surgery; the idea that bariatric procedures should have a primary goal of inducing remission of metabolic diseases, such as diabetes. However, this concept remains controversial, and further data need to be collected to determine the benefits of this approach.

Finally, the goal of individualizing bariatric treatment and predicting response remains challenging. The work on genotyping and predictive models is ongoing but usable models remain elusive. Evidence to date suggests that the factors most predictive of weight loss may be psychological [32]. As genome association data are gathered we may identify genes that can allow us to tailor the bariatric approach to the individual [36,37,152,153]. However, given the expense associated with this technology, its clinical utility at present is low and clinical evaluation will remain the mainstay of pre-operative assessment and procedure selection.

14.4 CONCLUSIONS

Bariatric surgery should be considered in individuals with a BMI of greater than 40 kg/m^2 and in those with a BMI of more than 35 kg/m^2 and obesity related co- morbidities. In future, guidelines may recommend surgery for those with BMIs of less than 35 kg/m2 with diabetes or other metabolic disease.

Not all candidates are suitable to proceed to surgery, and an experienced multi- disciplinary assessment is essential to select the appropriate candidates. The choice of surgical modality should take the individual's goals, surgeon's experience and existing co-morbidities into account. Individualizing care is central to the assessment, and this is determined by clinical evaluation rather than using predictive models, genotyping or biomarkers at present.

Bariatric surgery performed in experienced centers has a low complication rate and leads to long-term weight loss, with associated functional, metabolic and psychological improvements. Bariatric procedures are effective in treating and preventing many obesity related co-morbidities. Long-term follow-up is mandatory to support a safe outcome.

REFERENCES

1. World Health Organization: Global Strategy on Diet, Physical Activity and Health. Geneva, Switzerland; 2011. [updated June 2012]; Available from: [http://www.who.int/dietphysicalactivity/publications/obesity/en/index.html]
2. Yan LL, Daviglus ML, Liu K, Stamler J, Wang R, Pirzada A, Garside DB, Dyer AR, Van Horn L, Liao Y, Fries JF, Greenland P: Midlife body mass index and hospitalization and mortality in older age. JAMA 2006, 295:190-198.
3. Vlad I: Obesity costs UK economy 2bn pounds sterling a year. BMJ 2003, 327:1308.
4. Sjostrom L, Lindroos AK, Peltonen M, Torgerson J, Bouchard C, Carlsson B, Dahlgren S, Larsson B, Narbro K, Sjostrom CD, Sullivan M, Wedel H, Swedish Obese Study Scientific Group: Lifestyle, diabetes, and cardiovascular risk factors 10 years after bariatric surgery. N Engl J Med 2004, 351:2683-2693.
5. O'Brien PE, Dixon JB, Laurie C, Skinner S, Proietto J, McNeil J, Strauss B, Marks S, Schachter L, Chapman L, Anderson M: Treatment of mild to moderate obesity with laparoscopic adjustable gastric banding or an intensive medical program: a randomized trial. Ann Intern Med 2006, 144:625-633.
6. Adams TD, Gress RE, Smith SC, Halverson RC, Simper SC, Rosamond WD, Lamonte MJ, Stroup AM, Hunt SC: Long-term mortality after gastric bypass surgery. N Engl J Med 2007, 357:753-761.
7. Sjostrom L, Narbro K, Sjostrom CD, Karason K, Larsson B, Wedel H, Lystig T, Sullivan M, Bouchard C, Carlsson B, Bengtsson C, Dahlgren S, Gummesson A, Jacobson P, Karlsson J, Lindroos AK, Lönroth H, Näslund I, Olbers T, Stenlöf K, Torgerson J, Agren G, Carlsson LM, Swedish Obese Subjects Study: Effects of bariatric surgery on mortality in Swedish obese subjects. N Engl J Med 2007, 357:741-752.
8. Buchwald H, Oien DM: Metabolic/bariatric surgery worldwide 2008. Obes Surg 2009, 19:1605-1611.

9. Smith BR, Schauer P, Nguyen NT: Surgical approaches to the treatment of obesity: bariatric surgery. Med Clin North Am 2011, 95:1009-1030.
10. Reoch J, Mottillo S, Shimony A, Filion KB, Christou NV, Joseph L, Poirier P, Eisenberg MJ: Safety of laparoscopic vs open bariatric surgery: a systematic review and meta-analysis. Arch Surg 2011, 146:1314-1322.
11. O'Brien PE, Dixon JB, Laurie C, Anderson M: A prospective randomized trial of placement of the laparoscopic adjustable gastric band: comparison of the perigastric and pars flaccida pathways. Obes Surg 2005, 15:820-826.
12. Scott WR, Batterham RL: Roux-en-Y gastric bypass and laparoscopic sleeve gastrectomy: understanding weight loss and improvements in type 2 diabetes after bariatric surgery. Am J Physiol Regul Integr Comp Physiol 2011, 301:R15-27.
13. Scopinaro N, Gianetta E, Pandolfo N, Anfossi A, Berretti B, Bachi V: [Bilio- pancreatic bypass. Proposal and preliminary experimental study of a new type of operation for the functional surgical treatment of obesity]. Minerva Chir 1976, 31:560-566.
14. Hess DS, Hess DW: Biliopancreatic diversion with a duodenal switch. Obes Surg 1998, 8:267-282.
15. Gersin KS, Rothstein RI, Rosenthal RJ, Stefanidis D, Deal SE, Kuwada TS, Laycock W, Adrales G, Vassiliou M, Szomstein S, Heller S, Joyce AM, Heiss F, Nepomnayshy D: Open-label, sham-controlled trial of an endoscopic duodenojejunal bypass liner for preoperative weight loss in bariatric surgery candidates. Gastrointest Endosc 2010, 71:976-982.
16. Espinet-Coll E, Nebreda-Duran J, Gomez-Valero JA, Munoz-Navas M, Pujol-Gebelli J, Vila-Lolo C, Martinez-Gomez A, Juan-Creix-Comamaia A: Current endoscopic techniques in the treatment of obesity. Rev Esp Enferm Dig 2012, 104:72-87.
17. Tarnoff M, Rodriguez L, Escalona A, Ramos A, Neto M, Alamo M, Reyes E, Pimentel F, Ibanez L: Open label, prospective, randomized controlled trial of an endoscopic duodenal-jejunal bypass sleeve versus low calorie diet for pre-operative weight loss in bariatric surgery. Surg Endosc 2009, 23:650-656.
18. Schouten R, Rijs CS, Bouvy ND, Hameeteman W, Koek GH, Janssen IM, Greve JW: A multicenter, randomized efficacy study of the EndoBarrier Gastrointestinal Liner for presurgical weight loss prior to bariatric surgery. Ann Surg 2010, 251:236-243.
19. Centre for Public Health Excellence at NICE (UK), National Collaborating Centre for Primary Care (UK): Obesity: The Prevention, Identification, Assessment and Management of Overweight and Obesity in Adults and Children. London. 2006.
20. NIH Consensus Development Conference Panel: Gastrointestinal surgery for severe obesity. Ann Intern Med 1991, 115:956-961.
21. Serrot FJ, Dorman RB, Miller CJ, Slusarek B, Sampson B, Sick BT, Leslie DB, Buchwald H, Ikramuddin S: Comparative effectiveness of bariatric surgery and nonsurgical therapy in adults with type 2 diabetes mellitus and body mass index < 35 kg/m^2. Surgery 2011, 150:684-691.
22. Ogden J, Avenell S, Ellis G: Negotiating control: patients' experiences of unsuccessful weight-loss surgery. Psychol Health 2011, 26:949-964.
23. Saltzman E, Anderson W, Apovian CM, Boulton H, Chamberlain A, Cullum-Dugan D, Cummings S, Hatchigian E, Hodges B, Keroack CR, Pettus M, Thomason P, Veglia L, Young LS: Criteria for patient selection and multidisciplinary evaluation and treatment of the weight loss surgery patient. Obes Res 2005, 13:234-243.

24. Catheline JM, Bihan H, Le Quang T, Sadoun D, Charniot JC, Onnen I, Fournier JL, Bénichou J, Cohen R: Preoperative cardiac and pulmonary assessment in bariatric surgery. Obes Surg 2008, 18:271-277.
25. Association of Anaesthetists of Great Britain and Ireland: Peri-operative Management of the Morbidly Obese Patient. London 2007. [cited 12 June 2012]; [http://www.aagbi.org/publications/guidelines/docs/Obesity07.pdf]
26. Ravesloot MJ, van Maanen JP, Hilgevoord AA, van Wagensveld BA, de Vrie N: Obstructive sleep apnea is underrecognized and underdiagnosed in patients undergoing bariatric surgery. Eur Arch Otorhinolaryngol 2012, 269:1865-1871.
27. Carneiro G, Florio RT, Zanella MT, Pradella-Hallinan M, Ribeiro-Filho FF, Tufik S, Togeiro SM: Is mandatory screening for obstructive sleep apnea with polysomnography in all severely obese patients indicated? Sleep Breath 2012, 16:163-168.
28. Weingarten TN, Flores AS, McKenzie JA, Nguyen LT, Robinson WB, Kinney TM, Siems BT, Wenzel PJ, Sarr MG, Marienau MS, Schroeder DR, Olson EJ, Morgenthaler TI, Warner DO, Sprung J: Obstructive sleep apnoea and perioperative complications in bariatric patients. Br J Anaesth 2011, 106:131-139.
29. Nguyen NT, Masoomi H, Laugenour K, Sanaiha Y, Reavis KM, Mills SD, Stamos MJ: Predictive factors of mortality in bariatric surgery: data from the Nationwide Inpatient Sample. Surgery 2011, 150:347-351.
30. Alvarado R, Alami RS, Hsu G, Safadi BY, Sanchez BR, Morton JM, Curet MJ: The impact of preoperative weight loss in patients undergoing laparoscopic Roux- en-Y gastric bypass. Obes Surg 2005, 15:1282-1286.
31. Alami RS, Morton JM, Schuster R, Lie J, Sanchez BR, Peters A, Curet MJ: Is there a benefit to preoperative weight loss in gastric bypass patients? A prospective randomized trial. Surg Obes Relat Dis 2007, 3:141-145.
32. Livhits M, Mercado C, Yermilov I, Parikh JA, Dutson E, Mehran A, Ko CY, Meehan MM: Preoperative predictors of weight loss following bariatric surgery: systematic review. Obes Surg 2012, 22:70-89.
33. Mul JD, Begg DP, Alsters SI, van Haaften G, Duran KJ, D'Alessio DA, le Roux CW, Woods SC, Sandoval DA, Blakemore AI, Cuppen E, van Haelst MM, Seeley RJ: Effect of vertical sleeve gastrectomy in melanocortin receptor 4-deficient rats. Am J Physiol Endocrinol Metab 2012, 303:E103-110.
34. Calton MA, Ersoy BA, Zhang S, Kane JP, Malloy MJ, Pullinger CR, Bromberg Y, Pennacchio LA, Dent R, McPherson R, Ahituv N, Vaisse C: Association of functionally significant Melanocortin-4 but not Melanocortin-3 receptor mutations with severe adult obesity in a large North American case- control study. Hum Mol Genet 2009, 18:1140-1147.
35. Ranadive SA, Vaisse C: Lessons from extreme human obesity: monogenic disorders. Endocrinol Metab Clin North Am 2008, 37:733-751.
36. Sarzynski MA, Jacobson P, Rankinen T, Carlsson B, Sjostrom L, Bouchard C, Carlsson LM: Associations of markers in 11 obesity candidate genes with maximal weight loss and weight regain in the SOS bariatric surgery cases. Int J Obes (Lond) 2011, 35:676-683.
37. Liou TH, Chen HH, Wang W, Wu SF, Lee YC, Yang WS, Lee WJ: ESR1, FTO, and UCP2 genes interact with bariatric surgery affecting weight loss and glycemic control in severely obese patients. Obes Surg 2011, 21:1758-1765.

38. Harvey SB, Zhang Y, Wilson-Grady J, Monkkonen T, Nelsestuen GL, Kasthuri RS, Verneris MR, Lund TC, Ely EW, Bernard GR, Zeisler H, Homoncik M, Jilma B, Swan T, Kellogg TA: O-glycoside biomarker of apolipoprotein C3: responsiveness to obesity, bariatric surgery, and therapy with metformin, to chronic or severe liver disease and to mortality in severe sepsis and graft vs host disease. J Proteome Res 2009, 8:603-612.
39. Kim K, Perroud B, Espinal G, Kachinskas D, Austrheim-Smith I, Wolfe BM, Warden CH: Genes and networks expressed in perioperative omental adipose tissue are correlated with weight loss from Roux-en-Y gastric bypass. Int J Obes (Lond) 2008, 32:1395-1406.
40. Kim K, Zakharkin SO, Allison DB: Expectations, validity, and reality in gene expression profiling. J Clin Epidemiol 2010, 63:950-959.
41. Piaggi P, Lippi C, Fierabracci P, Maffei M, Calderone A, Mauri M, Anselmino M, Cassano GB, Vitti P, Pinchera A, Landi A, Santini F: Artificial neural networks in the outcome prediction of adjustable gastric banding in obese women. PloS One 2010, 5:e13624.
42. Lee WJ, Chong K, Ser KH, Chen JC, Lee YC, Chen SC, Su YH, Tsai MH: C-peptide predicts the remission of type 2 diabetes after bariatric surgery. Obes Surg 2012, 22:293-298.
43. Dixon JB, Chuang LM, Chong K, Chen SC, Lambert GW, Straznicky NE, Lambert EA, Lee WJ: Predicting the glycemic response to gastric bypass surgery in patients with type 2 diabetes. Diabetes Care, in press.
44. Hayes MT, Hunt LA, Foo J, Tychinskaya Y, Stubbs RS: A model for predicting the resolution of type 2 diabetes in severely obese subjects following Roux-en Y gastric bypass surgery. Obes Surg 2011, 21:910-916.
45. Lee WJ, Hur KY, Lakadawala M, Kasama K, Wong SK, Chen SC, Lee YC, Ser KH: Predicting success of metabolic surgery: age, body mass index, C-peptide, and duration score. Surg Obes Relat Dis, in press.
46. le Roux CW, Welbourn R, Werling M, Osborne A, Kokkinos A, Laurenius A, Lönroth H, Fändriks L, Ghatei MA, Bloom SR, Olbers T: Gut hormones as mediators of appetite and weight loss after Roux-en-Y gastric bypass. Ann Surg 2007, 246:780-785.
47. Pournaras DJ, Glicksman C, Vincent RP, Kuganolipava S, Alaghband-Zadeh J, Mahon D, Bekker JH, Ghatei MA, Bloom SR, Walters JR, Welbourn R, le Roux CW: The role of bile after Roux-en-Y gastric bypass in promoting weight loss and improving glycaemic control. Endocrinology 2012, 153:3613-3619.
48. le Roux CW, Aylwin SJ, Batterham RL, Borg CM, Coyle F, Prasad V, Shurey S, Ghatei MA, Patel AG, Bloom SR: Gut hormone profiles following bariatric surgery favor an anorectic state, facilitate weight loss, and improve metabolic parameters. Ann Surg 2006, 243:108-114.
49. Borg CM, le Roux CW, Ghatei MA, Bloom SR, Patel AG, Aylwin SJ: Progressive rise in gut hormone levels after Roux-en-Y gastric bypass suggests gut adaptation and explains altered satiety. Br J Surg 2006, 93:210-215.
50. Angrisani L, Lorenzo M, Borrelli V: Laparoscopic adjustable gastric banding versus Roux-en-Y gastric bypass: 5-year results of a prospective randomized trial. Surg Obes Relat Dis 2007, 3:127-132.

51. Tice JA, Karliner L, Walsh J, Petersen AJ, Feldman MD: Gastric banding or bypass? A systematic review comparing the two most popular bariatric procedures. Am J Med 2008, 121:885-893.
52. O'Brien PE, McPhail T, Chaston TB, Dixon JB: Systematic review of medium-term weight loss after bariatric operations. Obes Surg 2006, 16:1032-1040.
53. Kehagias I, Karamanakos SN, Argentou M, Kalfarentzos F: Randomized clinical trial of laparoscopic Roux-en-Y gastric bypass versus laparoscopic sleeve gastrectomy for the management of patients with BMI < 50 kg/m2. Obes Surg 2011, 21:1650-1656.
54. Clinical Issues Committee of American Society for Metabolic and Bariatric Surgery: Sleeve gastrectomy as a bariatric procedure. Surg Obes Relat Dis 2007, 3:573-576.
55. Himpens J, Dobbeleir J, Peeters G: Long-term results of laparoscopic sleeve gastrectomy for obesity. Ann Sur 2010, 252:319-324.
56. Laurenius A, Taha O, Maleckas A, Lonroth H, Olbers T: Laparoscopic biliopancreatic diversion/duodenal switch or laparoscopic Roux-en-Y gastric bypass for super-obesity-weight loss versus side effects. Surg Obes Relat Dis 2010, 6:408-414.
57. Buchwald H, Avidor Y, Braunwald E, Jensen MD, Pories W, Fahrbach K, Schoelles K: Bariatric surgery: a systematic review and meta-analysis. JAMA 2004, 292:1724-1737.
58. Sovik TT, Aasheim ET, Taha O, Engstrom M, Fagerland MW, Bjorkman S, Kristinsson J, Birkeland KI, Mala T, Olbers T: Weight loss, cardiovascular risk factors, and quality of life after gastric bypass and duodenal switch: a randomized trial. Ann Intern Med 2011, 155:281-291.
59. Karamanakos SN, Vagenas K, Kalfarentzos F, Alexandrides TK: Weight loss, appetite suppression, and changes in fasting and postprandial ghrelin and peptide-YY levels after Roux-en-Y gastric bypass and sleeve gastrectomy: a prospective, double blind study. Ann Surg 2008, 247:401-407.
60. Prachand VN, Ward M, Alverdy JC: Duodenal switch provides superior resolution of metabolic comorbidities independent of weight loss in the super-obese (BMI > or = 50 kg/m2) compared with gastric bypass. J Gastrointest Surg 2010, 14:211-220.
61. Buchwald H, Estok R, Fahrbach K, Banel D, Jensen MD, Pories WJ, Bantle JP, Sledge I: Weight and type 2 diabetes after bariatric surgery: systematic review and meta-analysis. Am J Med 2009, 122:248-256.
62. Hedberg J, Sundbom M: Superior weight loss and lower HbA1c 3 years after duodenal switch compared with Roux-en-Y gastric bypass--a randomized controlled trial. Surg Obes Relat Dis 2012, 8:338-343.
63. Schauer PR, Kashyap SR, Wolski K, Brethauer SA, Kirwan JP, Pothier CE, Thomas S, Abood B, Nissen SE, Bhatt DL: Bariatric surgery versus intensive medical therapy in obese patients with diabetes. N Engl J Med 2012, 366:1567-1576.
64. Mingrone G, Panunzi S, De Gaetano A, Guidone C, Iaconelli A, Leccesi L, Nanni G, Pomp A, Castagneto M, Ghirlanda G, Rubino F: Bariatric surgery versus conventional medical therapy for type 2 diabetes. N Engl J Med 2012, 366:1577-1585.
65. Wei YF, Tseng WK, Huang CK, Tai CM, Hsuan CF, Wu HD: Surgically induced weight loss, including reduction in waist circumference, is associated with improved pulmonary function in obese patients. Surg Obes Relat Dis 2011, 7:599-604.

66. Gutschow CA, Collet P, Prenzel K, Holscher AH, Schneider PM: Long-term results and gastroesophageal reflux in a series of laparoscopic adjustable gastric banding. J Gastrointest Surg 2005, 9:941-948.
67. Prachand VN, Alverdy JC: Gastroesophageal reflux disease and severe obesity: Fundoplication or bariatric surgery? World J Gastroenterol 2010, 16:3757-3761.
68. Greenburg DL, Lettieri CJ, Eliasson AH: Effects of surgical weight loss on measures of obstructive sleep apnea: a meta-analysis. Am J Med 2009, 122:535-542.
69. Boulet LP, Turcotte H, Martin J, Poirier P: Effect of bariatric surgery on airway response and lung function in obese subjects with asthma. Resp Med 2012, 106:651-660.
70. Wilson PW, D'Agostino RB, Sullivan L, Parise H, Kannel WB: Overweight and obesity as determinants of cardiovascular risk: the Framingham experience. Arch Intern Med 2002, 162:1867-1872.
71. Sjostrom L, Peltonen M, Jacobson P, Sjostrom CD, Karason K, Wedel H, Ahlin S, Anveden Å, Bengtsson C, Bergmark G, Bouchard C, Carlsson B, Dahlgren S, Karlsson J, Lindroos AK, Lönroth H, Narbro K, Näslund I, Olbers T, Svensson PA, Carlsson LM: Bariatric surgery and long-term cardiovascular events. JAMA 2012, 307:56-65.
72. Hofso D, Nordstrand N, Johnson LK, Karlsen TI, Hager H, Jenssen T, Bollerslev J, Godang K, Sandbu R, Røislien J, Hjelmesaeth J: Obesity-related cardiovascular risk factors after weight loss: a clinical trial comparing gastric bypass surgery and intensive lifestyle intervention. Eur J Endocrinol 2010, 163:735-745.
73. Alpert MA, Lambert CR, Panayiotou H, Terry BE, Cohen MV, Massey CV, Hashimi MW, Mukerji V: Relation of duration of morbid obesity to left ventricular mass, systolic function, and diastolic filling, and effect of weight loss. Am J Cardiol 1995, 76:1194-1197.
74. Lakhani M, Fein S: Effects of obesity and subsequent weight reduction on left ventricular function. Cardiol Rev 2011, 19:1-4.
75. Ashrafian H, le Roux CW, Darzi A, Athanasiou T: Effects of bariatric surgery on cardiovascular function. Circulation 2008, 118:2091-2102.
76. Leibson CL, Williamson DF, Melton LJ, Palumbo PJ, Smith SA, Ransom JE, Schilling PL, Narayan KM: Temporal trends in BMI among adults with diabetes. Diabetes Care 2001, 24:1584-1589.
77. Benaiges D, Goday A, Ramon JM, Hernandez E, Pera M, Cano JF: Laparoscopic sleeve gastrectomy and laparoscopic gastric bypass are equally effective for reduction of cardiovascular risk in severely obese patients at one year of follow-up. Surg Obes Relat Dis 2011, 7:575-580.
78. MacDonald KG Jr, Long SD, Swanson MS, Brown BM, Morris P, Dohm GL, Pories WJ: The gastric bypass operation reduces the progression and mortality of non-insulin-dependent diabetes mellitus. J Gastrointest Surg 1997, 1:213-220.
79. Iaconelli A, Panunzi S, De Gaetano A, Manco M, Guidone C, Leccesi L, Gniuli D, Nanni G, Castagneto M, Ghirlanda G, Mingrone G: Effects of bilio-pancreatic diversion on diabetic complications: a 10-year follow-up. Diabetes Care 2011, 34:561-567.
80. Narbro K, Agren G, Jonsson E, Naslund I, Sjostrom L, Peltonen M: Pharmaceutical costs in obese individuals: comparison with a randomly selected population sample

and long-term changes after conventional and surgical treatment: the SOS intervention study. Arch Intern Med 2002, 162:2061-2069.
81. Wang YC, McPherson K, Marsh T, Gortmaker SL, Brown M: Health and economic burden of the projected obesity trends in the USA and the UK. Lancet 2011, 378:815-825.
82. Herpertz S, Kielmann R, Wolf AM, Langkafel M, Senf W, Hebebrand J: Does obesity surgery improve psychosocial functioning? A systematic review. Int J Obes Relat Metab Disord 2003, 27:1300-1314.
83. Narbro K, Agren G, Jonsson E, Larsson B, Naslund I, Wedel H, Sjostrom L: Sick leave and disability pension before and after treatment for obesity: a report from the Swedish Obese Subjects (SOS) study. Int J Obes Relat Metab Disord 1999, 23:619-624.
84. Cremieux PY, Buchwald H, Shikora SA, Ghosh A, Yang HE, Buessing M: A study on the economic impact of bariatric surgery. Am J Manag Care 2008, 14:589-596.
85. Neovius M, Narbro K, Keating C, Peltonen M, Sjoholm K, Agren G, Sjostrom L, Carlsson L: Healthcare use during 20 years following bariatric surgery. JAMA 2012, 308:1132-1141.
86. Wadden TA, Sarwer DB, Fabricatore AN, Jones L, Stack R, Williams NS: Psychosocial and behavioral status of patients undergoing bariatric surgery: what to expect before and after surgery. Med Clin North Am 2007, 91:451-469.
87. Peltonen M, Lindroos AK, Torgerson JS: Musculoskeletal pain in the obese: a comparison with a general population and long-term changes after conventional and surgical obesity treatment. Pain 2003, 104:549-557.
88. Traish AM, Feeley RJ, Guay A: Mechanisms of obesity and related pathologies: androgen deficiency and endothelial dysfunction may be the link between obesity and erectile dysfunction. FEBS J 2009, 276:5755-5767.
89. Kort HI, Massey JB, Elsner CW, Mitchell-Leef D, Shapiro DB, Witt MA, Roudebush WE: Impact of body mass index values on sperm quantity and quality. J Androl 2006, 27:450-452.
90. Bastounis EA, Karayiannakis AJ, Syrigos K, Zbar A, Makri GG, Alexiou D: Sex hormone changes in morbidly obese patients after vertical banded gastroplasty. Eur Surg Res 1998, 30:43-47.
91. Sermondade N, Massin N, Boitrelle F, Pfeffer J, Eustache F, Sifer C, Czemichow S, Levy R: Sperm parameters and male fertility after bariatric surgery: three case series. Reprod Biomed Online 2012, 24:206-210.
92. Boots C, Stephenson MD: Does obesity increase the risk of miscarriage in spontaneous conception: a systematic review. Sem Reprod Med 2011, 29:507-513.
93. Escobar-Morreale HF, Botella-Carretero JI, Alvarez-Blasco F, Sancho J, San Millan JL: The polycystic ovary syndrome associated with morbid obesity may resolve after weight loss induced by bariatric surgery. J Clin Endocrinol Metab 2005, 90:6364-6369.
94. Maggard MA, Yermilov I, Li Z, Maglione M, Newberry S, Suttorp M, Hilton L, Santry HP, Morton JM, Livingston EH, Shekelle PG: Pregnancy and fertility following bariatric surgery: a systematic review. JAMA 2008, 300:2286-2296.
95. Dalfra MG, Busetto L, Chilelli NC, Lapolla A: Pregnancy and foetal outcome after bariatric surgery: a review of recent studies. J Matern-fetal Neonatal Med 2012, 25:1537-1543.

96. Karlsson J, Taft C, Ryden A, Sjostrom L, Sullivan M: Ten-year trends in health-related quality of life after surgical and conventional treatment for severe obesity: the SOS intervention study. Int J Obes (Lond) 2007, 31:1248-1261.
97. de Zwaan M, Enderle J, Wagner S, Muhlhans B, Ditzen B, Gefeller O, Mitchell JE, Muller A: Anxiety and depression in bariatric surgery patients: a prospective, follow-up study using structured clinical interviews. J Affect Disord 2011, 133:61-68.
98. Hell E, Miller KA, Moorehead MK, Norman S: Evaluation of health status and quality of life after bariatric surgery: comparison of standard Roux-en-Y gastric bypass, vertical banded gastroplasty and laparoscopic adjustable silicone gastric banding. Obes Surg 2000, 10:214-219.
99. Hrabosky JI, Masheb RM, White MA, Rothschild BS, Burke-Martindale CH, Grilo CM: A prospective study of body dissatisfaction and concerns in extremely obese gastric bypass patients: 6- and 12-month postoperative outcomes. Obes Surg 2006, 16:1615-1621.
100. Ratcliff MB, Eshleman KE, Reiter-Purtill J, Zeller MH: Prospective changes in body image dissatisfaction among adolescent bariatric patients: the importance of body size estimation. Surg Obes Relat Dis 2012, 8:470-475.
101. Sarwer DB, Wadden TA, Moore RH, Eisenberg MH, Raper SE, Williams NN: Changes in quality of life and body image after gastric bypass surgery. Surg Obes Relat Dis 2010, 6:608-614.
102. Zeller MH, Reiter-Purtill J, Ratcliff MB, Inge TH, Noll JG: Two-year trends in psychosocial functioning after adolescent Roux-en-Y gastric bypass. Surg Obes Relat Dis 2011, 7:727-732.
103. Colles SL, Dixon JB, O'Brien PE: Grazing and loss of control related to eating: two high-risk factors following bariatric surgery. Obesity (Silver Spring) 2008, 16:615-622.
104. Wong A, Fitzgerald RC: Epidemiologic risk factors for Barrett's esophagus and associated adenocarcinoma. Clin Gastroenterol Hepatol 2005, 3:1-10.
105. Csendes A, Burgos AM, Smok G, Burdiles P, Henriquez A: Effect of gastric bypass on Barrett's esophagus and intestinal metaplasia of the cardia in patients with morbid obesity. J Gastrointest Surg 2006, 10:259-264.
106. Verhave JC, Fesler P, Ribstein J, du Cailar G, Mimran A: Estimation of renal function in subjects with normal serum creatinine levels: influence of age and body mass index. Am J Kidney Dis 2005, 46:233-241.
107. Turgeon NA, Perez S, Mondestin M, Davis SS, Lin E, Tata S, Kirk AD, Larsen CP, Pearson TC, Sweeney JF: The impact of renal function on outcomes of bariatric surgery. J Am Soc Nephrol 2012, 23:885-894.
108. Navarro-Diaz M, Serra A, Romero R, Bonet J, Bayes B, Homs M, Perez N, Bonal J: Effect of drastic weight loss after bariatric surgery on renal parameters in extremely obese patients: long-term follow-up. J Am Soc Nephrol 2006, 17:S213-217.
109. Afshinnia F, Wilt TJ, Duval S, Esmaeili A, Ibrahim HN: Weight loss and proteinuria: systematic review of clinical trials and comparative cohorts. Nephrol Dial Transplant 2010, 25:1173-1183.
110. Li Z, Clark J, Diehl AM: The liver in obesity and type 2 diabetes mellitus. Clin Liver Dis 2002, 6:867-877.
111. Chavez-Tapia NC, Tellez-Avila FI, Barrientos-Gutierrez T, Mendez-Sanchez N, Lizardi-Cervera J, Uribe M: Bariatric surgery for non-alcoholic steatohepatitis in obese patients. Cochrane Database Syst Rev 2010, (1):CD007340.

112. Sjostrom L, Gummesson A, Sjostrom CD, Narbro K, Peltonen M, Wedel H, Bengtsson C, Bouchard C, Carlsson B, Dahlgren S, Jacobson P, Karason K, Karlsson J, Larsson B, Lindroos AK, Lönroth H, Näslund I, Olbers T, Stenlöf K, Torgerson J, Carlsson LM, Swedish Obese Subjects Study: Effects of bariatric surgery on cancer incidence in obese patients in Sweden (Swedish Obese Subjects Study): a prospective, controlled intervention trial. Lancet Oncol 2009, 10:653-662.
113. Ashrafian H, Ahmed K, Rowland SP, Patel VM, Gooderham NJ, Holmes E, Darzi A, Athanasiou T: Metabolic surgery and cancer: protective effects of bariatric procedures. Cancer 2011, 117:1788-1799.
114. Longitudinal Assessment of Bariatric Surgery (LABS) Consortium, Flum DR, Belle SH, King WC, Wahed AS, Berk P, Chapman W, Pories W, Courcoulas A, McCloskey C, Mitchell J, Patterson E, Pomp A, Staten MA, Yanovski SZ, Thirlby R, Wolfe B: Perioperative safety in the longitudinal assessment of bariatric surgery. N Engl J Med 2009, 361:445-454.
115. Nguyen NT, Rivers R, Wolfe BM: Factors associated with operative outcomes in laparoscopic gastric bypass. J Am Coll Surg 2003, 197:548-555.
116. Smith MD, Patterson E, Wahed AS, Belle SH, Berk PD, Courcoulas AP, Dakin GF, Flum DR, Machado L, Mitchell JE, Pender J, Pomp A, Pories W, Ramanathan R, Schrope B, Staten M, Ude A, Wolfe BM: Thirty-day mortality after bariatric surgery: independently adjudicated causes of death in the longitudinal assessment of bariatric surgery. Obes Surg 2011, 21:1687-1692.
117. Carucci LR, Turner MA, Conklin RC, DeMaria EJ, Kellum JM, Sugerman HJ: Roux-en-Y gastric bypass surgery for morbid obesity: evaluation of postoperative extraluminal leaks with upper gastrointestinal series. Radiology 2006, 238:119-127.
118. Simon TE, Scott JA, Brockmeyer JR, Rice RC, Frizzi JD, Husain FA, Choi YU: Comparison of staple-line leakage and hemorrhage in patients undergoing laparoscopic sleeve gastrectomy with or without Seamguard. Am Surg 2011, 77:1665-1668.
119. Mitchell MT, Carabetta JM, Shah RN, O'Riordan MA, Gasparaitis AE, Alverdy JC: Duodenal switch gastric bypass surgery for morbid obesity: imaging of postsurgical anatomy and postoperative gastrointestinal complications. AJR Am J Roentgenol 2009, 193:1576-1580.
120. Cunneen SA: Review of meta-analytic comparisons of bariatric surgery with a focus on laparoscopic adjustable gastric banding. Surg Obes Relat Dis 2008, 4:S47-55.
121. Mehran A, Szomstein S, Zundel N, Rosenthal R: Management of acute bleeding after laparoscopic Roux-en-Y gastric bypass. Obes Surg 2003, 13:842-847.
122. Sakran N, Assalia A, Sternberg A, Kluger Y, Troitsa A, Brauner E, Van Cauwenberge S, De Visschere M, Dillemans B: Smaller staple height for circular stapled gastrojejunostomy in laparoscopic gastric bypass: early results in 1,074 morbidly obese patients. Obes Surg 2011, 21:238-243.
123. Rabl C, Peeva S, Prado K, James AW, Rogers SJ, Posselt A, Campos GM: Early and late abdominal bleeding after Roux-en-Y gastric bypass: sources and tailored therapeutic strategies. Obes Surg 2011, 21:413-420.
124. Frezza EE, Reddy S, Gee LL, Wachtel MS: Complications after sleeve gastrectomy for morbid obesity. Obes Surg 2009, 19:684-687.

125. Daskalakis M, Berdan Y, Theodoridou S, Weigand G, Weiner RA: Impact of surgeon experience and buttress material on postoperative complications after laparoscopic sleeve gastrectomy. Surg Endosc 2011, 25:88-97.
126. Dillemans B, Sakran N, Van Cauwenberge S, Sablon T, Defoort B, Van Dessel E, Akin F, Moreels N, Lambert S, Mulier J, Date R, Vandelanotte M, Feryn T, Proot L: Standardization of the fully stapled laparoscopic Roux-en-Y gastric bypass for obesity reduces early immediate postoperative morbidity and mortality: a single center study on 2606 patients. Obes Surg 2009, 19:1355-1364.
127. Nguyen NT, Wilson SE: Complications of antiobesity surgery. Nat Clin Pract Gastroenterol Hepatol 2007, 4:138-147.
128. Crea N, Pata G, Di Betta E, Greco F, Casella C, Vilardi A, Mittempegher F: Long-term results of biliopancreatic diversion with or without gastric preservation for morbid obesity. Obes Surg 2011, 21:139-145.
129. Rodriguez A, Mosti M, Sierra M, Perez-Johnson R, Flores S, Dominguez G, Sánchez H, Zarco A, Romay K, Herrera MF: Small bowel obstruction after antecolic and antegastric laparoscopic Roux-en-Y gastric bypass: could the incidence be reduced? Obes Surg 2010, 20:1380-1384.
130. Nguyen NT, Stevens CM, Wolfe BM: Incidence and outcome of anastomotic stricture after laparoscopic gastric bypass. J Gastrointest Surg 2003, 7:997-1003.
131. Mathew A, Veliuona MA, DePalma FJ, Cooney RN: Gastrojejunal stricture after gastric bypass and efficacy of endoscopic intervention. Dig Dis Sci 2009, 54:1971-1978.
132. Bolen SD, Chang HY, Weiner JP, Richards TM, Shore AD, Goodwin SM, Johns RA, Magnuson TH, Clark JM: Clinical outcomes after bariatric surgery: a five-year matched cohort analysis in seven US states. Obes Surg 2012, 22:749-763.
133. Csendes A, Torres J, Burgos AM: Late marginal ulcers after gastric bypass for morbid obesity. Clinical and endoscopic findings and response to treatment. Obes Surg 2011, 21:1319-1322.
134. Thornton CM, Rozen WM, So D, Kaplan ED, Wilkinson S: Reducing band slippage in laparoscopic adjustable gastric banding: the mesh plication pars flaccida technique. Obes Surg 2009, 19:1702-1706.
135. Bernante P, Francini Pesenti F, Toniato A, Zangrandi F, Pomerri F, Pelizzo MR: Obstructive symptoms associated with the 9.75-cm Lap-Band in the first 24 hours using the pars flaccida approach. Obes Surg 2005, 15:357-360.
136. Allen JW: Laparoscopic gastric band complications. Med Clin North Am 2007, 91:485-497.
137. O'Brien PE, Dixon JB: Weight loss and early and late complications--the international experience. Am J Surg 2002, 184:42S-45S.
138. Favretti F, Segato G, Ashton D, Busetto L, De Luca M, Mazza M, Ceoloni A, Banzato O, Calo E, Enzi G: Laparoscopic adjustable gastric banding in 1,791 consecutive obese patients: 12-year results. Obes Surg 2007, 17:168-175.
139. Chakravarty PD, McLaughlin E, Whittaker D, Byrne E, Cowan E, Xu K, Bruce DM, Ford JA: Comparison of laparoscopic adjustable gastric banding (LAGB) with other bariatric procedures; a systematic review of the randomised controlled trials. Surgeon 2012, 10:172-182.

140. Ziegler O, Sirveaux MA, Brunaud L, Reibel N, Quilliot D: Medical follow up after bariatric surgery: nutritional and drug issues. General recommendations for the prevention and treatment of nutritional deficiencies. Diabet Metab 2009, 35:544-557.
141. Fujioka K: Follow-up of nutritional and metabolic problems after bariatric surgery. Diabetes Care 2005, 28:481-484.
142. Roberson EN, Gould JC, Wald A: Urinary and fecal incontinence after bariatric surgery. Dig Dis Sci 2010, 55:2606-2613.
143. Poylin V, Serrot FJ, Madoff RD, Ikramuddin S, Mellgren A, Lowry AC, Melton GB: Obesity and bariatric surgery: a systematic review of associations with defecatory dysfunction. Colorectal Dis 2011, 13:e92-103.
144. Tack J, Arts J, Caenepeel P, De Wulf D, Bisschops R: Pathophysiology, diagnosis and management of postoperative dumping syndrome. Nat Rev Gastroenterol Hepatol 2009, 6:583-590.
145. Goldfine AB, Mun EC, Devine E, Bernier R, Baz-Hecht M, Jones DB, Schneider BE, Holst JJ, Patti ME: Patients with neuroglycopenia after gastric bypass surgery have exaggerated incretin and insulin secretory responses to a mixed meal. J Clin Endocrinol Metab 2007, 92:4678-4685.
146. Rabiee A, Magruder JT, Salas-Carrillo R, Carlson O, Egan JM, Askin FB, Elahi D, Andersen DK: Hyperinsulinemic hypoglycemia after Roux-en-Y gastric bypass: unraveling the role of gut hormonal and pancreatic endocrine dysfunction. J Surg Res 2011, 167:199-205.
147. Spanakis E, Gragnoli C: Successful medical management of status post-Roux-en-Y-gastric-bypass hyperinsulinemic hypoglycemia. Obes Surg 2009, 19:1333-1334.
148. Patti ME, McMahon G, Mun EC, Bitton A, Holst JJ, Goldsmith J, Hanto DW, Callery M, Arky R, Nose V, Bonner-Weir S, Goldfine AB: Severe hypoglycaemia post-gastric bypass requiring partial pancreatectomy: evidence for inappropriate insulin secretion and pancreatic islet hyperplasia. Diabetologia 2005, 48:2236-2240.
149. Boza C, Gamboa C, Perez G, Crovari F, Escalona A, Pimentel F, Raddatz A, Guzman S, Ibáñez L: Laparoscopic adjustable gastric banding (LAGB): surgical results and 5-year follow-up. Surg Endosc 2011, 25:292-297.
150. Hamdan K, Somers S, Chand M: Management of late postoperative complications of bariatric surgery. Br J Surg 2011, 98:1345-1355.
151. Shimizu H, Timratana P, Schauer PR, Rogula T: Review of metabolic surgery for type 2 diabetes in patients with a BMI < 35 kg/m(2). J Obes 2012, 2012:147256.
152. Mirshahi UL, Still CD, Masker KK, Gerhard GS, Carey DJ, Mirshahi T: The MC4R(I251L) allele is associated with better metabolic status and more weight loss after gastric bypass surgery. J Clin Endocrinol Metab 2011, 96:E2088-2096.
153. Potoczna N, Branson R, Kral JG, Piec G, Steffen R, Ricklin T, Hoehe MR, Lentes KU, Horber FF: Gene variants and binge eating as predictors of comorbidity and outcome of treatment in severe obesity. J Gastrointest Surg 2004, 8:971-981.

AUTHOR NOTES

CHAPTER 1

Funding

This work was supported by the National Institute of Aging (P01 AG031093, Christakis, PI), the National Heart, Lung, and Blood Institute (R01 HL109263, O'Malley, PI) and by a contract from the National Heart, Lung, and Blood Institute (N01-HC-25195) to the Framingham Heart Study. Jason P. Block received support from the National Heart, Lung, and Blood Institute (P30 HL101312, Gillman, PI) and was supported by the Robert Wood Johnson Health and Society Scholars Program at the Harvard School of Public Health. S. V. Subramanian was supported by a National Heart, Lung, and Blood Institute Career Development Award (K25 HL081275) and the Robert Wood Johnson Foundation Investigator Award in Health Policy Research. The funders had no role in study design, data analysis, decision to publish, or preparation of the manuscript.

Competing Interests

The authors have declared that no competing interests exist.

Acknowledgments

We thank Rebecca Joyce and Laurie Meneades for the expert assistance required to build the data set.

Author Contributions

Conceived and designed the experiments: JPB SVS NAC AJO. Analyzed the data: JPB SVS AJO. Wrote the paper: JPB SVS NAC AJO.

CHAPTER 2

Conflict of Interest Statement

The authors declare that there are no conflicts of interest.

Acknowledgments

This research was supported by a grant to the African American Collaborative Obesity Research Network from the Robert Wood Johnson Foundation. Dr. Renzaho's participation in this project was supported, in part, by a Future Fellowship from the Australian Research Council.

CHAPTER 3

Funding

"This work was supported in part by NIH grants R01DK44073, R01DK56210, and R01DK076023 to R.A.P. and a Scientist Development Grant (0630188N) from the American Heart Association to W.D.L. Genome-wide genotyping was funded in part by an Institutional Development Award to the Center for Applied Genomics (H.H.) from the Children's Hospital of Philadelphia. Follow-up genotyping after the initial GWAS was funded in part by the Center for Inherited Disease Research (CIDR). CIDR is funded through a federal contract from the U.S. National Institutes of Health to The Johns Hopkins University, contract number HHSN268200782096C. No additional external funding was received for this study. The funders had no role in study design, data collection and analysis, decision to publish, or preparation of the manuscript."

Competing Interests

The authors have declared that no competing interests exist.

Acknowledgments

We thank all the patients and control subjects who donated blood samples for genetic research purposes.

Author Contributions

Conceived and designed the experiments: RAP. Performed the experiments: JTG SFG HH. Analyzed the data: KW W-DL CZ AW JTG HZ. Contributed reagents/materials/analysis tools: SFAG HH. Wrote the paper: KW RAP.

CHAPTER 4

Funding
No current external funding sources for this study.

Competing Interests
The authors have declared that no competing interests exist.

Acknowledgments
The authors acknowledge the examination participants, as well as the extraordinary efforts of the field staff, laboratory personnel, and statisticians who collected and processed the information in NHANES III and the National Death Index. The findings and conclusions in this article are those of the authors and do not necessarily reflect the official position of the Centers for Disease Control and Prevention.

Author Contributions
Conceived and designed the experiments: HSK KMB. Analyzed the data: KMB. Wrote the paper: HSK. Refined concept and design: LEB GI. Critical intellectual revision: LEB GI.

CHAPTER 5

Funding
The authors have no funding or support to report.

Competing Interests
JCK is employed by commercial company "Middletown Medical". This does not alter the authors' adherence to all the PLoS ONE policies on sharing data and materials.

Acknowledgments
We thank Steven Heymsfield, Michael Kleerekoper, James Levine, and Tom Rifai for valuable discussions and encouragement.

Author Contributions
Conceived and designed the experiments: NYK JCK. Performed the experiments: NYK JCK. Analyzed the data: NYK JCK. Contributed reagents/materials/analysis tools: NYK JCK. Wrote the paper: NYK JCK.

CHAPTER 6

Competing Interests

The authors declare that they have no competing interests.

Author Contributions

EKH, SKK, HO, LN, TS, JTS, JS, MV, MU and MP all had an important role in designing and conducting the FIN-D2D survey. PP wrote the first version of the manuscript. MP participated in the design of the study and performed the statistical analysis. AK, EKH, SKK, HO, LN, TS, JS, MV, MU and MP critically revised the manuscript for important intellectual content. All authors read and approved the final manuscript.

Acknowledgements and Funding

FIN-D2D was supported by financing from hospital districts of Pirkanmaa, Southern Ostrobothnia, North Ostrobothnia, Central Finland and Northern Savo, the Finnish National Public Health Institute, the Finnish Diabetes Association, the Academy of Finland (grant number 129293), Commission of the European Communities, Directorate C-Public Health (grant agreement no. 2004310), the Ministry of Social Affairs and Health in Finland and Finland's Slot Machine Association in cooperation with the FIN-D2D Study Group, and the Steering Committee: Huttunen J, Kesäniemi A, Kiuru S, Niskanen L, Oksa H, Pihlajamäki J, Puolakka J, Puska P, Saaristo T, Vanhala M, and Uusitupa M. Pia Pajunen was supported by the Finnish Medical Foundation. We thank Professor Aarne Pajunen for technical assistance.

CHAPTER 7

Funding

This study was supported by a grant: PTDC/SAU-OSM/100878/2008, from FCT, Portugal. The funders had no role in study design, data collection and analysis, decision to publish, or preparation of the manuscript.

Competing Interests

The authors have declared that no competing interests exist.

Author Contributions

Conceived and designed the experiments: MVM HCP TE CR. Performed the experiments: MVM DF RC ARS TE JC FC AC CR HCP. Analyzed the data: MVM HCP. Contributed reagents/materials/analysis tools: MVM DF RC ARS TE JC FC AC CR HCP. Wrote the paper: MVM HCP DF RC CR.

CHAPTER 8

Funding

A. Karlamangla is supported by the National Institute on Aging under grants 5R01AG26105-3 (PI: Karlamangla) and 5P30 AG028748 (PI: Reuben). P. Srikanthan is supported by the Multiethnic Study on Atherosclerosis by contracts N01-HC-95159 through N01-HC-95165 and N01-HC-95169 from the National Heart, Lung, and Blood Institute. A. Hevener is supported by the National Institutes of Health (DK060484, DK073227). The funding sources had no role in the design and conduct of the study; in the collection, management, analysis, and interpretation of the data; or in the preparation, review, or approval of the manuscript.

Competing Interests

The authors have declared that no competing interests exist.

Author Contributions

Conceived and designed the experiments: PS. Analyzed the data: PS ASK. Wrote the paper: PS. Reviewed and revised the manuscript: AH ASK. Aided in data analysis: ASK.

CHAPTER 9

Competing Interests

The authors declare that they have no competing interests.

Author Contributions

FJF participated in the design of the study and wrote the manuscript. MG performed the statistical analysis and participated in the manuscript writing. JMB participated in the design of the study and in the data collection. The other authors provided data and participated in the critical appraisal of the manuscript. All authors read and approved the final manuscript.

Acknowledgments

The authors wish to thank Jaume Marrugat for the expert revision of the manuscript content and Susanna Tello, Marta Cabañero and Leny Franco for their contribution to the data management of this project. We also appreciate the revision of the English text by Elaine Lilly, PhD, of Writer's First Aid.

This study was financed in its entirety with unconditional support from AstraZeneca. Data from the original component studies was obtained with financial support from: FEDER, Ministerio de Ciencia e Innovación, Instituto de Salud Carlos III (Programa HERACLES RD12/0042; Fondos para investigación. Acuerdo del Consejo Interterritorial de 8 de abril de 2003; EMER07/046 RCESP C3/09); Fondo de Investigación Sanitaria (FIS-FEDER) (PI01/0711, PI02/1158, PI02/1179, PI02/1717, PI03/20471, PI05/2364, PI05/2751, PI07/040, PI07/0934, PI07/1213, G03-045, FIS ETES 2007, CP06/00100, CM12/03287); Ministerio de Sanidad y Consumo, Plan Nacional I+D+i 2004–7 (IP071218); Agència de Avaluació de Tecnologia i Recerca Mèdica (034/33/02); Agència de Gestió d'Ajuts Universitaris i de Recerca (2005SGR00577); Departament de Salut de la Generalitat de Catalunya; Fundación Canaria de Investigación y Salud (45/98); Departamento de Salud del Gobierno de Navarra; Junta de Castilla y León; Beca Intensificación de la investigación (INT 07/289); Subdirección General de Promoción de la salud y Prevención. Consejería de Sanidad de la Comunidad de Madrid; Govern Balear; Servicio Andaluz de Salud; Programa de Iniciativa Comunitaria INTERREG IIIA (SP5.E51); Consejería de Salud de la Junta de Andalucía, Ayuda a Proyectos de Investigación (290/04 y 036/06); Sociedad Andaluza de Medicina Familiar y Comunitaria (SAMFYC 2008); Sociedad Española de Medicina de Familia y Comunitaria (semFYC 2009); Consejería de Sanidad y Consumo de la Región de Murcia; Consejería de Salud y Bienestar Social, Junta de Comunidades de Castilla-La Mancha.

CHAPTER 10

Funding

This study was fully supported by the National Institutes of Health (NIH), Intramural Research Program: National Institute of Diabetes and Digestive and Kidney Diseases (NIDDK). The funders had no role in study design, data collection and analysis, decision to publish, or preparation of the manuscript.

Competing Interests

The authors have declared that no competing interests exist.

Acknowledgments

We would like to thank in alphabetical order the following colleagues for their scientific advice and critical suggestions in the development and conduct of the study protocol: Karim Calis, Janet Gershengorn, Gregor Hasler, Emmanuel Mignot, Susan Redline, Nancy Sebring, Terry Phillips, Duncan Wallace, Robert Wesley, Elizabeth Wright, Xiong-ce Zhao. We would also like to thank the members of the study team: Peter Bailey, Laide Bello, Meredith Coyle, Paula Marincola, Patrick Michaels, Svetlana Primma, Angela Ramer, Rebecca Romero, Megan Sabo, Tanner Slayden, Sara Torvik, Elizabeth Widen, Lyda Williams and Sam Zuber. We would like to thank Dr. Alex Ling (NIH CC) for analysis of the computer tomography measurements. The bioinformatics support of Frank Pierce (Esprit Health) is gratefully acknowledged. Finally we are grateful to all of our enthusiastic study subjects.

Author Contributions

Conceived and designed the experiments: G. Cizza HK G. Csako KIR. Performed the experiments: MSM HK G. Cizza MW. Analyzed the data: PP LdJ EL. Wrote the paper: PP LdJ AP FS G. Cizza G. Csako KIR EL.

CHAPTER 11

Funding

Funding: National Institutes of Health (HL090982, AI070140, RR025011, RR025780, HL074227, HL074231, HL074204, HL074212, HL074073,

HL074206, HL074208, HL074225, HL074218). The funders had no role in study design, data collection and analysis, decision to publish, or preparation of the manuscript.

Competing Interests

Dr. Sutherland has read the journal's policy and has the following conflicts: Consultant: Forest Laboratories, GlaxoSmithKline, Merck, Novartis, Dey. Grants unrelated to the current study: Boehringer Ingelheim, Novartis. Educational presentation: Genentech. There are no patents, products in development or marketed products to declare. This does not alter the authors' adherence to all the PLoS ONE policies on sharing data and materials, as detailed online in the guide for authors.

Author Contributions

Conceived and designed the experiments: ERS EG TSK EL DYM. Performed the experiments: ERS EG ADS LPJ. Analyzed the data: ERS TSK EL. Contributed reagents/materials/analysis tools: ERS DYML. Wrote the paper: ERS EG TSK JVF DYML. Substantial contributions to analysis and interpretation of data: ERS EG ARS JVF DYML.

CHAPTER 12

Competing Interests

The authors declare that they have no competing interests.

Author Contributions

JRC, KS, KO and AHO designed and concepted the study. JRC designed the diet and the physical exercise protocol. JRC and AF together designed the cognitive behavioral training protocol. JRC was responsible for the work place, participant recruitment, intervention, test sessions, data collection and statistical analyses and together with DEK performed the data processing. All authors were involved in data interpretation. JRC wrote the first draft, and all authors read and approved the final manuscript.

Acknowledgements

This study was supported by The Ministry of Culture Committee on Sports Research, Denmark, and the Danish Working Environment Research

Foundation and conducted as a part of the FINALE program. We kindly thank the participating workplaces at Randers Municipality and their employees, without whom this study would not have been possible.

CHAPTER 13

Acknowledgments

We would like to acknowledge all SCOP members and the study participants for their participation in this research. We thank Tomoko Yasuda for her assistance.

Author Contributions

Conceived and designed the experiments: MG AM AG MN SW. Performed the experiments: MG AM AG KD SS NA MM MN. Analyzed the data: MG AG TS. Contributed reagents/materials/analysis tools: MG AG MN. Wrote the paper: MG AG YT MN.

CHAPTER 14

Competing interests

The authors declare that they have no competing interests.

Author Contributions

KJN reviewed the published literature for this review and drafted the manuscript. TO contributed to the content and structure of the article and, in particular, to the sections on surgical technique and complications. CWleR was invited to submit this review, and conceived the design and structure of the article. All authors edited, read and approved the final manuscript.

Author Information

KJN is a research fellow in metabolic medicine and has a clinical background in endocrinology and diabetes. His special interests include obesity and the metabolic effects of bariatric surgery, and the effects of the incretin system in obesity and diabetes.

CleR is the Professor of Experimental Pathology at University College Dublin with a special interest in the mechanisms and clinical application of bariatric surgery. His work has focused on how the operations allow long-term weight loss maintenance and metabolic benefit.

TO is a specialist bariatric surgeon who has performed more than 3,000 bariatric procedures. His practice is focused on laparoscopic gastric bypass, sleeve gastrectomy and duodenal switches. He completed his PhD at Sahlgrenska University Hospital in Sweden, and then became the director of the bariatric surgical unit at Carlanderska Hospital in Gothenburg. He is currently leader of a research group in the field of mechanisms and impact of bariatric surgery.

INDEX

A

A Body Shape Index (ABSI), xi, xxvii, 102, 104–121
adiponectin, xxxii, 89, 142, 148, 152–154, 159, 162, 168, 173, 235–241
adrenocorticotropic hormone (ACTH), xii, xxxi, 217, 224, 226, 228
age, xxiv, xxvi–xxvii, xxix–xxx, xxxii, 1, 5–12, 14–15, 22–25, 28, 41, 47, 62, 65–66, 72, 74, 77–81, 87, 90–92, 94, 102–112, 114, 118–119, 122, 124, 128, 133–134, 136, 146, 152–154, 170–171, 175–188, 194–198, 200–202, 204–206, 209–210, 219, 225, 228, 233, 236–242, 244, 254, 256–257, 259–262, 264, 271, 280–283, 299, 304, 310, 316, 319, 323
Akaike Information Criterion, 109
alcohol, 3, 5, 7–10, 68, 131, 136–137, 145, 147, 258
American Heart Association, 50, 71, 91, 94, 142, 209, 328
amputation, 177
analysis of covariance (ANCOVA), 131, 150, 218, 261, 270
anastomotic stricture, 311, 325
anthropology, 29, 44, 48, 50–51, 53, 121
arrhythmia, 298
arthritis, 251
Asia, xxxiv–xxxv, 21–22, 24–26, 28, 42, 48, 50, 54, 87, 90, 288
asthma, xii, xxxi–xxxii, 219, 233–250, 302, 304, 321
Australia, xix, 17, 20–21, 23, 27, 29, 36, 42, 46–47, 52–54, 87, 272

B

bariatric surgery, ix, xii, xix, xxviii, xxxiv, 146–147, 291–293, 295–326, 335–336
  adjustable gastric banding (AGB), 292, 294, 301–306, 308, 311–313, 316, 319, 321, 324–326
  biliopancreatic diversion, 292, 297, 317, 320, 325
  Roux-en-Y gastric bypass (RYGB), 292–293, 301–306, 308–313, 317, 319–320, 323–326
  sleeve gastrectomy (SG), 98, 292, 295–297, 302–306, 308, 310–313, 317–318, 320–321, 324–325, 336
bimodality, 59
bioelectric impedance (BI), xxxv, 65, 95–96, 123–124, 177–178, 188
blood pressure, xxvii, xxx, xxxiii–xxxiv, 101, 104, 108, 111, 118, 127, 129, 133, 137, 147–148, 193, 196–202, 259–260, 262, 264, 266–270, 273, 275, 277–278, 280–281, 283–285, 288

body
body composition, 65, 94, 97, 119, 122, 124, 140–141, 178, 190, 206, 210–211, 215
body image dysphoria, 308
bowel
obstruction, 311, 325
perforation, 310

C

C-peptide, 301, 319
C-reactive protein (CRP), xxxi–xxxii, 130, 136–137, 139, 179–180, 186, 188, 192, 217, 223, 225, 227, 230, 232, 235
caffeine, 214
calories, xxiii, xxv, 20, 31, 36, 38, 121, 256–257, 296, 317
Canada, 20, 22, 29, 42, 49, 54
Canadian Fitness Survey, 89
cancer, xxiii, 19, 57, 72, 90, 122, 251, 277, 291, 310, 324
capital, 35, 38, 40, 46
cardiomyopathy, 298, 305
cardiovascular disease, xxx, xxxiii, xxxv, 19, 57, 96–98, 123, 125, 127, 141–143, 176, 189, 191–194, 205, 209–211, 226, 269–270, 275, 277, 304
cell adhesion, 61
census, xxiv, 3, 5, 9, 12, 15–16, 45, 47
Centers for Disease Control and Prevention (CDC), xvi, 25, 28, 39, 94–96, 123, 190, 229, 329
children, xv–xvi, xxii, xxiv, xxxv, 2, 14, 20, 25–28, 38–39, 43, 46, 48–49, 51–54, 66, 175, 188, 248, 250, 317, 328
cholangitis, 147
cholesterol, xii, xxvii, xxx, 89, 98, 104, 108, 111, 118, 129–130, 133, 135–137, 142, 147–148, 152, 162, 171, 193–202, 205, 273, 278–279, 283
hypercholesterolemia, xii, xxx–xxxi, 75, 193, 195–202, 205, 207–208, 273
cirrhosis, 145, 147, 149, 151, 309
cognitive behavioral training (CBT), xxxiii, 251–253, 257–259, 267–268, 270, 334
communities, xi, xviii, xxv, 17, 19, 22, 29, 30–39, 42–43, 45, 47, 49–50, 52–54, 87, 92, 129, 175, 194, 206, 209, 330
Community Energy Balance, xxv, 19, 29, 32, 45
coronary
disease, xxxv, 191–192, 204–206, 211
risk, xii, xxx–xxxi, 194–195, 200–203, 205–207
cortisol, 217, 224, 226, 231
cotinine, 75
culture, xi, xxv, 19–21, 23, 25, 27, 29–37, 39–55, 300, 334

D

DARIOS, 191–192, 195, 204–206, 209
DARIOS study, 191–192, 206, 209
death, xxiii, xxvii, xxxv, 19, 75–76, 96–98, 101–103, 108–111, 113, 115, 118, 122, 124, 143, 191, 206, 211, 271, 324, 329
death rate, xxvii, 108–111, 113, 115, 118
deltoid, xxviii, 149, 154, 156, 260
demographic, xxiv, 9, 103, 218–219
diabetes, xii–xxi, xxiii, xxvi–xxxi, xxxv, 19, 46–47, 51, 53, 57, 68, 73–75, 87–88, 92–93, 95–98, 104,

108, 111, 118, 123, 127–128, 130, 134–143, 146–148, 151–152, 154, 159, 162, 165–166, 169–173, 175–176, 179–190, 193, 195–202, 205, 207–211, 213–214, 217, 226, 228–229, 231–232, 251, 270–271, 274–277, 279–280, 284–289, 291, 296, 298, 301–303, 305–306, 309, 311, 315–317, 319–321, 323, 326, 330, 333, 335
diabetes mellitus, xxxv, 96, 136, 142, 146–148, 151–152, 154, 159, 162, 165–166, 169, 171, 179, 232, 287, 289, 296, 298, 309, 311, 317, 321, 323
diet, xii, xxxiv, 49, 51–52, 55, 93, 125, 143, 166–168, 172, 176, 187, 251–253, 255, 257, 259, 261, 263, 265, 267–274, 277, 287, 296, 299, 316–317, 334
disability, xxiii, 19, 53, 189–190, 272, 306, 322
discrimination, 42
dysglycemia, xxx, 175–176, 179–188
dyslipidemia, xxiii, 147, 154, 210, 275, 305, 309

E

eating disorder, 308
economic development, 33
education, xvii, xix, xxix, 5, 7–9, 12, 34, 36, 38–39, 42, 74–75, 77, 80, 85, 90, 148, 171, 179–185, 219, 246, 250, 252, 261–262, 264, 269, 271, 273, 334
elderly, 11, 67, 71–72, 76–77, 81, 87, 89–92, 116, 119, 122, 124, 189–190, 192, 204, 208, 210–211, 254, 271, 273
employment, xxvi, 7–9, 12, 71, 76, 103, 108, 254, 256, 271, 301, 329
energy
balance, xxv, 19, 29, 31–32, 36, 45, 50–51
expenditure, 31, 43, 122, 210
food, 32
intake, 31, 36
metabolism, 252
enzymelinked immunosorbent assay (ELISA), 148, 217, 227, 235
estrogen, 147
ethnicity, xi, xxv, xxvii, xxix, xxxiv, 19–22, 24–25, 28–33, 35–36, 40--49, 51, 53–54, 66, 72, 98, 102–103, 108–109, 111–112, 118, 179, 181, 210, 229–230
exercise, xi–xii, xxxiii, 11, 44, 46–47, 53, 121, 125, 131, 146, 170, 172, 190, 251–253, 255–259, 261, 263, 265, 267–273, 277, 287, 296, 299, 334
extramyocellular lipids (EMCL), 146, 154, 157–158, 162

F

families, xviii, xxi, xxv, 5, 17, 34, 36–39, 44, 52–53, 58–59, 61–67. 77, 98, 210
family dynamics, 34
family systems, 34
fatty acids, 89, 93, 120, 146, 166–168, 171–172
fertility, 307, 322
fibrosis, xii, xxix, 148–149, 153–157, 159, 161–162, 165–167, 169, 309
Finland, xvii–xxi, 91, 127–128, 139–140, 142–143, 271, 330
food, xi–xii, xvii, xxiv–xxv, 19–20, 29, 31–32, 34, 36–40, 42–43, 46–54, 209, 258–259, 312
energy, 32
insecurity, 19, 32, 43

Framingham Heart Study (FHS), xxiv, 1–4, 7–8, 11–17, 142, 205, 327
fruit, xxiii, 131, 140

G

gender, 6, 22, 24–25, 28, 34, 41, 128, 180–181, 183, 207, 210, 225, 228, 230, 252, 257, 259, 269, 299, 310
genetic, xxiii, xxxiv, 20, 51, 57–58, 67–68, 93, 139, 143, 187, 206, 299–300, 328
genome, xi, xxv–xxvi, 57–61, 63, 65–69, 315, 328
  genome-wide association studies (GWAS), xi, xxv–xxvi, 57–67, 328
genotype, 58, 66–67, 300
geographic, 2, 98, 210
globalization, 33
glucose
  metabolism, xii, xxx–xxxi, 128, 134–135, 165, 176, 213–217, 219, 221, 223, 225–227, 229–232, 304
  tolerance, xxxi, xxxv, 50, 130, 141, 176, 216, 220–221, 232, 279–280, 284, 286–287, 289
  fasting, xii, xxviii, xxxi, 138, 147–148, 178–179, 182, 184–185, 190, 211, 218, 220, 222–226, 228–229, 279
glycogen, 149, 156, 158
growth hormone (GH), 141, 217, 224, 226, 228–229, 232, 248, 317

H

habitus, 35
hazard modeling, 108–114, 117–118
hazard ratio (HR), 77, 79–84, 86, 88, 111–113, 118, 211
health care, xii–xiii, xix, xxi, xxiii–xxiv, xxxi–xxxii, 19, 39, 47, 50, 175, 234, 251–255, 261–262, 268–269
health care systems, 19
health care workers, xii, xxxii, 251–254, 261–262, 268–269
health values, 32, 43
hemochromatosis, 147
hemoglobin, xxix, 75, 179, 181–185, 288, 301
hemorrhage, 311, 324
hepatic dysfunction, 277
hepatitis B, 147
hernias, 292, 311–312
high-performance liquid chromatography (HPLC), 179, 217, 278
Hispanic, 20, 22, 25, 42, 45, 47–48, 50, 54, 64, 66, 72, 74, 77, 91, 93, 103, 179–181
histology, xxix, 151, 153–157, 162, 164–165, 168
homeostasis, xxix, xxxiii, 136, 147, 170–171, 178, 217, 279–280, 282, 288
  homeostasis model assessment of insulin resistance (HOMA-IR), xxviii, xxix–xxx, 134–136, 138, 147, 53–155, 162, 165, 178–187, 279–280, 282, 284–285, 287
hormone, 173, 217–218, 226, 232, 296, 319, 322, 337
housing, 36
hunger, 19, 32, 43, 258, 314
hydrofluoroalkane beclomethasone dipropionate (HFA-BDP), 235–241
hypercholesterolemia, xxx–xxxi, 75, 193, 195–202, 205, 207–208, 273, 339

hyperglycemia, 183, 232
hypertension, xvi, xxx–xxxi, 75, 98, 129, 142, 147, 151–152, 154, 170, 193, 195–202, 205, 207–208, 251, 273, 305, 309
hypoxia, 226–227, 232

I

immigrant, 20–21, 42, 48, 52–54
income, xxv, 17, 20, 22, 25, 31, 34, 41–42, 52–53, 74–75, 77, 79, 84–85, 96, 101, 103
inflammation, xii, xxix, xxxi, 98, 139, 141, 148–149, 154–159, 162–163, 165, 167, 169, 173, 176, 180, 186–188, 190, 233–235, 238, 240, 242, 244–245, 247–249
insulin
  resistance, xii, xxviii–xxix, xxxi, 73, 93, 95, 98–99, 136, 141–143, 145–148, 151–155, 159, 162, 166–173, 175–190, 213–214, 217, 226–227, 229–230, 232, 249, 276, 279, 281–282, 285–288, 314
  sensitivity, xxix, xxxiii–xxxiv, 89, 97, 146, 166, 169–171, 176, 187, 213, 227, 231–232, 275, 279, 282, 284–285, 287–289
intervention, xi–xii, xxv, xxx, xxxii–xxxiii, 2, 14, 16, 21, 29–31, 33, 36–37, 41, 43–45, 47, 49–51, 53–55, 120, 146, 188, 214, 230, 232, 251–259, 261–274, 277, 280–283, 285, 287, 321–325, 334
intramyocellular lipids (IMCL), xxix, 146, 154, 156–158, 162, 165–167, 169–170

J

Japan, xii–xv, xviii, xx–xxii, xxxiii, 123, 275–279, 284–289

K

kidney, xiv, xviii, xx–xxi, 309, 323, 333
  function, 309

L

leisure time, xxxiii, 39, 131, 136–137, 139, 256, 258, 270
lifestyle modification, 275
linear regression, 66, 110, 119, 179–180, 186, 236, 279, 281–283
lipid accumulation product, (LAP) xxvi, 73, 76–77, 79–80, 85, 87, 91–95, 98, 325
lipotoxicity, 94, 97–98, 165, 169
liver, xii, xxviii–xxix, 93–95, 98, 127–128, 131, 134–138, 140–141, 143, 145–149, 151, 153–155, 157, 159, 161, 163, 165, 167–173, 227, 309, 319, 323
  biopsies, 148, 168
  fat, xxviii, 128, 136–138, 140, 143
  lesion, 159
lobular inflammation, 148, 154–157, 159, 162–163, 165
lung, xxxi–xxxii, 121, 142, 209, 234, 238, 240, 242, 244, 248–250, 261, 321, 327, 331

M

marital status, 5, 9

marketing, xxiv, 29, 38–39, 44, 48–49, 54
Markov Chain Monte Carlo (MCMC), 6, 17
metabolic syndrome (MetS), xxvii–xxviii, 48, 94, 97, 122, 128–129, 131–135, 137–143, 148, 151–154, 159, 162, 170, 208–209, 211, 232
migrant, 29, 41–42, 47–48, 51–52
migration, xix, 40–42, 53, 296, 312
mortality, xi–xii, xxvi–xxvii, xxxv, 71–77, 79–93, 95–99, 101–105, 107–125, 145, 171, 191–192, 205–208, 211, 251, 273, 291, 299, 302, 304–306, 310, 316, 318–319, 321, 324–325
  hazard, vii, xxvii, 101, 103, 105, 107–121, 123, 125
MQLS, 59, 64, 66–67
muscle, vxii, xxviii–xxx, xxxiii, 11, 93–94, 102, 119, 121, 145–147, 149–151, 153–173, 175–176, 178, 181, 187–190, 206, 258, 266, 268, 272–273
  mass, xxix–xxx, 11, 102, 176, 178, 187–190, 206, 258, 268
  musculoskeletal pain, xxxii–xxxiii, 251–253, 258, 261, 265–267, 270, 272, 322
  protein, 176
myogenesis, 176
myokines, 176, 189

N

National Center for Health Statistics (NCHS), 16, 75–76, 94–96, 103–104, 123, 177, 189–190
National Death Index, 75, 103, 329
National Health and Nutrition Examination Survey (NHANES), xi, xxvi–xxvii, xxix, 15, 22, 25, 72, 74–76, 87, 89–91, 93–96, 103–106, 108, 118–121, 123–124, 141, 175, 177, 180–181, 188–190, 204, 249, 329
National Institute of Clinical Excellence (NICE), 298, 317
National Institutes of Health (NIH), xiv, 101, 121, 170, 214, 233–234, 250, 298, 317, 328, 331, 333
Native American, 20
necrosis, 149, 156, 158, 165, 167–169, 172, 235
neighborhood, xxiv, 2–3, 5–9, 15–16, 37, 42
neurexins, 61
New Zealand, 19–20, 24, 28–29, 42, 50–51
non-alcoholic fatty liver disease (NAFLD), xii, xxviii–xxix, 98, 131, 136–138, 143, 145–146, 148–149, 151, 153–154, 156, 158–159, 167–169, 170–173
nonalcoholic steatohepatitis (NASH), xii, xxviii–xxix, 145, 148–154, 156, 158–159, 165–169, 171, 309, 323
nutrition, viii, xi, xiii, xv, xvii–xviii, xxi–xxii, xxvi–xxvii, xxix, xxxv, 15, 19, 22, 25–27, 29, 38–39, 46, 49, 51, 53–54, 72, 74, 94–96, 103, 122–124, 172, 175, 177, 189–190, 204, 249, 272–273, 276

O

obesity
  abdominal. xii, xxx–xxxi, 97, 125, 191–195, 201–202, 204–207, 209, 211
  paradox, 92
osteoporosis, 178, 190

P

pacemakers, 177
peripheral blood mononuclear cells (PBMC), 235, 242–243, 245 249
phenotype, xxvi–xxviii, xxxii, 58–59, 62, 65–67, 73, 94–95, 127–129, 131, 133–135, 137–143, 202, 211, 233–235, 237, 239, 241–247, 249, 299–300
physical activity, xi, xxiii–xxv, xxxv, 20, 27, 29–32, 35–47, 50–55, 93, 131, 136–137, 139, 171, 210, 252, 257, 272–273, 277–278, 280–283, 316
physiology, xxvii, xxxiv, 71, 118
polysomnography, 216, 229, 318
population dynamics, 33
Portugal, xiii–xv, xviii, xx, 146, 330
poverty, xxiv, 5, 7–9, 12, 15–16, 42, 54, 74–75, 77, 79, 84–85
pregnancy, xxvii, xxix, 72, 103–104, 177, 180–181, 261, 307, 322
psychologist, 29, 257, 298
public health, xvii–xxi, xxxiv, 29–31, 46–48, 51–54, 95–96, 124, 127, 141, 191, 207, 209, 211, 251, 271–272, 274, 317, 327, 330
public transportation, 15, 37

R

radioimmunoassay (RIA), 148, 178
ragged red fibers (RRF), 149, 158
regression, xxvii–xxix, 14, 66, 87, 104–105, 109–110, 118–119, 131, 151, 179–180, 186, 194, 210, 218, 225–226, 236, 279, 281–283, 308–309, 343
retirement, xxxii, 251, 271
rituals, 34

S

sarcopenia, viii, xii, xxix–xxx, 175–190
sedentary, xxiii, xxxv, 43, 52, 166, 170–171, 205–206, 210
segregation, 40, 42
sex, xi, xxiv, xxvi–xxvii, xxix, 6, 10, 66, 72, 75–78, 87, 89–92, 94, 97, 102–103, 105–112, 114, 118–119, 133, 136, 152, 178–179, 181–185, 194, 196, 198, 200–202, 205, 210, 233–234, 236–237, 240–242, 244, 256, 261, 264, 280–284, 322
single nucleotide polymorphism (SNP), xi, xxv, 58–61, 63–68
sleep, xii, xxiii, xxxi, 122, 131, 137, 147, 152, 213–217, 219–223, 225–232, 298–299, 302, 304, 318, 321
  apnea, xii, xxiii, xxxi, 122, 147, 152, 213, 215, 217–232, 298–299, 302, 304, 318, 321
  duration, xxxi, 213, 216, 222, 225, 228–229, 231
  efficiency, 216, 222
  sleep fragmentation, 214, 226, 231
  Sleep Extension Study, 213–214
smoking, xii, xxvii, 3, 5, 9–10, 68, 75, 93, 98, 102, 104, 108, 111, 118, 136–137, 152, 193, 195, 219, 257, 261, 264, 272, 286–287
social arenas, 34–36
social status, 40, 43
socioeconomic, xxvi, 2, 16–17, 30, 45, 50, 74–75, 81, 84–85, 139, 204, 210, 246, 251
sociology, 29, 35, 44, 46
Spain, xii–xvi, xviii–xxi, xxx–xxxi, 191–192, 194, 202, 204–210
sports, xx, 39, 44, 47, 125, 256, 258, 273, 334
standard deviation, xxiv, xxvii, 6–11, 13, 105–107, 110–112, 118, 121, 150, 197, 199, 218, 236–237, 241

steatosis, xxix, 73, 93, 95, 145, 148, 151–157, 159–160, 162, 165–168, 173, 249
stratification, 33, 42, 252, 280
stroke, xxiii, 98, 193, 275, 277
suicide, 298
synapse, 61

T

tobacco, xxvi, 74–75, 77, 79–81, 85–86, 90, 92–93, 96, 101
triglyceride (TG), 73, 93, 130, 137, 146, 169–170, 278–279, 281, 283–285
tumor necrosis factor-alpha (TNF-α), 167–168, 235

U

underemployment, 42
United States, xii–xxii, xxv, xxxv, 1, 16–17, 20–21, 29, 42, 52–54, 71, 95–96, 98, 122, 175, 189, 210
urban development, 36

V

variance, xxiv, xxxii, 3, 5, 9–11, 14–17, 151, 229, 236, 241
vegetables, xxiii–xxiv, 38, 131, 136–137, 140
vitamin B12, 313
vitamin D, 242, 245, 247, 249–250, 313

W

waist circumference (WC), xi–xii, xxvi–xxvii, xxx–xxxi, xxxiii, xxxv, 19, 59, 65, 68, 71–73, 76–81, 85, 87, 89–92, 98, 102–125, 129, 141, 148, 189–198, 201–204, 206–208, 211, 215, 219, 247–248, 259, 262, 266–267, 269, 271, 276–277, 280–281, 284–287, 289, 320, 324
waist to hip ratio (WHR), xxvi, 59, 61–62, 65, 73, 76–80, 85, 87, 120, 154
weight
- change, xxxv, 2, 120, 124, 131, 136, 261, 299
- classification, xxiv, 2, 6, 11–14, 16
- gain, 2, 10–11, 14, 20, 31, 36, 43, 97, 122, 246, 314
- loss, xii, 48, 97, 120–121, 125, 169–170, 172, 189–190, 252–253, 256–258, 261, 266–275, 285, 287–289, 296, 298–305, 308, 310, 312–323, 325–326, 336
- underweight, xi–xii, xxiii–xxiv, xxvi–xxviii, xxx–xxxv, 1–3, 6–7, 10–14, 16–17, 20, 22–24, 28, 31, 36, 39, 43, 48, 50–51, 54, 57, 61–62, 65, 67, 71, 73, 90, 95, 97, 101–106, 112, 115, 118–125, 128–129, 131, 133–134, 136–142, 147, 169–170, 172, 177–178, 189–190, 193–197, 202, 207, 211, 213, 215, 218–219, 246, 251–253, 256–262, 264, 266–275, 277, 285–289, 296, 298–305, 307–308, 310, 312–323, 325–326, 336

workplace, xxxiii, 251, 253, 255, 257–259, 261–263, 265, 267–273
World Health Organisation (WHO), xi, xxiii, xxxiv–xxxv, 2, 11, 14, 19–21, 30, 32–34, 36, 41–42, 44, 54–55, 58, 64, 72–73, 87, 90, 93–94, 101–102, 111, 118–121, 123–124, 129–130, 137, 141–142, 177, 181, 188, 190, 207, 209–210, 213–214, 226, 231, 242–243, 246–248, 254, 277, 280,

284, 286, 288–289, 296, 298, 303, 305–307, 316, 328–329, 336

X

X-ray absorptiometry, 124, 215

Y

young adult, 11, 16, 14, 175, 178, 188